TREATING PTSD IN MILITARY PERSONNEL

TREATING PTSD IN MILITARY PERSONNEL

A CLINICAL HANDBOOK

edited by
Bret A. Moore
Walter E. Penk

Foreword by Matthew J. Friedman

THE GUILFORD PRESS
New York   London

Last digit is print number: 9 8 7 6 5 4 3 2

The authors have checked with sources believed to be reliable in their efforts to provide information
that is complete and generally in accord with the standards of practice that are accepted at the time
of publication. However, in view of the possibility of human error or changes in behavioral, mental
health, or medical sciences, neither the authors, nor the editors and publisher, nor any other party
who has been involved in the preparation or publication of this work warrants that the information contained herein is in every respect accurate or complete, and they are not responsible for any
errors or omissions or the results obtained from the use of such information. Readers are encouraged to confirm the information contained in this book with other sources.

The views expressed in this book are those of the authors and do not reflect the official policy or
position of the Department of the Army, Department of the Navy, Department of the Air Force,
Department of Defense, or the United States Government. All case vignettes used in this volume are
either fictitious or have been disguised to protect confidentiality.

Library of Congress Cataloging-in-Publication Data

Treating PTSD in military personnel / edited by Bret A. Moore and Walter E. Penk.
   p. cm.
  Includes bibliographical references and index.
  ISBN 978-1-60918-635-7 (hbk. : alk. paper)
  1. Post-traumatic stress disorder—Treatment—United States.   2. Soldiers—United States—
Psychology.   3. Veterans—United States—Psychology.   4. Soldiers—Mental health—
United States.   5. Veterans—Mental health—United States.   6. War neuroses—Prevention.
I. Moore, Bret A.   II. Penk, Walter.   III. Title: Treating PTSD in military personnel.
  RC552.P67T7655 2011
  616.85′21—dc23

2011023300

*To all the selfless men and women in uniform
serving around the world*

To Lori and Kaitlyn

—B. A. M.

To Mark, Janice, Erica, and Danielle

—W. E. P.

About the Editors

Bret A. Moore, PsyD, ABPP, is founder of Military Psychology Consulting and a board-certified clinical psychologist in San Antonio, Texas. He is a former active-duty Army psychologist and two-tour veteran of Iraq. Dr. Moore is coauthor of *Wheels Down: Adjusting to Life after Deployment, The Veterans and Active Duty Military Psychotherapy Treatment Planner,* and *Veterans and Active Duty Military Psychotherapy Homework Planner,* editor of *Handbook of Counseling Military Couples,* and coeditor of *Living and Surviving in Harm's Way: A Psychological Treatment Handbook for Pre- and Post-Deployment of Military Personnel, Pharmacotherapy for Psychologists: Prescribing and Collaborative Roles,* and the forthcoming *Psychopharmacology for Psychologists.* He also writes a biweekly newspaper column titled "Kevlar for the Mind" for *Military Times.* In 2007, Dr. Moore received the American Psychological Association's Arthur W. Melton Award for Early Career Achievement in Military Psychology from Division 19, and, in 2011, the Early Career Achievement Award from Division 18. He is also a Fellow of the American Psychological Association.

Walter E. Penk, PhD, ABPP, is Professor of Psychiatry and Behavioral Sciences at Texas A&M College of Medicine and consultant to the Veterans Health Administration's VISN 17 VA Center of Excellence in Stress Disorders Research and VA Rehabilitation Research and Development in Washington, DC. Dr. Penk's research has been funded by the Department of Veterans Affairs, the National Institute on Drug Abuse, and the National Institute of Mental Health to validate treatments for co-occurring posttraumatic stress disorder, addictions, and other mental disorders. He has published more than 135 articles in peer-reviewed journals, including findings from randomized clinical trials for cognitive-behavioral therapy and vocational rehabilitation, and he coedited *Returning Wars' Wounded, Injured, and Ill: A Reference Handbook.* Awards for his contributions include a Presidential Citation, the Division 18 Harold Hildreth Award from the American Psychological Association, a VA Distinguished Career Award, and recognition from the American Rehabilitation Counseling Association. Dr. Penk is also a Fellow of the American Psychological Association.

Contributors

Nathan Ainspan, PhD, Civilian Personnel Evaluation Agency, U.S. Army, Alexandria, Virginia

Jean C. Beckham, PhD, Department of Psychiatry and Behavioral Sciences, Duke University School of Medicine, and VA Mid-Atlantic Health Care Network (VISN 6) Mental Illness Research, Education and Clinical Center–Durham VA Medical Center, Durham, North Carolina

William L. Brim, PhD, Center for Deployment Psychology, Department of Medical and Clinical Psychology, Uniformed Services University of the Health Sciences, Bethesda, Maryland

Nigel Bush, PhD, National Center for Telehealth and Technology, Tacoma, Washington

Frank Castro, PhD, National Center for PTSD, VA Boston Healthcare System, and Department of Psychiatry, Boston University School of Medicine, Boston, Massachusetts

Kevin M. Connolly, PhD, G. V. (Sonny) Montgomery VA Medical Center, VA South Central Health Care Network (VISN 16) Mental Illness Research, Education and Clinical Center, and Division of Psychology, Department of Psychiatry and Human Behavior, University of Mississippi Medical Center, Jackson, Mississippi

Kent D. Drescher, PhD, National Center for PTSD, Menlo Park, California

Eric B. Elbogen, PhD, Department of Psychiatry, University of North Carolina at Chapel Hill School of Medicine, and VA Mid-Atlantic Health Care Network (VISN 6) Mental Illness Research, Education and Clinical Center–Durham VA Medical Center, Durham, North Carolina

Charles Figley, PhD, Traumatology Institute, Tulane University, New Orleans, Louisiana

Edna B. Foa, PhD, Center for the Treatment and Study of Anxiety, Department of Psychiatry, University of Pennsylvania School of Medicine, Philadelphia, Pennsylvania

David W. Foy, PhD, Graduate School of Education and Psychology, Pepperdine University, Malibu, California

Tara E. Galovski, PhD, Center for Trauma Recovery, University of Missouri–St. Louis, St. Louis, Missouri

Suzy Bird Gulliver, PhD, VA Heart of Texas Health Care Network (VISN 17) Center of Excellence for Research on Returning War Veterans, and Department of Psychiatry and Behavioral Sciences, College of Medicine, Texas A&M Health Science Center, Waco, Texas

Jasmeet P. Hayes, PhD, National Center for PTSD, VA Boston Healthcare System, and Department of Psychiatry, Boston University School of Medicine, Boston, Massachusetts

Kevin M. Holloway, PhD, National Center for Telehealth and Technology, Tacoma, Washington

Sally C. Johnson, MD, Department of Psychiatry, University of North Carolina at Chapel Hill School of Medicine, Durham, North Carolina

Karen A. Kattar, PhD, Phoenix VA Health Care System, Phoenix, Arizona

Terence M. Keane, PhD, National Center for PTSD, VA Boston Healthcare System and Department of Psychiatry, Boston University School of Medicine, Boston, Massachusetts

Nathan A. Kimbrel, PhD, VA Heart of Texas Health Care Network (VISN 17) Center of Excellence for Research on Returning War Veterans, and Department of Psychiatry and Behavioral Sciences, Texas A&M Health Science Center, Waco, Texas

Marc I. Kruse, PhD, VA Heart of Texas Health Care Network (VISN 17) Center of Excellence for Research on Returning War Veterans, and Department of Psychiatry and Behavioral Sciences, Texas A&M Health Science Center, Waco, Texas

Harold Kudler, MD, VA Mid-Atlantic Health Care Network (VISN 6) Mental Illness Research, Education and Clinical Center, Durham VA Medical Center, and Department of Psychiatry, Duke University, Durham, North Carolina

Howard Lipke, PhD, Department of Psychology, Rosalind Franklin University of Medicine and Science, Chicago, Illinois

Dolores Little, PhD, U.S. Department of Veterans Affairs, Washington, DC (retired)

David D. Luxton, PhD, National Center for Telehealth and Technology, Tacoma, Washington

Judith A. Lyons, PhD, G. V. (Sonny) Montgomery VA Medical Center, VA South Central (VISN 16) Health Care Network Mental Illness Research, Education and Clinical Center, and Division of Psychology, Department of Psychiatry and Human Behavior, University of Mississippi Medical Center, Jackson, Mississippi

Danielle J. Maack, PhD, G. V. (Sonny) Montgomery VA Medical Center, and Department of Psychiatry and Human Behavior, University of Mississippi Medical Center, Jackson, Mississippi

Susan M. McGlynn, PhD, Psychology Service, VA Boston Healthcare System, and Department of Psychiatry, Boston University School of Medicine, Boston, Massachusetts

Donald Meichenbaum, PhD, Department of Psychology, University of Waterloo, Waterloo, Ontario, Canada, and the Melissa Institute for Violence Prevention and Treatment, Miami, Florida

Eric C. Meyer, PhD, VA Heart of Texas Health Care Network (VISN 17) Center of Excellence for Research on Returning War Veterans, and Department of Psychiatry and Behavioral Sciences, Texas A&M Health Science Center, Waco, Texas

Bret A. Moore, PsyD, ABPP, Military Psychology Consulting, San Antonio, Texas

Sandra B. Morissette, PhD, VA Heart of Texas Health Care Network (VISN 17) Center of Excellence for Research on Returning War Veterans, and Department of Psychiatry and Behavioral Sciences, Texas A&M Health Science Center, Waco, Texas

Walter E. Penk, PhD, ABPP, Department of Psychiatry and Behavioral Sciences, Texas A&M College of Medicine, New Braunfels, Texas

Alan L. Peterson, PhD, Department of Psychiatry, School of Medicine, University of Texas Health Science Center at San Antonio, San Antonio, Texas

Greg M. Reger, PhD, National Center for Telehealth and Technology, Tacoma, Washington

Patricia A. Resick, PhD, National Center for PTSD, VA Boston Healthcare System, and College of Arts and Sciences, Boston University, Boston, Massachusetts

David S. Riggs, PhD, Center for Deployment Psychology, Department of Medical and Clinical Psychology, Uniformed Services University of the Health Sciences, Bethesda, Maryland

Iya Ritchie, MA, Graduate School of Education and Psychology, Pepperdine University, Malibu, California

Michael Ritter, PhD, G. V. (Sonny) Montgomery VA Medical Center, and Division of Psychology, Department of Psychiatry and Human Behavior, University of Mississippi Medical Center, Jackson, Mississippi

M. David Rudd, PhD, College of Social and Behavioral Science, University of Utah, Salt Lake City, Utah

Mark C. Russell, PhD, School of Applied Psychology, Counseling, and Family Therapy, Antioch University, Seattle, Washington

William M. Sauvé, MD, Clinical Director, Military Program, Poplar Springs Hospital, Petersburg, Virginia

Nancy A. Skopp, PhD, National Center for Telehealth and Technology, Tacoma, Washington

Julia C. Smith, PsyD, VA North Texas Health Care System, and Department of Psychiatry, University of Texas Southwestern Medical Center, Dallas, Texas

Stephen M. Stahl, MD, PhD, Department of Psychiatry, University of California, San Diego, California, and Department of Psychiatry, University of Cambridge, Cambridge, United Kingdom

Laurie E. Steffen, BA, VA Heart of Texas Health Care Network (VISN 17) Center of Excellence for Research on Returning War Veterans, and Department of Psychiatry and Behavioral Sciences, Texas A&M Health Science Center, Waco, Texas

Alina M. Surís, PhD, VA North Texas Health Care System, and Department of Psychiatry, University of Texas Southwestern Medical Center, Dallas, Texas

Matthew T. Tull, PhD, Department of Psychiatry and Human Behavior, Division of Psychology, University of Mississippi Medical Center, Jackson, Mississippi

Jennifer J. Vasterling, PhD, Psychology Service and VA National Center for PTSD, VA Boston Healthcare System, and Department of Psychiatry, Boston University School of Medicine, Boston, Massachusetts

Mieke Verfaellie, PhD, Memory Disorders Research Center, VA Boston Healthcare System, and Department of Psychiatry, Boston University School of Medicine, Boston, Massachusetts

Patricia J. Watson, PhD, National Center for PTSD, White River Junction, Vermont

Amy M. Williams, PhD, private practice, Flower Mound, Texas

Foreword

Although most men and women deployed to Iraq and Afghanistan have coped successfully with the sometimes extreme psychological stressors encountered in the war zone, a significant number have not. The risk of post-traumatic stress disorder (PTSD) and related problems has been amplified by increased exposure to such events through multiple deployments. From a clinical perspective, PTSD is rarely the only problem that must be addressed. Indeed, complicated clinical presentations are generally the rule rather than the exception. PTSD is often comorbid with depression, substance use disorders, traumatic brain injury (TBI), insomnia, aggressive behaviors, chronic pain, and other medical and/or surgical complaints.

Considering the clinical options available to Vietnam veterans in the 1970s and 1980s, the current changes are monumental. There have been remarkable advances in our understanding of the etiology and pathophysiology of PTSD through a synthesis of theory and evidence from behavioral science, neuroscience, and more recent research on resilience. Indeed, we now have a much deeper appreciation of the impact of traumatic stress on cognition, memory, emotions, neurocircuitry, neuroplasticity, psychobiological mechanisms, and, of course, behavior. From a clinical perspective, practitioners are now equipped with very sensitive assessment tools and evidence-based treatments. Clinicians in the Department of Defense (DoD) and Department of Veterans Affairs (VA) systems of care have unprecedented institutional support to offer a wide spectrum of services from community-based clinics to highly specialized inpatient tertiary care.

In short, the quality and quantity of clinical options available to service members and veterans have never been better. But many challenges remain. First, most military and VA practitioners have not been trained in evidence-based cognitive-behavioral therapies. That problem has been addressed head-on, especially in the VA, where over 3,000 clinicians have received such training in recent years. Second, most civilian (e.g., VA or private sector) practitioners are unfamiliar with military culture, seriously compromising their capacity to achieve credibility and rapport with recently deployed clientele. Third, lessons learned with Vietnam veterans, who were usually in their 30s at the time they sought treatment, are not always applicable to currently serving 18- to 25-year-olds, who often present maturational and motivational challenges along with the usual diagnostic and therapeutic issues. Fourth, there is considerable inexperience in many quarters regarding the treatment of female service members and veterans. Since the number of women in the armed forces and veteran population continues to grow, improving care for servicewomen and veterans is an urgent priority. Fifth, National Guard troops and military reservists, especially those from rural areas, are a high-risk cohort who lack the social support available to active-duty personnel. Finally, there are major gaps in the clinical body of knowledge needed to inform treatment decisions for many patients with complicated conditions. For example, although there are evidence-based practice guidelines for separate disorders such as PTSD, depression, substance use disorders, or TBI, there is very little rigorous empirical evidence to guide treatment decisions when any of these disorders occur in combination.

Bret A. Moore and Walter E. Penk have assembled a very distinguished panel of contributors to produce a book that addresses all of these concerns. They set the stage in Part I with a thoughtful and practical chapter titled "Understanding and Working within the Military Culture." This initial chapter should be mandatory reading for any nonveteran civilian practitioner who hopes to achieve meaningful engagement with previously deployed men and women. Having established this crucial context, the authors develop this perspective through each succeeding chapter so that, for example, a discussion of a particular treatment approach is presented quite specifically within a postdeployment framework. There is great overlap, to be sure, between the provision of a cognitive-behavioral treatment to civilians and to veterans, but there are also important and uniquely military contextual issues that must be incorporated into treatment delivery and the therapeutic relationship.

The book is both comprehensive and specific in scope. Each important PTSD treatment currently in use—prolonged exposure, cognitive processing therapy, eye movement desensitization and reprocessing, virtual reality exposure therapy, psychodynamic psychotherapy, group therapy, couple/family therapy, psychopharmacotherapy, and psychosocial rehabilitation—is covered in separate chapters. The book is also quite practical in focus, providing specific assessment tools and treatment approaches, when indicated.

Part II, with its eight chapters that address the complex clinical presentations mentioned earlier, is a unique contribution of this book. Moore and

Penk have wisely dedicated specific chapters to a number of co-occurring diagnoses (e.g., affective and anxiety disorders, substance use disorders, TBI, and sleep disorders) and co-occurring clinical problems that are often encountered along with PTSD, such as suicidal ideation, sexual assault, anger, aggression, and violence. Each chapter is addressed to the clinician in the trenches and provides a thorough review of whatever literature might be available, as well as thoughtful practical guidance regarding the best clinical management of these typically difficult patients.

The final chapter focuses on one of my favorite areas, building resilience in order to prevent PTSD and related disorders. Although our scientific understanding of resilience, at both the individual and public health level, is at a relatively early stage, the DoD has already implemented pre- and post-deployment programs designed to fortify resilience to prevent PTSD among soldiers, marines, and navy and air force personnel. It is a thoughtful and, I hope, prophetic note on which to end this book. Should there be future wars, and therefore a need for another book of this sort, I hope that any sequel will include several chapters on evidence-based resilience techniques that effectively prevent the onset of PTSD and related disorders.

Moore and Penk have produced a unique book that covers the full range of effective treatments for PTSD and related disorders without ever losing its specific focus on military personnel and veterans. Although each chapter includes a scholarly review of its designated topic, its major value is as a practical resource for practitioners that provides sound clinical advice, a guide to the best assessment instruments and treatment manuals, and thoughtful clinical vignettes to drive home major points. In short, whatever you know, or think you know, about treatment of PTSD among military and veteran clientele will be challenged and enriched by this important book.

MATTHEW J. FRIEDMAN, MD, PhD
National Center for PTSD,
U.S. Department of Veterans Affairs,
and Dartmouth Medical School

Acknowledgments

Without the support of many people in our lives, this book would not have been possible. We would like to thank our families for their encouragement and patience. We are grateful for the professionalism and dedication of the publishing staff at The Guilford Press, specifically Jim Nageotte, Senior Editor, and Jane Keislar, Senior Assistant Editor. And, finally, we are indebted to the many experts who agreed to participate in this volume.

Contents

PTSD in the Military

Bret A. Moore
Walter E. Penk

Throughout the centuries, philosophers, historians, researchers, and clinicians have given many names to the invisible wounds of combat. In the fifth century, Herodotus wrote of a brave warrior from the battle of Marathon who was rendered blind "without blow of sword or dart" as a fellow warrior next to him was struck down by the enemy (Waterfield, 2008). In the mid-18th century, the term "Swiss disease" was used to describe unexplained physical and psychological symptoms in Swiss villagers who were forced to serve in rogue armies (Jones et al., 1995). During the American Civil War, the Army physician J. M. Da Costa wrote of "irritable heart," which included symptoms we now label as panic (Da Costa, 1871). Other terms such as "shell shock," "war neurosis," "battle fatigue," and "post-Vietnam syndrome" have followed.

It was not until 1980 that the American Psychiatric Association adopted the current term, posttraumatic stress disorder (PTSD), into its third edition of the *Diagnostic and Statistical Manual of Mental Disorders*. This is the term we continue to use today, and the disorder on which this book is based. It is unlikely that any other psychiatric disorder in the last half century has received so much attention, debate, and controversy. In part, the focus on PTSD arose from political pressures to label and categorize the psychological symptoms that Vietnam veterans were struggling with on their return home (Keane, 2009). It was also due in part to our inability to fully understand the differences in how individuals interpreted and reacted to trauma, as well as the concept of resiliency that has gained prominence in the field today.

Today, we have found new PTSD controversies to combine with the old, particularly with veterans of Operation Enduring Freedom and Operation Iraqi Freedom. Some of the current debate continues to be political (e.g., loosening disability compensation requirements to minimize false negatives), but the discourse also originates from scientific inquiry and a genuine desire to provide for those who have sacrificed for their country. The latter is the focus of this book.

In this volume, the reader will find a compilation of chapters from top experts on the study and treatment of PTSD in service members and veterans. Many issues relevant to this area will be covered in detail throughout the chapters. However, there are two salient points we feel deserve brief attention at the outset: the prevalence and significance of PTSD in the military and the need for better treatments.

Prevalence and Significance

It has been known for some time that service members and veterans are at increased risk of stress disorders due to their exposure to combat (Kessler, Sonnega, Bromet, Hughes, & Nelson, 1995; Prigerson, Maciejewski, & Rosenheck, 2002). Estimates of lifetime prevalence of PTSD for Vietnam veterans has been shown to be around 30% using broad criteria (Kulka et al., 1988) and approximately 19% when stricter criteria were applied (Dohrenwend et al., 2006).

Studies of veterans of the combat operations in Iraq and Afghanistan are showing significant levels of PTSD as well; however, there is some variability in prevalence reports. In a seminal study by Hoge and colleagues (2004) from the Walter Reed Army Institute of Research, four U.S. combat infantry units were given an anonymous survey either before their deployment to Iraq ($n = 2,530$) or, in a different cohort of troops, 3–4 months after their return from combat duty in Iraq or Afghanistan ($n = 3,671$). Results indicated that service members deployed to Iraq screened positive for PTSD at rates of 18–20% and those from Afghanistan at approximately 12%. Using the Post-Deployment Health Assessment, Hoge, Auchterlonie, and Milliken (2006) found that approximately 10% of Iraq veterans and 5% of Afghanistan veterans screened positive for PTSD. A particularly strong aspect of this latter study is that it utilized the records of nearly a quarter of a million troops. A follow-up study by Milliken, Auchterlonie, and Hoge (2007), which included active-duty, National Guard, and reserve soldiers, revealed that approximately 17% of active-duty soldiers screened positive for PTSD at 3–6 months postdeployment. Levels for National Guard and reserve soldiers reached nearly 25%. However, a more recent study has shown rates of approximately 7% in active-duty service members and 11% in National Guard service members at 12 months postdeployment (Thomas et al., 2010).

Although variation exists in the estimated prevalence rates of PTSD in veterans of the Iraq and Afghanistan wars, the level of PTSD in returning troops is significant and translates into thousands of service members being affected. Furthermore, millions of loved ones are also affected by this disorder, and billions of dollars are spent each year in the attempt to better understand and prevent PTSD, as well as to rehabilitate those service members and veterans living with the disorder. It has rightly been placed at the top of the priority lists by the Departments of Defense and Veterans Affairs.

Need for Better Treatments

The evidence base for effective treatments for PTSD is lagging behind our knowledge about the mechanisms associated with the development, maintenance, and course of the disorder. In essence, a 2007 report by the Institute of Medicine (IOM) supported this claim.

After being commissioned by the Department of Veterans Affairs, the IOM was asked to review the current efficacy research on psychological and pharmacological treatments for PTSD. The IOM reviewed 90 randomized clinical trials (53 psychotherapeutic interventions and 37 pharmacological interventions) that focused on PTSD outcomes. The committee concluded that, based on their criteria, there was insufficient evidence to support the efficacy of pharmacological intervention for PTSD. Furthermore, exposure therapy was the only psychotherapeutic treatment modality shown to have sufficient evidence to support its use for PTSD.

Does this mean exposure therapy is the only treatment that works? In our opinion, the answer is no. It does, however, highlight an important issue in the field of PTSD research. The evidence for both pharmacological and psychotherapeutic treatments is lacking, particularly in active-duty and veteran populations. Consequently, too often clinical work is based on clinician preference or prior training, marketing from pharmaceutical companies, and alliances with specific theoretical "camps" rather than on data from scientific studies. In other words, it may not be in the best interest of the patient.

Fortunately, PTSD research is moving at an accelerated pace. Dozens of drug and psychotherapeutic trials are currently under way. The greatest promise appears to be in the psychotherapeutic realm, with treatments such as prolonged exposure and cognitive processing therapy. However, pharmacological studies utilizing atypical antipsychotics, mood stabilizers, and various corticotropin modulators also show promise. We hope the chapters in this volume will spark interest in PTSD research that will translate to the clinical setting.

The Current Volume

This volume provides a snapshot of the most common, as well as emerging, treatments for service members and veterans suffering from PTSD. It will be of use to the student as well as the seasoned clinician.

Part I covers important cultural issues regarding working with military personnel (Chapter 1), effective assessment strategies (Chapter 2), and different treatment approaches (Chapters 3–11). Part II covers specific clinical issues associated with PTSD, such as co-occurring affective and anxiety and substance use disorders, traumatic brain injury, sexual assault suicidal ideation (Chapters 12–18), and resiliency building as a means to prevent PTSD (Chapter 19). Finally, the Appendices provide readers with various resources for gaining competence and fluency in working with military service members, including relevant training programs, journal articles, book chapters and books; a list of key supportive military organizations and programs; and a brief review of common military abbreviations.

Although much of the material in this volume is exclusively related to the U.S. military, the information will likely be beneficial to clinicians, researchers, and students from different nations who work with service members and veterans. Our focus on the U.S. military is a direct consequence of our limited exposure to other national forces and not a lack of appreciation of the need to provide effective care for all men and women in uniform.

References

Da Costa, J. M. (1871). Membranous enteritis. *American Journal of Medicine, 124,* 321–338.

Dohrenwend, B. P., Turner, J. B., Turse, N. A., Adams, B. G., Koenen, K. C., & Marshall, R. (2006). The psychological risks of Vietnam for U.S. veterans: A revision with new data and methods. *Science, 313,* 979–982.

Hoge, C. W., Auchterlonie, J. L., & Milliken, C. S. (2006). Mental health problems, use of mental health services, and attrition from military service after returning from deployment to Iraq or Afghanistan. *Journal of the American Medical Association, 295*(9), 1023–1032.

Hoge, C. W., Castro, C. A., Messer, S. C., McGurk, D., Cotting, D. I., & Koffman, R. L. (2004). Combat duty in Iraq and Afghanistan, mental health problems, and barriers to care. *New England Journal of Medicine, 351*(1), 13–22.

Institute of Medicine. (2007). *Treatment of posttraumatic stress disorder: An assessment of the evidence.* Washington, DC: National Academies Press.

Jones, F. D., Sparacino, L. R., Wilcox, V. L., Rothberg, J. M. & Stokes, J. W. (1995). *War psychiatry.* Washington, DC: Department of the Army.

Keane, T. (2009). Improving models, methods, and measures: Contributions of CITRM to the field of psychological trauma. *Journal of Traumatic Stress, 22*(6), 632–633.

Kessler, R. C., Sonnega, A., Bromet, E., Hughes, M., & Nelson, C. B. (1995). Posttraumatic stress disorder in the National Comorbidity Survey. *Archives of General Psychiatry, 52,* 1048–1060.

Kulka, R. A., Schlenger, W. E., Fairbank, J. A., Hough, R. L., Jordan, B. K., Marmar, C. R., et al. (1988). *National Vietnam Veterans Readjustment Study (NVVRS): Description, current status, and initial PTSD prevalence estimates.* Washington, DC: Veterans Administration.

Milliken, C. S., Auchterlonie, J. L., & Hoge, C. W. (2007). Longitudinal assessment of mental health problems among active and reserve component soldiers returning from the Iraq war. *Journal of the American Medical Association, 298*(18), 2141–2148.

Prigerson, H. G., Maciejewski, P. K., & Rosenheck, R. A. (2002). Population attributable fractions of psychiatric disorders and behavioral outcomes associated with combat exposure among U.S. men. *American Journal of Public Health, 92,* 59–63.

Thomas, J. L., Wilk, J. E., Riviere, L. A., McGurk, D., Castro, C. A., & Hoge, C. W. (2010). Prevalence of mental health problems and functional impairment among active component and National Guard Soldiers 3 and 12 months following combat in Iraq. *Archives of General Psychiatry, 67,* 614–623.

Waterfield, R. (2008). *Herodotus: The histories.* Oxford, UK: Oxford University Press.

PART I

TREATMENT APPROACHES FOR PTSD IN MILITARY PERSONNEL

CHAPTER 1

Understanding and Working within the Military Culture

Bret A. Moore

Over the past decade, the field of psychology has placed a great emphasis on the importance of practicing from a culturally competent framework. In 2002, the American Psychological Association adopted the *Guidelines on Multicultural Education, Training, Research, Practice, and Organizational Change for Psychologists* (2002b). Currently, its accreditation process for doctoral and internship programs in professional psychology ensures that certain levels of cultural competence are met.

Although much of the emphasis on cultural competency has focused on racial and ethnic minorities, the field of psychology has recognized the importance of being inclusive of all unique and diverse groups (e.g., gay and lesbian, different religions). However, one group that has received little attention in the psychological literature, with regard to issues of culture and values as related to practice, is the military.

Is the military a unique cultural entity about which clinicians should have a fundamental working knowledge of the customs, values, and traditions in order to practice competently? A 2008 paper by Reger, Etherage, Reger, and Gahm posited that the military is indeed a unique culture: "To the extent that a culture includes a language, a code of manners, norms of behavior, belief systems, dress, and rituals, it is clear that the Army represents a unique cultural group" (p. 22). Furthermore, citing the American Psychological Association's ethical code of conduct (2002a), Reger et al. contended that psychologists unfamiliar with the military culture were ethically bound to obtain education, training, supervision, and/or consultation in order to provide the most competent clinical services possible:

> Where scientific or professional knowledge in the discipline of psychology establishes that an understanding of factors associated with age, gender, gender identity, race, ethnicity, culture, national origin, religion, sexual orientation, disability, language, or socioeconomic status is essential for effective implementation of their services or research, psychologists have or obtain the training, experience, consultation, or supervision necessary to ensure the competence of their services, or they make appropriate referrals, except as provided in Standard 2.02, Providing Services in Emergencies. (American Psychological Association, 2002a, §2.01b)

The ability to understand and appreciate the military culture and to tailor clinical practices based on that understanding and appreciation is imperative for clinicians working with service members. Like Reger and colleagues (2008), we recognize that the military shares a unique language, as well as common norms of behavior, customs, and traditions. Clinicians treating service members thus need training, education, and supervision that will make them "culturally competent."

The goals of the current chapter are to (1) provide a brief background on what draws men and women to the military; (2) review the various norms, behaviors, values, and traditions of the military culture and applicable clinical implications; and (3) provide recommendations for improving clinical practice through training, education, and supervision.

Throughout this chapter we use many generalizations, primarily because of scope and page constraints and not a lack of recognition that there are variations among the different branches of the military (i.e., Army, Navy, Air Force, Marine Corps, Coast Guard), as well as within each branch itself. However, it is generally agreed upon by those knowledgeable about military culture that many cultural characteristics are transferable between branches (Christian, Stivers, & Sammons, 2009; Hall, 2008; Matthews, 2009; Reger et al., 2008).

Reasons for Joining the Military

As of December 31, 2009, 1,421,668 people were on active duty (Department of Defense, 2009) in the military, with an additional 848,000 people in the various reserve components (U.S. Congress, 2008). The majority of the force is under the age of 40, married with children, and falls within the designation of "middle class." Across all branches, approximately 15% of the active-duty force is female (the percentage is slightly higher in the reserves;

Kennedy & Malone, 2009), and every major race, religion, and ethnicity is represented. However, even with the tremendous diversity in today's military, service members share many traits and characteristics that lead them down the path of service.

Patriotism

The term "patriotism" has taken on several connotations since the beginning of the wars in Iraq and Afghanistan. It has been used to describe those who are supportive of a particular political party or viewpoint ("unpatriotic" has been used to describe those who dissent from a particular party or viewpoint), as well as to demean classes of people—both those who openly show signs of strong nationalism and those who believe that strong displays of nationalism detract from the need to have rational debates on important political issues.

These issues are of little relevance to the service member while he or she is serving, and likely had no relevance prior to joining. For the service member, patriotism is more in line with *Merriam-Webster's* (2010) definition, "love for or devotion to one's country." The service member's perception of what it means to be an American and how it is connected to self-sacrifice in relation to military and national service has been a primary motivating factor in the decision to serve since the Revolutionary War (Burke, 1992; Doob, 1964; Shaffer, 2007). This perception is also an important variable with regard to choosing to remain in the military (Griffith, 2008, 2010). In short, for service members, patriotism is more than just a word or a springboard to contentious political debate. It is a core and prominent value directly tied to their identity that greatly influences their lives and career decisions.

A Sense of Belonging

Whether it comes from social, religious, occupational, or other types of groups, humans need to feel a sense of acceptance and belonging. Abraham Maslow clearly stated this in his influential paper, "A Theory of Human Motivation," in 1943. For many people, joining the military is a way to develop a sense of belonging and connection with others. The military is a massive "club" that lets in many but retains only those who are able to function within its prescribed rules and boundaries. It promotes comradery, cohesion, unity, and reliance on others, all of which are conducive to giving one a sense of connectedness. Moreover, the military promotes in its members self-esteem and self-worth, and it provides them protection.

There can, however, be drawbacks for those whose identity and sense of belonging are too bound to the military culture. Like those of any other group, members of the military become distrustful of outsiders. If they are not careful, service members can disconnect from the civilian world, which leads to problems once they leave service. Difficulty adjusting to civilian life after many years of service is not uncommon for senior enlisted members and officers (Moore, 2010). Civilian clinicians need to be aware of this when providing care.

Family Tradition

Parental and family variables are strong influences on children's career choices. This is true for civilian children (Bryant, Zvonkovic, & Reynolds, 2006; Chope, 2005; Dietrich & Kracke, 2009), as well as for those in military families (Bachman, Segal, Freedman-Doan, & O'Malley, 2000; Legree et al., 2000). However, following in the career footsteps of the parent, sibling, or grandparent is much more likely for those in military families than it is for kids from nonmilitary families (Gegax & Thomas, 2005).

In her book *Counseling Military Families* (2008), Hall writes about the strong influence of the "family tradition" regarding the choice to join and remain in the military. She writes of a personal conversation with an airman that elucidates the significance of the tradition:

> So I asked what drew him into the military. He said he grew up as a military brat because his dad was career enlisted military. He was born in Japan, had lived in Spain, Panama, and England.... He said being in the military was just a "family thing," and even though his father had actually discouraged him from carrying on the military tradition, it was all he knew. (p. 35)

Hall also makes the point that the fear of living and working in the civilian world is a strong motivating factor for some military children to serve. Just as it is for adults, adjusting to civilian life can be difficult for children who are raised within the military culture. The unknown and untested civilian world can be anxiety provoking. This is not unlike an immigrant who longs for his native country as he finds the customs, traditions, and norms of his new culture strange, confusing, and frightening.

Looking for a Better Life

In general, service members do not come from families of privilege or high financial means. Most come from the working or lower middle class scattered throughout small towns around the country. For many, the values that families in these towns hold revolve around hard work, and less emphasis is placed on education and climbing the "white-collar ladder."

Financial, occupational, and social opportunities are often limited (Henderson, 2006).

The military is an attractive opportunity for those who feel they have limited choices. At the time of this writing, the lowest ranking enlisted member can start out earning over $35,000 a year once base pay, housing and subsistence allowances, and tax advantages are factored into the equation. The salary for a new college graduate entering as an officer is nearly $55,000. Other benefits include free comprehensive medical and dental care, tax-free purchases on base or post, and various other discounts and incentives in the civilian world. These figures are quite impressive if you compare them against the average compensation of a high-school-educated 18-year-old and a college-educated 22-year-old in the civilian world.

Although many service members join the military for the financial benefits, the opportunities for travel to distant and exotic lands is also enticing. Service members have the potential to serve at numerous bases and posts in places such as Germany, Japan, Korea, England, and Italy. Although duty stations vary by branch, stateside bases can also be attractive (e.g., San Diego, Honolulu, San Antonio). And then there are some who join looking for a way to escape from their world and start over (Hall, 2008, p. 39). Whether it be poverty, abuse, discrimination, or interpersonal problems, the military can be an effective escape route for the weary.

Norms, Values, and Traditions of the Military Culture

Group over Individuality

Arguably, the starkest contrast between the civilian and military cultures is the importance placed on individualism versus collectivism, respectively (Christian et al., 2009). McGurk, Colting, Britt, and Adler (2006) discuss three core components of this collective tendency seen in military culture: viewing self as part of the group, placing greater emphasis on group goals than on personal goals, and being emotionally invested in the group.

Although independence and individuality of the person are the cornerstones of today's American culture, these traits are counterproductive in the military for a variety of reasons. In order to function as an effective team and accomplish difficult and complex tasks, a collectivistic approach is required. Individualism fragments the group, which creates an excess of "moving parts" leading to uncertain outcomes. Consider a standard combat infantry platoon. In a combat environment, a common mission would be to breach, clear, and search an unfamiliar home in a known hostile neighborhood. In order to accomplish this task and minimize risk to the team, platoon members must work together on a unified plan. They must know each other's role during the mission, protect themselves as well as their team members, and respond and react collectively if the mission does not go according to plan.

Collectivism also promotes morale and unit cohesion. In my (B. A. M.) experience in providing consultation to commanders in Iraq regarding behavioral problems among service members, poor morale resulting from a lack of unit cohesion was invariably one of the primary culprits. Problem units tended to have leaders who did not appreciate the importance of group cohesion and how it affected a service member's job satisfaction, belief in the mission, and level of stress. They were more likely to put their needs ahead of those of their team members and either consciously or unconsciously splintered the unit by forming and promoting competing alliances. Consequently, morale would diminish, and those service members who felt neglected or marginalized would become more self-focused and rebel against any perceived injustices. In a combat environment, this type of unit atmosphere can have dire consequences.

A collectivistic approach may also function as a protective factor against stress (Christian et al., 2009; Department of the Army, 1994; Mareth & Brooker, 1985). A well-functioning unit with relatively low levels of personal and unit stress had leaders who promoted cohesion and were perceived by subordinates as fair, inclusive, and focused on team and mission.

Implications for the Clinician

It is important for the clinician working with service members to appreciate and understand the emphasis placed in the military on group versus individual interests. Considering that individualism is a treasured and pervasive value in American culture, it is reasonable to assume that a clinician not familiar with the military may unintentionally impose the value of individualism onto the service member during treatment. Consequently, the service member may become defensive and resistant. The service member may also view the clinician as possessing a selfish attitude and may be convinced of any preexisting perceptions that the nonmilitary clinician is an outsider who can't fully appreciate what the service member is going through. An unintended consequence of such a knowledge gap on the clinician's part may be a difficult and unproductive therapeutic relationship.

Hierarchical Class System

The military is built on a rigid and unambiguous hierarchical system. By definition, it would be considered a class system (i.e., the arrangement of people within specific social and economic groups). It is likely one of the most open and transparent cultural class systems in the world, and it ascribes its success and survival to maintaining this structure.

The most glaring example of the military class system is rank. In general, the military is divided into two groups: officers and enlisted. Officers are college-educated men and women who are placed in the highest leadership positions within the military. Within the officer corps, there are various ranks, each related to experience, type of job, and success in past positions. Officers are compensated at a higher level than enlisted members and are discouraged from interacting with enlisted members in social settings (e.g., going to dinner on the weekends). Within the officer corps a similar class system exists. For example, in the Army it would be unusual for a senior officer (colonel) to fraternize with a junior officer (first lieutenant). This hierarchical mindset extends to the family members of the officers as well. It would be unusual for the wives of a colonel and a first lieutenant to be close friends. Although some enlisted members have college degrees, most that enter the service as enlisted men or women do not.

Enlisted members hold various leadership positions but are always under the direction of an officer. The enlisted group also has a separate class system within its ranks. It is made up of junior enlisted members (e.g., private first class, specialist) and senior enlisted members, or noncommissioned officers (NCO; e.g., staff sergeant, master sergeant). Similar to the officer corps, the fraternization between junior- and senior-ranking enlisted members is discouraged. The taboo of interaction between family members is still present; however, it is less pronounced than it is among members of the officer corps. In both groups, there is a tremendous power and influence differential among ranks. Deference must always be paid to those of higher rank. Disrespect is not tolerated and can even be grounds for punishment under the Uniform Code of Military Justice, which consists of the legal rules that govern the military.

The basis for maintaining such a rigid hierarchical class structure is not to create the "haves" and "have nots" but to support a system in which responsibilities are easily delegated and accountability is transparent. If this type of structure is not in place, then little would be accomplished, and it would be difficult to find people to "volunteer" for difficult and dangerous tasks, which are common in the military.

Implications for the Clinician

It is important for the clinician to understand that the service member's status may have some connection to his or her presenting problem. A junior enlisted member or officer is more likely to present with problems associated with lack of autonomy, independence, and overall adjustment to the military culture. For the senior enlisted member or officer seeking psychiatric services, it is likely that the presenting problem is of a more serious nature (Axis I disorders, marital or occupational problems, substance abuse/

dependence). The reason is what I (B. A. M.) refer to as "double stigma": Not only is the senior service member faced with the general stigma associated with seeking psychiatric help in the military, but he or she is also faced with the stigma of showing weakness as a senior person. As a result, he or she will likely be reluctant to seek help until functioning is dramatically reduced. The clinician needs to be sensitive to these issues and consistently reinforce the service member's decision to seek help.

Other issues to be aware of are that the nonmilitary clinician may be viewed by the junior enlisted member as an "officer equivalent" and be treated accordingly (e.g., calling the clinician "sir" or "ma'am," standing at attention when the clinician walks in); senior service members may feel disrespected if not referred to by their rank; and junior service members may be under pressure from superiors to seek help. The latter has considerable implications for treatment outcome, particularly as related to compliance and attitude toward the therapist. Furthermore, there are a number of ethical issues to be considered, not the least of which is the issue of voluntary consent to treatment.

A Language of Their Own

Each culture has its own unique and distinct language, and the military culture is no different. The language of the military is filled with acronyms, abbreviations, and unique words that are used for the primary purpose of relaying important information in an expedient manner, while minimizing confusion and verbal communication errors. Moreover, much of the military common language is nonverbal (e.g., hand signals) and subtle (e.g., head nodding). For the clinician unfamiliar with the military language, there can be much confusion and frustration. The case example borrowed from Reger, Etherage, Reger, and Gahm (2008, p. 23) illustrates this point:

> Dr. Smith had trained at a VA during graduate school and his father had volunteered for the Army during the Vietnam Conflict. He now wanted to serve those in uniform as a civilian psychologist and accepted a position at an Army MTF. However, he wondered if he had made a mistake as he listened, confused, to his first patient. Specialist Johnson entered Dr. Smith's office and stoically explained that his wife encouraged him to come to the clinic due to a variety of stressors associated with his recent arrival at his new assignment. He alleged that DFAS had cheated him out of some money related to his recent partial DITY and that his new platoon SGT was a "POG" who, he was told, was nothing but a FOBIT on the last deployment. Now in garrison, the platoon SGT was employing his troops in "fulltime PMCS. I never get to do my job." Nonetheless, he had gotten into trouble for missing a formation and had just had his first reading for an Article 15. Dr. Smith was caught off guard when the Soldier referred to

him constantly as "Sir" and rose formally when Dr. Smith stood. Specialist Johnson hesitated to commit to any treatment plan, saying he wasn't sure about coming in today and he certainly was not sure he would come back. He joked, "I don't think I need to be here. Pain is just weakness leaving the body."[1]

Implications for the Clinician

The clinician unfamiliar with military language who tries to treat a service member faces the same challenges one would face working with clients from any other unfamiliar cultural group. To provide the most effective services possible, a basic understanding of military jargon and idioms is required. Clinicians lacking this understanding who encounter clients from the military should ask what a particular term or phrase means if he or she doesn't understand it. An attempt to "fake it" during the therapy by pretending to understand something will be detected by most service members. In contrast, acknowledging a lack of understanding about a military concept or term allows the service member to educate the clinician, which can strengthen the therapeutic alliance, particularly for the service member who is unsure and hesitant regarding treatment. In addition to improving the therapeutic alliance, understanding military terminology will help the clinician avoid missing important information regarding the service member's presenting problem, views about mental health treatment, and overall functioning.

Strong Values of Service

As Matthews (2009) recently pointed out, one cannot fully understand the motivation and mind-set of the solider without understanding the value-based system of the military culture. Adhering to strong values is a way of life for service members, and none are excused from exemplifying these values daily. For example, Army doctrine lists seven core values (loyalty, respect, duty, honor, integrity, selfless service, and personal courage) that are assumed to be necessary for developing strong leaders and soldiers. The Marine Corps and Navy define their core values as honor, courage, and commitment. The Air Force lists integrity, selfless service, and excellence as its value base. And the Coast Guard puts forth honor, respect, and devotion to duty as its core.

---

[1]Definitions for acronyms and terms: MTF, military or medical treatment facility; DFAS, defense finance and accounting service; DITY, do it yourself move; POG, person other than grunt; FOBIT, someone who doesn't leave the base in a combat zone; garrison, nondeployed duty station; PMCS, preventive maintenance checks and services (vehicle maintenance); Formation, gathering of service members in an organized fashion; Article 15, nonjudicial military punishment; SGT, sergeant.

The value-laden culture of the military is driven by practical need. High moral and ethical standards exist in the military not for the purpose of giving members a sense of superiority but to foster commitment, unity, collectivism, nationalism, and sacrifice—qualities that are necessary for the greater mission of protecting the nation and its citizens.

Implications for the Clinician

To be effective, the clinician must appreciate and acknowledge the value-based life of the service member. Failing to do so jeopardizes the therapeutic relationship. However, this appreciation should not require any special skills or training, as respect for any patient's values is imperative when providing therapy (Bergin, 1980; Holmes, 1997; Kelly, 1990). What it does require, however, is an understanding that many service members consider values daily and are acutely aware of how not exemplifying them can bring about ridicule, harassment, and guilt, as well as reduce force effectiveness and put their teammates at risk. There are even potential career and legal consequences for not adhering to key values (e.g., having an extramarital affair).

Considering the sanctity of the core values among service members, it's also important for the clinician to be aware of how his or her own personal values, ethics, and beliefs may affect the relationship. The clinician may have strong views about war and violence or what it means to have integrity and honor. Obviously, the therapy session is not the place for debating these issues. Moreover, under no circumstances should the service member be criticized or judged for his or her actions while serving in a deployed setting. This will only reinforce any preexisting guilt and shame the service member may have and all but guarantee a poor outcome in treatment.

Solution Focused

During the initial weeks of recruit training, service members are taught how to be problem solvers. This is evidenced by the Military Problem Solving Process (Department of the Army, 1999) and the Military Decision Making Process (Department of the Army, 2010; see Tables 1.1 and 1.2), which are taught to soldiers during the early stages of training.

In general, service members are required to be solution focused and are taught that every problem can be solved given enough time, thought, resources, and effort. A common phrase used in the military to highlight this point is "adapt and overcome," referring to the need to be flexible and to find a solution when one is not immediately apparent. Taken to the extreme, a service member who is not solution oriented but focuses on the problem instead may be seen as inept, unmotivated and lazy, or whining.

TABLE 1.1. Military Problem-Solving Process

1. Recognize and define the problem.
2. Gather facts and make assumptions.
3. Define end states and establish criteria.
4. Develop possible solutions.
5. Analyze and compare possible solutions.
6. Select and implement solution.
7. Analyze solution for effectiveness.

Implications for the Clinician

For the therapist who is comfortable being directive and prescriptive, the service member's solution-focused mind-set can be a tremendous asset in treatment. In concert with the therapist, the service member will generate and implement strategies for change. Moreover, the therapist can be confident that cognitive and behavioral homework assignments will be completed and that attendance at scheduled sessions will be consistent. For those therapists uncomfortable with a directive and prescriptive approach, effective treatment is still possible. However, the service member may become uncomfortable with a passive and Socratic approach, leading to impatience, resistance, inadequate rapport, and inconsistent attendance.

Show No Weakness

Stoicism is a valued trait in the military (Sherman, 2005). It is associated with strength, emotional control, and calmness under pressure. Although useful in a deployed setting, this characteristic promotes the stigma that seeking mental health services is a sign of weakness and lack of dependability. As has been noted elsewhere, stigma is one of the largest impediments

TABLE 1.2. Military Decision-Making Process

1. Receipt of mission.
2. Mission analysis.
3. Course of action development.
4. Course of action analysis.
5. Course of action comparison.
6. Course of action approval.
7. Orders production.

to service members and veterans getting the psychological care they need (Hoge et al., 2004; Pietrzak et al., 2010; Wright et al., 2009).

Implications for the Clinician

The clinician must be cognizant that the stoic mind-set is highly adaptive in the military environment. If not, the clinician unfamiliar with military culture may perceive the service member's stoicism as resistance, prompting a possible countertransference reaction. In my (B. A. M.) experience, it is productive to address the issue of stigma early in treatment, as well as to reinforce the service member's courage in seeking help. Accepting that stigma is a normal aspect of military culture only reinforces the problem.

Conclusion

The military is a unique culture that possesses its own set of norms, values, and customs, as well as its own language and class structure. To be effective, the clinician must be aware of these cultural issues. Not to be will affect individual treatment outcome and potentially have a significant effect on the military unit.

Gaining military cultural awareness is no different from gaining cultural awareness of any other group. It is a matter of taking time, making an effort, and applying what is learned to practice. For a list of resources regarding gaining military cultural competence, see Appendix A in this volume.

References

American Psychological Association. (2002a). Ethical principles of psychologists and code of conduct. *American Psychologist, 57*(12), 1060–1073.

American Psychological Association. (2002b). *Guidelines on multicultural education, training, research, practice, and organizational change for psychologists.* Washington, DC: Author.

Bachman, J., Segal, D., Freedman-Doan, P., & O'Malley, P. (2000). Who chooses military service? Correlates of propensity and enlistment in the U.S. Armed Forces. *Military Psychology, 12*(1), 1–30.

Bergin, A. (1980). Psychotherapy and religious values. *Journal of Consulting and Clinical Psychology, 48*(1), 95–105.

Bryant, B., Zvonkovic, A., & Reynolds, P. (2006). Parenting in relation to child and adolescent vocational development. *Journal of Vocational Behavior, 69*(1), 149–175.

Burke, J. S. (1992). *The persistence and importance of patriotism in the all volunteer force.* Columbus, OH: Battelle Memorial Institute.

Chope, R. (2005). Qualitatively Assessing Family Influence in Career Decision Making. *Journal of Career Assessment, 13*(4), 395–414.

Christian, J., Stivers, J., & Sammons, M. (2009). Training to the warrior ethos: Implications for clinicians treating military members and their families. In S. Morgillo-Freeman, B. A. Moore, & A. Freeman (Eds.), *Living and surviving in harm's way: A psychological treatment handbook for pre- and postdeployment of military personnel* (pp. 27–49). New York: Routledge/Taylor & Francis.

Department of the Army. (1994). *Field manual no. 22-51: Leader's manual for combat stress control.* Washington, DC: Author.

Department of the Army. (1999). *Field manual no. 22-100: Army leadership.* Washington, DC: Author.

Department of the Army. (2010). *Field manual no. 5-0: The operations process.* Washington, DC: Author.

Department of Defense. (2009, December 31). *Active duty military personnel strengths by regional area and by country.* Retrieved July 27, 2010, from *siadapp.dmdc.osd.mil/personnel/MILITARY/history/hst0912.pdf.*

Dietrich, J., & Kracke, B. (2009). Career-specific parental behaviors in adolescents' development. *Journal of Vocational Behavior, 75*(2), 109–119.

Doob, L. W. (1964). *Patriotism and nationalism: Their psychological foundations.* New Haven, CT: Yale University Press.

Gegax, T. T., & Thomas, E. (2005, June 20). The family business. *Newsweek, 145*(25), 24–31.

Griffith, J. (2008). Institutional motives for serving in the U.S. Army National Guard: Implications for recruitment, retention, and readiness. Armed Forces and Society, 34, 230–258.

Griffith, J. (2010). When does soldier patriotism or nationalism matter?: The role of transformational small-unit leaders. *Journal of Applied Social Psychology, 40*(5), 1235–1257.

Hall, L. (2008). *Counseling military families: What mental health professionals need to know.* New York: Routledge/Taylor & Francis

Henderson, K. (2006). *While they're at war: The true story of American families on the homefront.* New York: Houghton Mifflin.

Hoge, C., Castro, C., Messer, S., McGurk, D., Cotting, D., & Koffman, R. (2004). Combat duty in Iraq and Afghanistan, mental health problems, and barriers to care. *New England Journal of Medicine, 351*(1), 13–22.

Holmes, J. (1997). Values in psychotherapy. *Australian and New Zealand Journal of Psychiatry, 31*(3), 331–339.

Kelly, T. (1990). The role of values in psychotherapy: A critical review of process and outcome effects. *Clinical Psychology Review, 10*(2), 171–186.

Kennedy, C. H., & Malone, R. C. (2009). Integration of women into the modern military. In S. Morgillo-Freeman, B. A. Moore, & A. Freeman (Eds.), *Living and surviving in harm's way: A psychological treatment handbook for pre- and postdeployment of military personnel* (pp. 67–81). New York: Routledge/Taylor & Francis.

Legree, P., Gade, P., Martin, D., Fischl, M., Wilson, M., Nieva, V., et al. (2000). Military enlistment and family dynamics: Youth and parental perspectives. *Military Psychology, 12*(1), 31–49.

Mareth, T. R., & Brooker, A. E. (1985). Combat stress reaction: A concept in evolution. *Military Medicine, 150*(4), 186–190.

Maslow, A. H. (1943). A theory of human motivation. *Psychological Review, 50*(4), 370–396.

Matthews, M. (2009). The soldier's mind: Motivation, mindset, and attitude. In S. Morgillo-Freeman, B. A. Moore, & A. Freeman (Eds.), *Living and surviving in harm's way: A psychological treatment handbook for pre- and postdeployment of military personnel* (pp. 9–26). New York: Routledge/Taylor & Francis.

McGurk, D., Cotting, D., Britt, T., & Adler, A. (2006). Joining the ranks: The role of indoctrination in transforming civilians to service members. In T. W. Britt, A. B. Adler, & C. A. Castro (Eds.), *Military life: The psychology of service in peace and combat: Vol. 2. Operational stress* (pp. 13–31). Westport, CT: Praeger.

Merriam-Webster's online dictionary. Retrieved July 28, 2010, from *www.merriam-webster.com/dictionary/patriotism.*

Moore, B. A. (2010, August 2). Patience, restraint can help you cope with civilians. *Army Times,* p. B13.

Pietrzak, R., Goldstein, M., Malley, J., Rivers, A., Johnson, D., & Southwick, S. (2010). Risk and protective factors associated with suicidal ideation in veterans of operations Enduring Freedom and Iraqi Freedom. *Journal of Affective Disorders, 123*(1–3), 102–107.

Reger, M., Etherage, J., Reger, G., & Gahm, G. (2008). Civilian psychologists in an Army culture: The ethical challenge of cultural competence. *Military Psychology, 20*(1), 21–35.

Shaffer, J. (2007). Performing patriotism: National identity in the colonial and revolutionary American theater. Philadelphia: University of Pennsylvania Press.

Sherman, N. (2005). *Stoic warriors: The ancient philosophy behind the military mind.* New York: Oxford University Press.

U.S. Congress. (2008). S. 3001 [Report No. 110-335]. Retrieved July 27, 2010, from *frwebgate.access.gpo.gov/cgibin/getdoc.cgi?dbname=110_cong_bills&docid =f:s3001pcs.txt.pdf.*

Wright, K., Cabrera, O., Bliese, P., Adler, A., Hoge, C., & Castro, C. (2009). Stigma and barriers to care in soldiers postcombat. *Psychological Services, 6*(2), 108–116.

CHAPTER 2

Issues in Assessment of PTSD in Military Personnel

Frank Castro
Jasmeet P. Hayes
Terence M. Keane

Compared with individuals in the general population, men and women who participate in military combat are at greater risk for the development of posttraumatic stress disorder (PTSD). The National Vietnam Veterans Readjustment Study (NVVRS; Kulka et al., 1990a, 1990b) suggests that approximately 30% percent of Vietnam theater males and 27% of females met criteria for lifetime PTSD, whereas overall lifetime prevalence rates for PTSD in the general population range from 7.8 to 9.5% (Breslau, Davis, Andreski, & Peterson, 1991; Kessler, Sonnega, Bromet, Hughes, & Nelson, 1995), with PTSD being more prevalent in women (rates range from 10.4 to 12%) than in men (5.0 to 9.5%; Resnick, Kilpatrick, Dansky, Saunders, & Best, 1993). Current estimates for the prevalence of PTSD in veterans of Operation Enduring Freedom (OEF) and Operation Iraqi Freedom (OIF) vary widely. In a recent review, Ramchand and colleagues (2010) examined PTSD prevalence rates for previously deployed personnel across 29 studies. Prevalence rates for personnel not seeking treatment generally ranged from 5 to 20%. Across the ten studies examining OEF/OIF veterans seeking treatment, prevalence rates ranged from 4 to 50%. The authors attribute the wide range of estimates to a number of factors, including multiple methods of assessment and criteria used to determine a positive PTSD screen/diagnosis. Veterans Affairs (VA) estimates that approximately 26% of veterans seeking treatment at VA facilities meet criteria for PTSD (U.S. Department of Veterans Affairs, Veterans Health Administration, Office of Public Health and Environmental Hazards, 2010), which we believe is a more representative estimate of treatment-seeking OEF/OIF veterans.

Despite the long association between military combat and the development of PTSD, the assessment and treatment of PTSD in military personnel continue to present a unique series of challenges to mental health professionals. The goal of the present chapter is twofold. First, we aim to highlight a number of the most salient barriers to accurate assessment of PTSD in military populations. Second, we provide a robust assessment plan that takes into account these barriers in order to increase the likelihood of accurate case conceptualization and treatment planning.

Assessment Barriers

Accurate assessment of PTSD is necessary for many reasons: (1) to aid in treatment planning, (2) to permit progress in research of the disorder, (3) to present systematic information for policy decisions, and (4) to determine disability benefits. To be truly useful, the assessment approach must measure the diagnosis accurately and be sensitive and specific to the diagnosis. However, there are several obstacles that may arise that challenge the accuracy of the PTSD and other mental health assessments in military populations.

One significant barrier to PTSD assessment is underreporting of mental health symptoms due to stigma (Corrigan, 2004). Stigma associated with psychiatric illness is often exacerbated in military culture, which often prides itself on a stoic response to extreme duress, and emotional responses such as hyperarousal and nightmares may be considered a significant frailty (see Chapter 1, this volume). For example, 65% of a sample of OEF/OIF military personnel who screened positive for a mental health disorder feared being perceived as "weak," and 63% feared adverse treatment from their superiors (Hoge et al., 2004). Military personnel may also discount their symptoms out of guilt or shame. In the aftermath of war, bullet wounds, amputations, burns, and other visible injuries serve as a physical, tangible, and often noble reminder of the war experience. These reminders are often officially recognized by the military in the form of medals such as the Purple Heart. Veterans suffering from psychological symptoms may feel that their trauma does not merit the same attention and respect as a physical ailment and may be disinclined to report their symptoms. Clearly, the stigma surrounding emotional distress in the military may prevent soldiers and veterans from receiving the care they need causing them to avoid appointments or simply underreport their current level of distress.

Limits in confidentiality are additional barriers that may prevent military personnel from disclosing a traumatic event. Depending on the index trauma, patients can experience feelings of shame, guilt, fear, and anger associated with their perceived actions or inactions during the event. They may privilege disclosing or endorsing one set of experiences as their index trauma over another for reasons of social desirability. Admission of traumatic events such as military sexual trauma (e.g., rape) or participating in atrocities could adversely affect a person's military career or lead to other serious consequences, including criminal charges and even imprisonment. Further, being diagnosed with PTSD or other mental illnesses could prevent an individual from being deployed or continuing his or her current mission. As many military personnel highly value their jobs, their comrades, and their units, they may be more willing to suffer in silence than risk nondeployment or removal from active duty. Therefore, trust and confidentiality during the assessment session become key factors in order for an individual to reveal his or her role in a distressing event. However, depending on the assessment context, complete confidentiality often cannot be guaranteed (Michaels, 2006). This risk is particularly salient for active-duty personnel.

For example, although the Military Rules of Evidence (MRE) includes a statute protecting psychotherapist–patient privilege of confidentiality (Rule 513), an exception can be made to this privilege when the information is "necessary to ensure the safety and security of military personnel, military dependents, military property, classified information, or the accomplishment of a military mission" (Manual for Courts-Martial, United States, Military Rules of Evidence 513[d], 2008). In addition, if a service member is referred for a mental health assessment by a commanding officer, information regarding his or her diagnosis and treatment can be disclosed (Department of Defense 1997, 1998). Given these statutes, providers can be compelled to break confidentiality. (For an in-depth review of the ethical obligations and limits of confidentiality in the military see Howe, 1989, or Warner, Appenzeller, Grieger, Benedek, & Roberts, 2009.) Reticence to disclose traumatic events can also occur when an individual is seeking care in an outpatient setting, such as a VA facility. Although uncommon, medical records for National Guard, reservists, or other personnel likely to be redeployed may be reviewed by the Department of Defense (DoD). In addition, if a veteran believes his or her trauma can be classified as a war crime, they may fear possible prosecution, as war crimes do not have a statute of limitations (War Crimes Act of 1996).

Underreporting of symptoms presents a great challenge for clinicians in the accurate assessment of PTSD, but an equally challenging assessment barrier is overreporting of symptoms or questionable veracity of military and veterans' self-reports. In particular, compensation-seeking (CS) veterans have been singled out for possible symptom malingering or exaggeration for secondary gain.

VA Disability Compensation is a tax-free benefit paid to a veteran for injuries or diseases that developed while on active duty or that were exacerbated by active military service. In addition to the monthly stipend (in some cases totaling $3,000 a month or more), a veteran may also be eligible for free VA healthcare and other ancillary benefits, depending on the rating of his or her disability (often referred to as his or her level of service connection). Studies comparing CS and non-compensation-seeking (NCS) veterans observed that CS veterans are more likely to report elevated rates of PTSD symptoms but are less likely to be diagnosed with PTSD, indicative of a possible overreporting bias for CS veterans (DeViva & Bloem, 2003; Frueh, Gold, & de Arellano, 1997; Frueh, Smith, & Barker, 1996; Gold & Frueh, 1999; Jordan, Nunley, & Cook, 1992; Smith, & Frueh, 1996). Alternatively, Tolin and colleagues (2004) found that CS veterans reported increased symptoms and were more likely to be diagnosed with PTSD than NCS veterans. Each of these studies employed convenience samples rather than representative ones, and so strong conclusions cannot yet be drawn.

At this time, there is little systematic available evidence that documents the rates of malingered PTSD in the interest of procuring service-connected benefits. PTSD, being an invisible wound of war (much like mild traumatic brain injury [TBI]), lends itself to both over- and underendorsement of symptoms. Most experts believe, however, that the rates of PTSD found in the NVVRS represent true rates of the condition following that war, because the data in that study were collected anonymously without the possibility of directly influencing eligibility for financial or healthcare benefits for participants.

It is also notable that a veteran's CS status can affect a clinician's attitude about the veteran. Sayer and Thuras (2002) found that VA clinicians in PTSD programs were more likely to have a more negative view of the treatment engagement and therapeutic alliance of compensation seekers than non-compensation seekers, and that this view increased as a function of the time a clinician worked with PTSD patients. Overall, determining the etiology and magnitude of symptom elevation or overreporting bears critical impact on a clinician's case conceptualization and the client's prognosis.

A final notable barrier in the assessment of PTSD for military personnel relates to safety (e.g., suicidal/homicidal ideation and attempts). Although of concern during any mental health assessment, attention to issues of safety is especially warranted when dealing with clients with possible PTSD. In a recent meta-analysis of the general population, Krysinska and Lester (2010) found PTSD to be associated with an increase in previous suicide attempts, as well as current and previous suicidal ideation. Veterans with PTSD are likely to manifest several risk factors that increase the probability of suicidal thinking and suicide attempts, including depression and feelings of hopelessness, substance abuse, estrangement from social supports, chronic anxiety and anger, and employment or financial difficulties (Chiles & Strosahl, 2005). Vietnam combat veterans with PTSD appear to own a large number of weapons (Freeman, Clothier, Thornton, & Keesee, 1994) and to engage in problematic behaviors such as suicide attempts, suicidal ideation, threatening family members, and assault with these weapons (Freeman & Roca, 2001). Importantly, this concern applies equally to male and female veterans. Although women in the general population are more likely to use less lethal means (e.g., drug overdose) during a suicide attempt, female military personnel are more likely to mirror their male counterparts and use more lethal means, such as firearms, during a suicide attempt (Kaplan, McFarland, & Huguet, 2009).

Assessment Recommendations

Accurate assessment of PTSD for military personnel is a multifaceted process that includes orienting the client to the assessment process, creating a comfortable environment in which patients feel at ease to share their experiences, and engaging in a multimethod approach to the assessment of PTSD that includes structured diagnostic interviews, self-report psychological questionnaires, and medical record review, particularly when self-report may not be reliable (Keane, Fairbank, Caddell, Zimering, & Bender, 1985). This approach is recommended to overcome assessment barriers that may potentially interfere with accurate case conceptualization. First, we present general recommendations that help to orient the client to assessment and, second, present a variety of measures from which clinicians can choose that constitute an evidence-based evaluation approach for the assessment of PTSD.

General Recommendations

Establish Rapport and Engage in Psychoeducation

During assessment cases in which the patient appears reluctant to disclose his or her traumatic event, the clinician can strive toward reducing stigma by expressing genuine empathy and recognition of the difficulty inherent in discussing a personally traumatic event (Keane et al., 1985). For patients experiencing feelings of guilt and shame surrounding their trauma, the clinician can acknowledge that there are certain contexts in which people engage in acts that they would normally never do. Additionally, normalizing combat stress reactions (e.g., explaining how hypervigilance was adaptive in a combat situation but is problematic in the civilian world), providing clients with specific readjustment resources, and informing clients of empirically supported interventions for PTSD and other mental health concerns have great value in reducing stigma surrounding mental health symptoms. When the stigma associated with their symptoms is reduced, clients may be more inclined to accurately report their index traumas, as well as their current symptomatology.

Know and Convey the Limits of Confidentiality

During the assessment process, clients are asked to disclose highly sensitive information, which may raise questions for the patient, such as how the sensitive information will be handled, who will have access to it, and whether the patient has any control over the information once it is disclosed. Explaining the limits of confidentiality can reduce the patient's anxiety over personal disclosure by promoting openness, trust, and rapport with the clinician and providing a sense of empowerment for the patient in his or her decision of what information to disclose. Prior to the assessment, clinicians who know the answers to the following questions will be able to provide crucial information and assurance to the patient:

1. What are the explicit limits to confidentiality for the client given his or her active-duty status?
2. What are the limits to confidentiality for the client at the current setting (e.g., DoD, Vet Center versus VA)?
3. What are the limits of confidentiality as determined by the clinician's professional governing body?
4. What are the clinician's personal ethics regarding confidentiality, and are they in line with questions 1 and 2?
5. What are the possible ramifications for the client if the clinician breaks confidentiality?
6. What are the possible ramifications for the clinician if confidentiality is broken?

Importantly, the clinician has the responsibility to discuss the limits of confidentiality with the client and to provide written documentation, as well as verbal instruction, as to the limits of their confidentiality. By knowing the real risks involved, clients can decide for themselves what risks, if any, they are willing to take for the sake of their mental health.

Plan for Multiple Assessment Sessions

When feasible, scheduling multiple assessment sessions will greatly enhance accurate case conceptualization and overcome assessment barriers in military populations. Multiple sessions become particularly necessary when there is a question of under- or overreporting of symptoms, comorbid substance abuse problems, or endorsement of homicidal or suicidal ideation. In addition, it may take time to adequately develop enough rapport with the client to facilitate his or her disclosure of certain traumatic events. The amount of time necessary for an accurate assessment depends on a number of factors, including the purpose of the assessment outcome, clinical complications, severity of the case, and number and type of assessment measures used. Although there are no established guidelines, when time permits, best-practice models of assessment might involve the use of structured diagnostic interviews, the administration of psychological tests and questionnaires, and even measures of psychophysiological reactivity (Keane, Silberbogen, & Weierich, 2008).

Evidence-Based Assessment Measures

Many approaches are available for the assessment of PTSD, but the International Society for Traumatic Stress Studies (ISTSS; Foa, Keane, Friedman, & Cohen, 2009) presented one approach to best practices that incorporates the use of important evidence-based measures that are keyed to the diagnostic criteria for PTSD (cf., Keane, Weathers, & Foa 2000; Weathers, Keane, & Foa, 2009). Our approach here mirrors that described in the ISTSS guidelines and reflects the inaugural work completed by our group in the earliest stages of assessment development (e.g., Keane et al., 1985; Keane & Kaloupek, 1982).

Structured Diagnostic Interviews

Although the use of structured diagnostic interviews requires more investment of clinic resources than self-report questionnaires, their use in clinical settings is highly recommended in order to improve diagnostic accuracy and aid in treatment planning for PTSD (Keane, Wolfe, & Taylor, 1987). In particular, we recommend the use of clinical interviews to clearly establish a Criterion A event to anchor subsequent symptom endorsement. Next we highlight a brief list of structured diagnostic interviews that we recommend be used in practice.

CLINICIAN-ADMINISTERED PTSD SCALE

Developed by the National Center for PTSD (Blake et al., 1990), the Clinician-Administered PTSD Scale (CAPS) is the most widely used structured interview for diagnosing and measuring PTSD severity (Weathers, Keane, & Davidson, 2001). The CAPS assesses all DSM-IV (American Psychiatric

Association, 1994) diagnostic criteria for PTSD, as well as the associated symptoms of guilt and dissociation. Importantly, the CAPS provides separate ratings for the frequency and intensity of each symptom, which permits flexibility in scoring and analysis. It also promotes uniform administration and scoring through carefully phrased prompt questions and explicit rating scale anchors with clear behavioral referents. There is also flexibility built into the administration of the CAPS. Interviewers can administer only the 17 core symptoms, all DSM-IV criteria, and/or the associated symptoms. Administration time is approximately 30 minutes to an hour, depending on the severity of the client's PTSD symptoms and the sections that the interviewer chooses to utilize. Once trained, interviewers are able to ask their own follow-up questions and use clinical judgment in arriving at a diagnosis.

Weathers, Ruscio, and Keane (1999) examined the reliability and validity data of the CAPS across five samples of male Vietnam veterans interviewed at the National Center for PTSD. Robust estimates were found for interrater reliability over a 2- to 3-day interval for each of the three symptom clusters and all 17 symptoms. Test–retest reliability for a CAPS-based PTSD diagnosis was also excellent. Thus the data indicate that trained raters can achieve a high degree of consistency in using the CAPS to rate symptom severity and diagnose PTSD. Weathers et al. (1999) also found excellent internal consistency across all 17 items in research and clinical samples, which supports the use of the CAPS in both settings.

There is strong evidence for validity of the CAPS. Weathers et al. (1999) reported that the CAPS total severity score correlated highly with other measures of PTSD, such as the Mississippi Scale, the Minnesota Multiphasic Personality Inventory (MMPI) PTSD Scale, the number of PTSD symptoms endorsed on the Structured Clinical Interview for DSM-IV (SCID-IV), and the PTSD Checklist (Weathers, Litz, Herman, Huska, & Keane, 1993). They also found strong evidence for the diagnostic utility of the CAPS using three different CAPS scoring rules for predicting a SCID-based PTSD diagnosis (Weathers et al., 2001).

STRUCTURED CLINICAL INTERVIEW FOR DSM-IV

The SCID-IV (First, Spitzer, Williams, & Gibbon, 2000) assesses a broad range of Axis I and II psychiatric conditions. It is divided into separate modules corresponding to DSM-IV diagnostic criteria, with each module providing the interviewer with prompts and follow-up inquiries intended to be read verbatim to respondents. The SCID can be administered by clinicians and highly trained interviewers.

Although the administration of the full SCID-IV can be time-consuming, the modular structure allows clinicians to tailor their assessment appropriately. Within the context of a trauma clinic, it is recommended that the anxiety disorder, affective disorder, and substance use disorder modules be administered in order to rule out any comorbid diagnoses. Administration of the psychotic screen will also help to rule out psychiatric conditions that require a different set of treatment interventions (Keane & Barlow, 2002).

The SCID-PTSD module is considered to be psychometrically sound. Keane et al. (1998) reported that the SCID-PTSD had adequate reliability, and McFall, Smith, Roszell, Tarver, and Malas (1990) reported evidence of convergent validity, finding significant correlations between the SCID-PTSD and other measures of PTSD, including the Mississippi Scale (Keane, Caddell, & Taylor, 1988) and the Keane PTSD (PK) scale of the MMPI-2 (Keane, Malloy, & Fairbank, 1984). The SCID-PTSD module also had good diagnostic utility when used in the clinical subsample of the NVVRS (Kulka et al., 1988).

Although the SCID is a good diagnostic tool, several limitations exist. First, the SCID permits only dichotomous ratings of PTSD symptoms (e.g., presence or absence of symptoms), whereas most clinicians agree that psychological symptoms occur in a dimensional rather than dichotomous fashion (Keane, Weathers, & Foa, 2000). Second, the SCID does not assess for the frequency or severity of symptoms. Finally, only those symptoms associated with the "worst event" are assessed, and the effects of other traumas are not evaluated.

PTSD SYMPTOM SCALE INTERVIEW

Developed by Foa, Riggs, Dancu, and Rothbaum (1993), the PTSD Symptom Scale Interview (PSS-I) is a structured interview designed to assess symptoms of PTSD. Using a Likert scale, interviewers rate the severity of 17 symptoms corresponding to the DSM-III-R criteria for PTSD. One limitation of the PSS-I is that it measures symptoms over the preceding 2 weeks, rather than the 1 month that the DSM criteria specify as necessary for a diagnosis of PTSD (Cusak, Falsetti, & de Arellano, 2002). The PSS-I is brief (administration time is approximately 20 minutes) and can be administered by novice clinical interviewers who are trained to work with trauma patients.

The PSS-I was originally tested in a sample of women with a history of rape and nonsexual assault (Foa et al., 1993) and found to have strong psychometric properties. Foa et al. reported good internal consistency, test–retest reliability over a 1-month period, and interrater agreement for a PTSD diagnosis. The PSS-I is significantly correlated with other measures of traumatic stress, such as the Impact of Events Scale (IES) Intrusion score (Horowitz, Wilner, & Alvarez, 1979) and the Rape Aftermath Symptom Test total score (Kilpatrick, 1988). In addition, it has demonstrated good diagnostic utility when compared with a SCID-PTSD diagnosis. The PSS-I appears to possess many strong features that warrant its consideration for clinical use, especially with sexual assault survivors.

Self-Report Measures

Self-report measures provide information on the presence or absence of PTSD, trauma symptoms, and their severity. Many of these measures provide specific cutoffs that are indicative of a diagnosis of PTSD, whereas the majority of measures incorporate continuous indicators of symptom severity. As an actuarial method of assessment, self-report measures complement clinical judgments made during the structured diagnostic interview. Self-report measures with validity scales, such as the MMPI-2, are especially useful in the assessment process, as they can help determine possible malingering or underreporting. In addition, many of these measures were normed on veteran rather than civilian populations, thereby providing the assessing clinician with an expected range of symptomatology. The following list of self-report measures provides the assessing clinician with a wide selection of assessment tools from which to choose.

MINNESOTA MULTIPHASIC PERSONALITY INVENTORY— SECOND EDITION

Created as an updated version of the original MMPI (Hathaway & McKinley, 1951), the MMPI-2 (Butcher et al., 2001) is one of the most widely used assessment tools. It provides comprehensive psychological assessment across a variety of domains and a set of validity and response-bias scales that are particularly useful in the assessment of malingering and underreporting of symptomatolgy. In particular, the F_p scale is effective in determining overreporting with respect to veterans being assessed for PTSD (Tolin et al., 2004).

In addition to the validity and response-bias scales, subscales of the MMPI-2 can be used as a direct assessment tool of the presence of PTSD. Originally derived from the MMPI Form R (Keane et al., 1984), the Keane PTSD scale (PK) consists of 46 items empirically drawn from the MMPI-2 (Lyons & Keane, 1992). The scale is typically administered as part of the full MMPI-2, but it can be useful as a stand-alone scale. The embedded and stand-alone versions are highly correlated (.90; Herman, Weathers, Litz, & Keane, 1996). The PK scale yields a total score that reflects the presence or absence of PTSD. The stand-alone scale takes 15 minutes to administer.

Psychometric data on the embedded and stand-alone versions of the PK scale are excellent. Herman et al. (1996) reported evidence from a veteran sample of strong internal consistency of the embedded and stand-alone versions of the PK scale and high test–retest reliability coefficients for the stand-alone version over 2–3 days. With regard to validity, the embedded and stand-alone versions of the PK scale were correlated with other self-report measures of PTSD, including the Mississippi Scale, the IES, the PTSD Checklist (PCL), and a diagnostic interview (CAPS). The embedded and stand-alone versions of the PK scale differed slightly in their optimally efficient cutoff score, but both demonstrated good clinical utility as compared with a CAPS diagnosis.

MISSISSIPPI SCALE FOR COMBAT-RELATED PTSD

Developed by Keane et al. (1988), the 35-item Mississippi Scale is widely used to assess combat-related PTSD symptoms. The scale items were selected from an initial pool of 200 items generated by experts to reflect the disorder. Unlike other self-report measures of PTSD, the Mississippi Scale is a dimensional measure of PTSD and possesses a high degree of content validity, as its items were not restricted to the diagnostic criteria for the disorder but rather included items associated with the construct of the condition. Accordingly, the value of the Mississippi Scale continues across modifications of the DSM criteria. To complete this scale, respondents are asked to rate the severity of symptoms over the time period occurring "since the event" using a Likert scale. The Mississippi Scale yields a continuous score of symptom severity, as well as diagnostic information. It is available in several languages and takes 10–15 minutes to administer.

The Mississippi Scale has excellent psychometric properties. In Vietnam-era veterans seeking treatment, Keane et al. (1988) reported high internal consistency and test–retest reliability over a 1-week time interval. In a subsequent validation study, the authors found an overall hit rate of 90% when the scale was used to differentiate between a PTSD group and two non-PTSD comparison groups.

McFall, Smith, Mackay, and Tarver (1990) replicated these findings and further demonstrated that PTSD patients with and without substance use disorders did not differ on the Mississippi Scale. Given the high comorbidity between PTSD and substance use disorders, the authors felt it was important to demonstrate that the test assesses PTSD symptoms rather than effects associated with alcohol and drug use. McFall et al. (1990) also obtained information on convergent validity, finding significant correlations between the Mississippi Scale and other measures of PTSD, including the total number of SCID-PTSD symptoms, total IES score, and degree of traumatic combat exposure on the Vietnam Era Stress Inventory (Wilson & Krauss, 1984). These findings suggest that the Mississippi Scale is a valuable self-report tool in settings in which assessment of combat-related PTSD is needed.

POSTTRAUMATIC DIAGNOSTIC SCALE

Developed by Foa, Cashman, Jaycox, and Perry (1997), the Posttraumatic Diagnostic Scale (PDS) is a 49-item scale designed to measure DSM-IV PTSD criteria and symptom severity. The PDS is a revised version of an earlier self-report scale based on DSM-III-R, referred to as the PTSD Symptom Scale—Self-Report Version (PSS-SR; Foa et al., 1993). The PDS reviews trauma exposure and identifies the most distressing trauma. It also assesses Criterion A2 (physical threat or helplessness), Criteria B–D (intensity and frequency of all 17 symptoms), and functional impairment (Criterion F). This scale has been used with several populations, including combat veterans, accident victims, and sexual and nonsexual assault survivors and has been validated in other languages (e.g., German; Griesel, Wessa & Flor, 2006). The PDS can be administered in 10–15 minutes.

The psychometric properties of the PDS were evaluated among 264 volunteers recruited from several PTSD treatment centers, as well as from non-treatment-seeking populations at high risk for trauma (Foa et al., 1997). Investigators reported high internal consistency for the PTSD total score and subscales and adequate test–retest reliability coefficients for the total PDS score and for the symptom cluster scores. With regard to validity, the PDS total score correlated highly with other scales that measure traumatic responses, such as the IES. In addition, the measure yielded high levels of diagnostic agreement with a SCID diagnosis.

Most recently, Griffin, Uhlmansiek, Resick, and Mechanic (2004) compared the PDS with the CAPS in a population of female survivors of domestic violence. They found strong intercorrelations between the two measures, although the PDS tended to overdiagnose PTSD. These findings suggest that the PDS might serve as an acceptable screening device for identifying cases of PTSD in this population but that clinicians should be alerted to elevations in false positive rates.

PTSD CHECKLIST

Developed by researchers at the National Center for PTSD (Weathers et al., 1993), the PTSD Checklist (PCL) is a 17-item self-report measure of PTSD symptoms. Different scoring procedures may be used to yield either a continuous measure of symptom severity or a dichotomous indicator of diagnostic status. Dichotomous scoring methods include either an overall cutoff score or a symptom cluster scoring approach. The original scale was based on the DSM-III-R criteria for PTSD and has been updated to reflect the 17 diagnostic criteria outlined in DSM-IV. Respondents are asked to rate, on a Likert scale, "how much each problem has bothered them" during the past month. The time frame can be adjusted as needed to suit the goals of the assessment. There is a civilian (PCL-C) and a military version (PCL-M) of the measure. On the PCL-C, reexperiencing and avoidance symptoms apply to any lifetime stressful event, whereas for the PCL-M, reexperiencing and avoidance symptoms apply to stressful events that are military-related only. The PCL has been used extensively in both research and clinical settings and takes 5–10 minutes to administer. If needed, a 17-item Life Events Checklist, developed as a companion to the CAPS to identify potentially traumatic experiences, can be used with the PCL.

The PCL was validated in a sample of Vietnam and Persian Gulf War veterans and found to have strong psychometric properties (Weathers et al., 1993). Keen, Kutter, Niles, and Krinsley (2008) examined the psychometric properties of the updated PCL in veterans with both combat and noncombat traumas and found evidence for high internal consistency. Test–retest reliability was not examined, but the original study suggested that this was robust over a 2–3 day interval. Other investigators have also documented adequate test–retest reliability of this measure over a 2-week time frame (Ruggiero, Del Ben, Scotti, & Rabalais, 2003).

With respect to validity, Keen et al. (2008) found that the scale was highly correlated with other measures of PTSD, including the Mississippi Scale and the CAPS, and had good diagnostic power. Additionally, using the CAPS as the gold standard, Dobie et al. (2006) reported that the PCL had good diagnostic utility. In addition, there is evidence that different scoring options for the PCL (e.g., an absolute cutoff score vs. symptom cluster scoring) yield differences in sensitivity, specificity, and diagnostic efficiency. Keen et al. (2008) suggest that the selection of a scoring routine may depend on the goal of the assessment (e.g., symptom cluster scoring was associated with higher sensitivity and may be preferable when the goal is to identify all possible cases of PTSD, whereas the cutoff method was associated with higher specificity and may be preferable for research or when clinical resources are limited).

INVENTORY OF PSYCHOSOCIAL FUNCTIONING

The Inventory of Psychosocial Functioning (IPF; Marx et al., 2009) is a newly developed 87-item self-report measure designed to assess functional impairment across multiple domains experienced by active-duty service members and veterans. Respondents rate their functioning over the past 30 days on a 7-point scale ranging from 1 ("never") to 7 ("always"). The IPF yields a total score for each of seven subscales, including romantic relationships with a spouse or partner, family relationships, work, friendships and socializing, parenting, education, and day-to-day functioning. Subscale total scores are computed by taking the mean of the responses to each item within that subscale. An overall functional impairment score is also computed by calculating the mean of the scores for each completed subscale.

At this time, based on data collected from 169 veterans, the IPF subscales demonstrate strong internal consistency, with Cronbach's alpha ranging from .76 to .91. Additionally, nearly all items within each subscale correlate significantly with the mean of item responses for that corresponding subscale, with correlations ranging from $r = .36$ to $r = .86$.

The overall mean IPF score correlates significantly ($r = .54$) with PTSD symptom severity using the CAPS. Individuals meeting diagnostic criteria for PTSD had overall mean IPF scores of 3.86 ($SD = 1.06$), whereas individuals not meeting diagnostic criteria for PTSD had significantly lower overall mean IPF scores ($M = 2.85$, $SD = .85$) $t(167) = -6.74$, $p = .000$. The IPF represents an important new step forward in the assessment of trauma-exposed individuals as it appears to successfully quantify existing areas of impaired interpersonal functioning, a key feature of all psychological evaluations.

Conclusion

The current geopolitical climate suggests that U.S. military personnel and war veterans will continue to be exposed to life-altering traumatic events, making the accurate assessment of PTSD as important as ever. As we presented in this review, there are a number of barriers to the assessment process, in particular, stigma, possible overreporting, concerns about confidentiality, and the need to identify and assess the lethality of suicidal/homicidal ideation in a group at higher risk than the general population. In light of these concerns, we recommend the use of a multimethod assessment process consisting of structured clinical interviews and self-report measures to make the best use of clinical acumen and actuarial prediction. The review of assessment tools focused primarily on PTSD symptomatology; however, we suggest that the same multimethod approach be used when dealing with other aspects of the assessment process, including assessing lethality and the presence of other comorbid disorders such as depression, substance abuse, and other anxiety disorders.

Although this chapter is by no means exhaustive, our intention here is to provide the reader with a useful starting point from which to conduct a thorough assessment that is able to meet the needs of the client while gaining as much information as possible. We firmly believe case conceptualization and treatment planning are only as useful as the assessment from which they are derived. Given the nature of psychological trauma, an approach to assessment that optimizes disclosure of traumatic events and normalizes an individual's response to these events will yield therapeutic advances by itself. Identification of the key contributing factors surrounding the traumatic event will serve as important targets for treatment, whether exposure therapy, cognitive therapy, behavioral strategies, or pharmacological interventions will ultimately constitute the treatment provided.

References

American Psychiatric Association. (1994). *Diagnostic and statistical manual of mental disorders* (4th ed.). Washington, DC: Author.

Blake, D. D., Weathers, F. W., Nagy, L. M., Kaloupek, D. G., Charney, D. S., & Keane, T. M. (1990). *The Clinician-Administered PTSD Scale–IV*. Boston: National Center for PTSD, Behavioral Sciences Division.

Breslau, N., Davis, G. C., Andreski, P., & Peterson, E. (1991). Traumatic events and posttraumatic stress disorder in an urban population of young adults. *Archives of General Psychiatry, 48,* 216–222.

Butcher, J. N., Graham, J. R., Ben-Porath, Y. S., Tellegen, A., Dahlstrom, W. G., & Kaemmer, B. (2001). *MMPI-2 (Minnesota Multiphasic Personality Inventory—2): Manual for administration, scoring, and interpretation, revised edition*. Minneapolis: University of Minnesota Press.

Chiles, J. A., & Strosahl, K. D. (2005). *Clinical manual for assessment and treatment of suicidal patients*. Washington, DC: American Psychiatric.

Corrigan, P. (2004). How stigma interferes with mental health care. *American Psychologist, 59,* 614–625.

Cusack, K., Falsetti, S., & de Arellano, M. (2002). Gender considerations in the psychometric assessment of PTSD. In R. Kimerling, P. Ouimette, & J. Wolfe (Eds.), *Gender and PTSD* (pp. 150–176). New York: Guilford Press.

Department of Defense. (1997). Mental health evaluations of members of the armed forces (Directive 6490.1). Washington, DC: Author.

Department of Defense. (1998). Requirements for mental health evaluations of members of the armed forces (Instructions 6490.4). Washington, DC: Author.

DeViva, J., & Bloem, W. (2003). Symptom exaggeration and compensation seeking among combat veterans with posttraumatic stress disorder. *Journal of Traumatic Stress, 16,* 503–507.

Dobie, D. J., Maynard, C., Kivlahan, D. R., Johnson, K. M., Simpson, T., David, A. C., et al. (2006). Posttraumatic stress disorder screening status is associated with increased VA medical and surgical utilization in women. *Journal of General Internal Medicine, 21,* S58–S64.

First, M., Spitzer, R., Williams, J., & Gibbon, M. (2000). Structured Clinical Interview for DSM-IV AXIS I Disorders (SCID-I). In *American Psychiatric Association handbook of psychiatric measures* (pp. 49–53). Washington, DC: American Psychiatric Association.

Foa, E. B., Cashman, L., Jaycox, L., & Perry, K. (1997). The validation of a self-report measure of posttraumatic stress disorder: The Posttraumatic Diagnostic Scale. *Psychological Assessment, 9,* 445–451.

Foa, E. B., Keane, T. M., Friedman, M. J., & Cohen, J. (Eds.). (2009). *Effective treatments for PTSD* (2nd ed.). New York: Guilford Press.

Foa, E. B., Riggs, D. S., Dancu, C.V., & Rothbaum, B. O. (1993). Reliability and validity of a brief instrument for assessing posttraumatic stress disorder. *Journal of Traumatic Stress, 6,* 459–474.

Freeman, T., Clothier, J., Thornton, C., & Keesee, N. (1994). Firearm collection and use among combat veterans admitted to a posttraumatic stress disorder rehabilitation unit. *Journal of Nervous and Mental Disease, 182,* 592–594.

Freeman, T., & Roca, V. (2001). Gun use, attitudes toward violence, and aggression among combat veterans with chronic posttraumatic stress disorder. *Journal of Nervous and Mental Disease, 189,* 317–320.

Frueh, B. C., Gold, K. L., & de Arellano, M. A. (1997). Symptom overreporting in combat veterans evaluated for PTSD: Differentiation on the basis of compensation seeking status. *Journal of Personality Assessment, 68,* 369–384.

Frueh, B. C., Smith, D. W., & Barker, S. E. (1996). Compensation seeking status and psychometric assessment of combat veterans seeking treatment for PTSD. *Journal of Traumatic Stress, 9,* 427–439.

Gold, P. B., & Frueh, B. C. (1999). Compensation-seeking and extreme exaggeration of psychopathology among combat veterans evaluated for posttraumatic stress disorder. *Journal of Nervous and Mental Disease, 187,* 680–684.

Griesel, D., Wessa, M., & Flor, H. (2006). Psychometric qualities of the German version of the Posttraumatic Diagnostic Scale (PTDS). *Psychological Assessment, 18,* 262–268.

Griffin, M. G., Uhlmansiek, M. H., Resick, P. A., & Mechanic, M. B. (2004). Comparison of the Posttraumatic Stress Disorder Scale versus the Clinician-Administered Posttraumatic Stress Disorder Scale in domestic violence survivors. *Journal of Traumatic Stress, 17,* 497–503.

Hathaway, S. R., & McKinley, J. C. (1951). *Minnesota Multiphasic Personality Inventory; manual (Revised).* San Antonio, TX: Psychological Corporation.

Herman, D. S., Weathers, F. W., Litz, B. T., & Keane, T. M. (1996). Psychometric properties of the embedded and stand-alone versions of the MMPI-2 Keane PTSD Scale. *Assessment, 3,* 437–442.

Hoge, C. W., Castro, C. A., Messer, S. C., McGurk, D., Cotting, D. I., & Koffman, R. L. (2004). Combat duty in Iraq and Afghanistan, mental health problems, and barriers to care. *New England Journal of Medicine, 351,* 13-22.

Horowitz, M. J., Wilner, N., & Alvarez, W. (1979). Impact of Event Scale: A measure of subjective stress. *Psychosomatic Medicine, 41,* 209–218.

Howe, E. G. (1989). Confidentiality in the military. *Behavioural Sciences and the Law, 7,* 317–337.

Jordan, R. G., Nunley, T. V., & Cook, R. R. (1992). Symptom exaggeration in a PTSD inpatient population: Response set or claim for compensation. *Journal of Traumatic Stress, 5,* 633–642.

Kaplan, M., McFarland, B., & Huguet, N. (2009). Characteristics of adult male and female firearm suicide decedents: Findings from the National Violent Death Reporting System. *Injury Prevention, 15,* 322–327.

Keane, T. M., & Barlow, D. H. (2002). Posttraumatic stress disorder. In D.H. Barlow (Ed.), *Anxiety and its disorders: The nature and treatment of anxiety and panic* (2nd ed., pp. 418–453). New York: Guilford Press.

Keane, T. M., Caddell, J. M., & Taylor, K. L. (1988). Mississippi Scale for combat-related posttraumatic stress disorder: Three studies in reliability and validity. *Journal of Consulting and Clinical Psychology, 56,* 85–90.

Keane, T. M., Fairbank, J. A., Caddell, J. M., Zimering, R. T., & Bender, M. E. (1985). A behavioral approach to assessing and treating post-traumatic stress disorder in Vietnam veterans. In C. R. Figley (Ed.), *Trauma and its wake* (pp. 257-294). New York: Brunner/Mazel.

Keane, T. M., & Kaloupek, D. G. (1982). Imaginal flooding in the treatment of a post-traumatic stress disorder. *Journal of Consulting and Clinical Psychology, 50,* 138–140.

Keane, T. M., Kolb, L. C., Kaloupek, D. G., Orr, S. P., Blanchard, E. B., Thomas, R. G., et al. (1998). Utility of psychophysiology measurement in the diagnosis of posttraumatic stress disorder: Results from a Department of Veterans Affairs cooperative study. *Journal of Consulting and Clinical Psychology, 66,* 914-923.

Keane, T. M., Malloy, P. F., & Fairbank, J. A. (1984). Empirical development of an MMPI subscale for the assessment of combat-related posttraumatic stress disorder. *Journal of Consulting and Clinical Psychology, 52,* 888–891.

Keane, T. M., Silberbogen, A., & Weierich, M. (2008) Assessment of posttraumatic stress disorder. In J. Hunsley & E. J. Mash (Eds.), *A guide to assessments that work* (pp. 293–315) New York: Oxford University Press.

Keane, T. M., Weathers, F. W., & Foa, E. B. (2000). Diagnosis and assessment. In E. B. Foa, T. M. Keane, & M. J. Friedman (Eds.), *Effective treatments for PTSD: Practice guidelines from the International Society for Traumatic Stress Studies* (pp. 18–36). New York: Guilford Press.

Keane, T. M., Wolfe, J., & Taylor, K. L. (1987). Post-traumatic stress disorder: Evidence for diagnostic validity and methods of psychological assessment. *Journal of Clinical Psychology, 43,* 32–43.

Keen, S. M., Kutter, C. J., Niles, B. L., & Krinsley, K. E. (2008). Psychometric properties of PTSD Checklist in sample of male veterans. *Journal of Rehabilitation Research and Development, 45,* 465–474.

Kessler, R. C., Sonnega, A., Bromet, E., Hughes, M., & Nelson, C. B. (1995). Post-traumatic stress disorder in the National Comorbidity Survey. *Archives of General Psychiatry, 52,* 1048–1060.

Kilpatrick, D. G. (1988). Rape aftermath symptom test. In M. Hersen & A. S. Bellack (Eds.), *Dictionary of behavioral assessment techniques* (pp. 658–669). Oxford, UK: Pergamon Press.

Krysinska, K., & Lester, D. (2010). Post-traumatic stress disorder and suicide risk: A systematic review. *Archives of Suicide Research, 14,* 1–23.

Kulka, R. A., Schlenger, W. E., Fairbank, J. A., Hough, R. L., Jordan, B. K., Marmar, C. R., et al. (1988). *National Vietnam Veterans Readjustment Study (NVVRS): Description, current status, and initial PTSD prevalence estimates.* Washington, DC: Veterans Administration.

Kulka, R. A., Schlenger, W. E., Fairbank, J. A., Hough, R. L., Jordan, B. K., Marmar, C. R., et al. (1990a). *The National Vietnam Veterans Readjustment Study: Tables of findings and technical appendices.* New York: Brunner/Mazel.

Kulka, R. A., Schlenger, W. E., Fairbank, J. A., Hough, R. L., Jordan, B. K., Marmar, C. R., et al. (1990b). *Trauma and the Vietnam War generation: Report of findings from the National Vietnam Veterans Readjustment Study.* New York: Brunner/Mazel.

Lyons, J. A., & Keane, T. M. (1992). Keane PTSD scale: MMPI and MMPI-2 update. *Journal of Traumatic Stress, 5,* 111–117.

Manual for Courts-Martial, United States, Military Rules of Evidence [513]. (2008).

Marx, B. P., Schnurr, P., Rodriguez, P., Holowka, D. H., Lunney, C., Weathers, F., et al. (2009, November). Development of a functional evaluation scale for active duty service members and veterans. In K. M. Lester (Chair), *Beyond PTSD symptom reduction: Social and health-related benefits of trauma focused treatment.* Symposium conducted at the meeting for the International Society for Traumatic Stress Studies, Atlanta, GA.

McFall, M. E., Smith, D. E., Mackay, P. W., & Tarver, D. J. (1990). Reliability and validity of Mississippi Scale for Combat-Related Posttraumatic Stress Disorder. *Journal of Consulting and Clinical Psychology, 2,* 114–121.

McFall, M. E., Smith, D. E., Roszell, D. K., Tarver, D. J., & Malas, K. L. (1990). Convergent validity of measures of PTSD in Vietnam combat veterans. *American Journal of Psychiatry, 147,* 645–648.

Michaels, M. H. (2006). Ethical considerations in writing psychological assessment reports. *Journal of Clinical Psychology, 62,* 47–58.

Ramchand, R., Schell, T., Karney, B., Osilla, K., Burns, R., & Caldarone, L. (2010). Disparate prevalence estimates of PTSD among service members who served in Iraq and Afghanistan: Possible explanations. *Journal of Traumatic Stress, 23,* 59–68.

Resnick, H. S., Kilpatrick, D. G., Dansky, B. S., Saunders, B. E., & Best, C. L. (1993). Prevalence of civilian trauma and PTSD in a representative national sample of women. *Journal of Clinical and Consulting Psychology, 61,* 984–991.

Ruggiero, K. J., Del Ben, K., Scotti, J. R., & Rabalais, A. E. (2003). Psychometric properties of the PTSD Checklist—Civilian Version. *Journal of Traumatic Stress, 16,* 495–502.

Sayer, N., & Thuras, P. (2002). The influence of patients' compensation-seeking status on the perceptions of Veterans Affairs clinicians. *Psychiatric Services, 53*(2), 210–212.

Smith, D. W., & Frueh, B. C. (1996). Compensation seeking, comorbidity, and apparent exaggeration of PTSD symptoms among Vietnam combat veterans. *Psychological Assessment, 8,* 3–6.

Tolin, D. F., Maltby, N., Weathers, F. W., Litz, B. T., Knight, J. A., & Keane, T. M. (2004). The use of the MMPI-2 Infrequency-Psychopathology Scale in the assessment of posttraumatic stress disorder in Vietnam veterans. *Journal of Psychopathology and Behavioral Assessment, 26,* 23–29.

U.S. Department of Veterans Affairs, Veterans Health Administration, Office of Public Health and Environmental Hazards. (2010). *Analysis of VA health care utilization among U.S. Global War on Terrorism (GWOT) veterans.* Unpublished quarterly report (cumulative through 4th quarter FY2009). Washington, DC: Author.

War Crimes Act of 1996, 18 U.S.C. § 2441 (1996).

Warner, C., Appenzeller, G., Grieger, T., Benedek, D., & Roberts, L. (2009). Ethical considerations in military psychiatry. *Psychiatric Clinics of North America, 32*(2), 271–281.

Weathers, F. W., Keane, T. M., & Davidson, J. R. T. (2001). The Clinician-Administered PTSD Scale (CAPS): A review of the first ten years of research. *Depression and Anxiety, 13,* 132–156.

Weathers, F. W., Keane, T. M., & Foa, E. (2009). Assessment and diagnosis of posttraumatic stress disorder. In E. Foa, T. M. Keane, M. J. Friedman, & J. Cohen (Eds.), *Effective treatments for PTSD* (2nd ed., pp. 23–61). New York: Guilford Press.

Weathers, F. W., Litz, B. T., Herman, D. S., Huska, J. A., & Keane, T. M. (1993, October). *The PTSD Checklist (PCL): Reliability, validity, and diagnostic utility.* Poster session presented at the annual meeting of the International Society for Traumatic Stress Studies, San Antonio, TX.

Weathers, F. W., Ruscio, A. M., & Keane, T. M. (1999). Psychometric properties of nine scoring rules for the Clinician-Administered PTSD scale (CAPS). *Psychological Assessment, 11,* 124–133.

Wilson, J. P., & Krauss, G. E. (1984, September). *The Vietnam Era Stress Inventory: A scale to measure war stress and post-traumatic stress disorder among Vietnam veterans.* Paper presented at the National Conference on Posttraumatic Stress Disorder, Baltimore, MD.

CHAPTER 3

Prolonged Exposure Therapy

Alan L. Peterson
Edna B. Foa
David S. Riggs

Prolonged exposure therapy (PE) is a cognitive-behavioral therapy (CBT) based on the integration of exposure therapy principles with the framework of emotional processing theory (Foa & Kozak, 1986). PE therapy is designed specifically to ameliorate posttraumatic stress disorder (PTSD) and related problems. Research supports the efficacy of exposure therapy with patients who suffer from PTSD (Institute of Medicine, 2008). The published research has found large effect sizes, and the majority of individuals either achieve remission (loss of diagnosis) or exhibit clinically significant symptom reduction (Bradley, Greene, Russ, Dutra, & Westen, 2005). Most randomized clinical trials (RCTs) have been conducted with civilian populations who have experienced civilian-type traumas such as sexual assault, physical assault, and motor vehicle accidents. By comparison, little research has been published on the treatment of combat-related PTSD in active-duty military or veteran populations, and the effect sizes from published studies have been much more modest.

Overview of PE

PE is a manualized treatment that includes four primary components: (1) repeated revisiting of the trauma memories (imaginal exposure), (2) repeated exposure to avoided situations (*in vivo* exposure), (3) education about common reactions to trauma, and (4) breathing retraining. The standard PE treatment program includes ten to twelve 90-minute individual treatment sessions conducted once or twice weekly, although clinical experience suggests a range of 8 to 15 sessions. The PE treatment program has been manualized on the basis of clinical studies, and a therapist guide includes complete details of the treatment program, including therapist and patient materials (Foa, Hembree, & Rothbaum, 2007).

Rationale for PE

When confronted with a dangerous situation, responding with fear is normal and adaptive. Fear activates a "fight or flight" response that helps the individual who faces danger to protect him- or herself by escaping or fighting. However, PTSD patients overgeneralize this fear response to the extent that they avoid or escape situations that are not dangerous. This often occurs in the context of reexperiencing symptoms (e.g., flashbacks and nightmares), which may themselves be cued by environmental reminders of the trauma. For example, the smell of diesel fuel, if it was present at the time of the trauma, might cue the trauma memory.

Two sets of negative cognitions are thought to underlie the excessive fear and other negative emotions associated with the trauma memory in patients suffering from PTSD: The world is an extremely dangerous place, and I am no longer competent to serve in the military. Examples of such cognitions are "the world is completely unpredictable," "I am a horrible person," and "what happened in Iraq is all my fault."

Confronting, rather than avoiding, the memory of the trauma and trauma reminders can assist patients in correcting their unrealistic, negative cognitions and reduce (habituate) their unrealistic fear. However, PTSD patients typically go to extreme measures to avoid the traumatic memory, and doing so only perpetuates PTSD symptoms. PE uses the techniques of imaginal and *in vivo* exposure to help the patient confront his or her traumatic memories and trauma reminders. Over the course of repeated imaginal and *in vivo* exposure exercises, the patients' anxiety and other negative emotions (guilt, shame, anger) typically decrease.

Confronting the traumatic memory by repeatedly retelling the trauma story (imaginal exposure) helps the individual with PTSD to process the memory and to change inaccurate, trauma-related cognitions. Across repetitions, the trauma story script often evolves to reflect a more realistic perspective of the trauma and a modification of inaccurate trauma-related cognitions, even without specifically targeting these thoughts. Also, imaginal exposure helps the patient realize that thinking about the trauma is not the same as being traumatized again and that engaging with the traumatic memory rather than avoiding or escaping it does not lead to loss of control or "going crazy." Through imaginal exposure the patient learns that anxiety does not stay forever but rather habituates during the exercise and across repetitions and, furthermore, that he or she is able to handle the distress associated with remembering the trauma.

In vivo exposure, real-life confrontation with trauma-related situations and objects, helps the patient realize that those situations are not dangerous, that the "disaster" he or she expects to happen (e.g., being attacked again) does not materialize, that anxiety decreases during exposure, and that he or she can handle the distress associated with confronting the situations that had been avoided. In concert, imaginal and *in vivo* exposure help patients correct their perceptions that the world is extremely dangerous and that they are incapable of coping effectively with it.

Psychoeducation

Treatment with PE involves a significant amount of psychoeducation about the rationale for treatment and common reactions to trauma. The primary goals of the psychoeducational component are (1) to normalize the patient's symptoms, (2) to gather information about the patients' experience of PTSD symptoms and related problems, (3) to instill hope that many of the patient's problems are related to PTSD and should improve with treatment, and (4) to promote communication between the patient and therapist to foster the therapeutic alliance needed for successful treatment.

Symptoms are normalized by describing common reactions to trauma and how they are related to the development of PTSD as an overgeneralization of an adaptive fear response. The therapist then outlines typical PTSD symptoms and gathers information by asking the patient whether he or she has had any similar experiences. Next, the therapist explains how avoidance can maintain PTSD and how confronting the memory through PE techniques can help eliminate anxiety.

Breathing Retraining

Breathing retraining involves teaching the patient a technique to reduce overall physiological arousal by focusing on slow, rhythmic, and relaxed breathing. This skill is taught early in PE treatment because it is a tool that patients can use immediately to help alleviate anxiety symptoms and create a sense of mastery over daily anxiety and distress. However, as a rule we do not recommend the use of breathing retraining during imaginal or *in vivo* exposure exercises because this can lead patients to attribute their success at confronting feared memories and situations to the use of special breathing rather than to their own inner strength. Furthermore, a certain level of anxiety and discomfort is necessary and expected during exposure.

In Vivo Exposure

In vivo exposure involves exposure to situations that the patient has been avoiding owing to irrational fear and anxiety. The therapist introduces *in vivo* exposure by describing the rationale for the exercise (i.e., breaking the habit of reducing distress through avoidance, realizing that the avoided situations are not dangerous, and habituation) and providing naturalistic examples of *in vivo* exposure. For example, many people are afraid of roller coasters at first but habituate to them after several safe roller coaster rides as they find out that nothing bad happens to them.

After explaining the rationale, the therapist works with the patient to identify situations that the patient has been avoiding because they cue trauma-related memories and emotions or because the patient simply feels that they are dangerous. Each avoided situation is ranked using a scale called the Subjective Units of Distress Scale (SUDS). Using the SUDS, a patient rates each avoided situation from 0 (not distressing at all) to 100 (extremely distressing). Based on the SUDS ratings, the avoided situations are arranged on a hierarchy, from least to most feared. Throughout PE, patients work their way up the hierarchy by repeatedly confronting situations on the hierarchy and remaining in each feared situation for 30 to 45 minutes or until their anxiety decreases by at least 50 percent.

Imaginal Exposure

Imaginal exposure (revisiting the traumatic memories) is essentially the repeated retelling of the traumatic event aloud. As with *in vivo* exposure, the therapist begins by describing the rationale for the exercise. Imaginal exposure helps the patient (1) process the traumatic memory, "make sense" of the trauma, and gain a new perspective on it, (2) distinguish between the trauma and the memory of the trauma, (3) come to realize that he or she will not "lose it" or "go crazy" as a consequence of recalling the memory, (4) habituate to the memory, and (5) gain a sense of mastery over the memory.

Patients are given instructions to retell the trauma story in present tense, while vividly picturing the events with closed eyes. They are encouraged to include as many details as possible, such as thoughts or sensations, to help them to fully engage in the memory. The memory is repeated for the full time allotted for imaginal exposure during the session, usually 30–40 minutes. During imaginal exposure exercises, therapists work to promote engagement in the memory by including details of the event, to provide encouragement, and to periodically ask their patients to rate their anxiety

on the SUDS scale to monitor distress. During the first few imaginal exposures, the therapist, with the help of the patient, identifies "hot spots" or
portions of the trauma memory that are particularly distressing. In later
sessions of PE these portions of the memory are targeted specifically by
focusing the imaginal exposure exercises on them. This is not to say that
other parts of the trauma memory are not important but to recognize more
distressing aspects of the memory that require greater attention.

Brief Outline of Sessions 1–10

After the completion of a clinical intake interview, including a thorough
trauma history and PTSD diagnostic evaluation, treatment session 1 includes
a general overview of PE, a discussion of the patient's trauma, and breathing
retraining. From this session forward, patients are assigned homework to
continue to practice calm breathing and to listen to the audio recording of
the session. Progress on homework is reviewed at the beginning of each subsequent session. During session 2, the therapist discusses common reactions
to trauma and the rationale and procedure for *in vivo* exposure. The SUDS
rating is introduced, and the therapist and patient collaboratively develop
an *in vivo* hierarchy. For homework, patients are instructed to complete at
least one *in vivo* exposure exercise for homework each day between treatment sessions and to add situations to the *in vivo* hierarchy.

Imaginal exposure exercises begin during session 3. The therapist
begins by reviewing the rationale and procedure for imaginal exposure, and
then the patient completes 30–40 minutes of imaginal exposure in session.
Afterward the therapist discusses and helps process the imaginal exposure
exercise with the patient. As homework, the therapist asks the patient to
listen to the audiotape of the imaginal exposure once a day and to continue
working through the *in vivo* hierarchy. Sessions 4 and 5 contain the same
content as session 3, except that the therapist does not need to review the
rationale again. During sessions 6–9, imaginal exposure is focused on "hot
spots," but otherwise the sessions are the same as 4 and 5. During session
10 (or the final session), the patient recounts the full trauma again during
an imaginal exposure exercise. The therapist concludes with a final review
of the patient's progress and all that was learned.

Research on PE with Civilian Populations

A comprehensive review of the research evidence on the treatment of PTSD
conducted by the Institute of Medicine (2008) concluded that exposure
therapy was the only treatment approach with sufficient scientific data to

support its efficacy. PE has been investigated in numerous randomized clinical trials in civilian populations (Foa, Rothbaum, Riggs, & Murdock, 1991; Foa et al., 1999, 2005; Resick, Nishith, Weaver, Astin, & Feuer, 2002; Bryant, Moulds, et al., 2008).

In one of the first studies to evaluate PE (Foa et al., 1991), rape victims with PTSD were randomly assigned to PE, stress inoculation training (SIT), supportive counseling (SC), or wait-list control (WL). The results indicated that immediately posttreatment, SIT produced significantly more improvement on PTSD symptoms than did SC and WL. However, at the 3½-month follow-up, PE produced superior outcome on PTSD symptoms.

Two studies evaluated whether the efficacy of PE might be enhanced by the addition of SIT (Foa et al., 1999) or cognitive therapy (Foa et al., 2005). In the first study, female victims of physical or sexual assault were randomly assigned to PE, SIT, combined PE/SIT, and a wait-list. At posttreatment, only 40% of PE participants met criteria for PTSD compared with 58% of those receiving SIT, 60% receiving PE/SIT, and all of the participants in the WL condition. In the second study (Foa et al., 2005) female assault survivors were randomly assigned to PE, PE plus cognitive restructuring (PE/CR) and WL control. The results indicated that both PE and PE/CR produced significant improvement in PTSD and that treatment gains were maintained over the 9-month follow-up period. As in the earlier study that combined PE with SIT, the addition of CR did not augment the efficacy of PE alone at the end of treatment or at follow-up. In another study, Resick et al. (2002) compared PE, cognitive processing therapy (CPT), and a minimal-attention control condition. Both treatments produced greater improvement than did the control condition at the end of treatment, and the gains were maintained up to 9 months posttreatment.

Bryant, Moulds, et al. (2008) compared the efficacy of the full PE treatment protocol with imaginal exposure alone, *in vivo* exposure alone, or the combination of imaginal exposure and *in vivo* exposure. At the 6-month follow-up assessment, there were fewer patients with PTSD in the group receiving the full PE treatment protocol (31%) as compared with the imaginal exposure alone (75%), *in vivo* exposure alone (69%), or the combined imaginal exposure and *in vivo* exposure condition (63%).

PE has also been demonstrated to be effective for the treatment of acute stress disorder (ASD) and the prevention of chronic PTSD. In a study of civilians with ASD (Bryant, Mastrodomenico, et al., 2008), 90 patients were randomly assigned to 5 weekly sessions of exposure therapy, cognitive restructuring, or a wait-list group. Intent-to-treat analyses indicated that at posttreatment, only 33% of patients in the exposure group had PTSD as compared with 63% in the cognitive restructuring and 77% in the wait-list group.

Research on PE with Military Populations

Only a limited amount of research has been conducted on the use of PE for treatment of combat-related PTSD in military populations. One of the first studies of an exposure therapy approach for combat-related PTSD included 24 Vietnam veterans randomized either to a treatment condition involving relaxation plus imaginal exposure or to a wait-list control condition (Keane, Fairbank, Caddell, & Zimering, 1989). Treated subjects showed decreases in reexperiencing symptoms, startle reactions, memory and concentration problems, impulsivity, and irritability, whereas numbing and avoidance symptoms did not significantly improve.

Two uncontrolled case studies evaluated PE for the treatment of combat-related PTSD in veterans who had previously served on active duty. Nacasch et al. (2007) reported on five Israeli veterans with severe and chronic combat-related PTSD treated after discharge from active duty 13–30 years after their combat-trauma exposure. The patients, all of whom had been unresponsive to previous treatments with medication and supportive therapy, were treated with 10–15 sessions of PE therapy. All five patients showed marked improvement with PE, with a mean decrease of 48% in PTSD symptoms. Four of the patients maintained treatment gains or kept improving 6–18 months after the treatment. In a similar study (Rauch et al., 2009) clinical treatment data were presented on 10 U. S. veterans with chronic PTSD treated in a Veterans Health Administration clinic. Symptoms of PTSD were reduced by about 50% from pre- to posttreatment. More recently, Nacasch et al. (2010) reported on results of an RCT in which veterans with combat-related PTSD who received 10–15 sessions of PE had significantly less severe PTSD and depression symptoms than those who received treatment as usual after treatment and at a 1-year follow-up. Treatment as usual did not result in symptom reduction.

There is one series of three case studies that evaluated the use of PE for combat-related trauma in an active-duty military population (Cigrang, Peterson, & Schobitz, 2005). Three active-duty U. S. military personnel with significant symptoms of ASD were treated during a combat deployment in Iraq. In each case the patient's symptoms were severe enough that his ability to perform military duties was significantly impaired and all three were considered for possible redeployment back to the United States for treatment. The treatment involved a modified four-session version of PE similar to that described by Bryant and colleagues (Bryant, Mastrodomenico, et al., 2008). The results indicated that symptoms were significantly reduced over a 5-week period by an average of 56% and were within normal ranges. All three patients were able to voluntarily remain in Iraq and resume their primary military duties.

The largest RCT conducted to date to evaluate the efficacy of PE in a military population did not actually target combat-related PTSD (Schnurr et al., 2007). It included 284 female veterans, but only a small percentage of the reported traumatic events (5%) were related to military combat. In addition, most of the women (97.5%) were veterans who had previously served in the military but were no longer on active duty. Participants were randomly assigned to receive 10 weekly 90-minute sessions of PE ($n = 141$) or present-centered therapy (PCT; $n = 143$). The results indicated that the women who received PE experienced greater reductions in PTSD symptoms relative to women who received present-centered therapy (effect size, 0.27; $P = .03$). In addition, the PE group was more likely to no longer meet PTSD diagnostic criteria (41% vs. 28%) and to achieve a total remission (15% vs. 7%). It should be noted that this effect size is smaller than the effect sizes reported in most studies of civilian patients (Foa et al., 1999; Foa et al., 2005; Resick et al., 2002).

It is currently not known whether the smaller effect sizes found in studies of combat-related PTSD result in differences between PTSD in military and civilian populations or whether the reason is that most studies of combat-related PTSD have been conducted decades after the combat trauma exposure. Comorbid conditions such as substance abuse, chronic medical problems, homelessness, unemployment, and PTSD disability compensation are all factors that may also be related to the more modest improvements found in studies targeting combat-related PTSD. To date, no randomized clinical trial has been published to evaluate the efficacy of any treatment approach for PTSD in an active-duty military population.

Strengths of PE with Military Personnel

The primary strength of PE is its overall effectiveness, as demonstrated by the numerous RCTs in civilians and preliminary studies in military personnel previously mentioned. PE has been successfully implemented across a wide variety of demographic populations, including patients of various cultures and socioeconomic statuses (Feske, 2008; Asukai, Saito, Tsuruta, Ogami, & Kishimoto, 2008). Research indicates that patients treated with exposure therapy are unlikely to relapse after treatment (Bradley et al., 2005; IOM, 2008) and experience improvement in other debilitating symptoms often associated with PTSD, such as poor work and social functioning, sleep problems, health-related concerns, and depression (Foa et al., 2005; Taylor et al., 2003; Rauch et al., 2009; Galovski, Monson, Bruce, & Resick, 2009).

Despite its solid empirical support, many therapists are hesitant to implement PE because of concerns that it might be intolerable for patients or exacerbate PTSD symptoms. Foa, Zoellner, Feeny, Hembree, and Alvarez-Conrad (2002) conducted a civilian study specifically investigating symptom exacerbation after the first imaginal exposure session and found that only 10% of sexual assault survivors engaging in PE or PE/CR experienced an exacerbation of PTSD symptoms. In addition, the exacerbation was only temporary and was not related to overall outcome measures or dropout rates. Similarly, Taylor et al. (2003) compared eye movement desensitization and reprocessing (EMDR), exposure therapy, and relaxation for PTSD and investigated symptom worsening across treatment and follow-up. Symptom worsening was rare in all three conditions and did not significantly differ among the conditions. Furthermore, Taylor and colleagues found that participants in the exposure therapy condition experienced a more rapid decrease in avoidance behavior than in the other two conditions and showed overall better improvement in reexperiencing and avoidance symptoms.

Research investigating dropout rates additionally confirms the tolerability of exposure therapy. A meta-analysis of 25 different studies conducted by Hembree et al. (2003) found that the dropout rate for exposure therapy without the addition of anxiety management or cognitive therapy components was about 20% and was not significantly different from the rates of dropout from exposure therapy plus anxiety management or cognitive therapy (27%) or from anxiety management or cognitive therapy alone (22%). These dropout rates compare favorably with dropout occurring during treatments for other diagnoses. Similarly, the dropout rates reported by Bradley et al. (2005) in their meta-analysis of psychotherapy for PTSD revealed no statistical differences between exposure alone (24.1%), exposure plus CBT (33%), and CBT without exposure (17.2%). Thus patients appear to tolerate exposure therapy at least as well as other forms of CBT. Civilian research even suggests that the majority of PTSD patients would select PE over some other treatments, such as the medication sertraline (Feeny, Zoellner, Mavissakalian, & Roy-Byrne, 2009).

In addition to being effective and tolerable, PE can be easily and effectively disseminated. Foa et al. (2005) directly compared the effectiveness of PE disseminated at an academic site by doctoral-level clinical psychologists with PE disseminated at a community site by master's-level therapists with no previous training in CBT. Clinicians from both sites attended a 5-day workshop in PE and received weekly supervision throughout the study. Analyses of the posttreatment outcome measures from both settings found no significant differences between the sites, and follow-up results even suggested that the community site had better outcomes in depression and social functioning. These results suggest that PE can be easily and effectively disseminated to communities.

Research has also found that PE can be implemented under circumstances that might be particularly advantageous to the military. For example, preliminary evidence from the previously mentioned case study by Cigrang et al. (2005) demonstrates that PE can be disseminated successfully in the deployment setting. This could be an excellent tool for preventing the onset of PTSD in at-risk patients and aeromedical evacuation for mental health reasons.

As well as being viable in the deployment setting, civilian research suggests that PE can also be used in patients with comorbid traumatic brain injury (TBI). Since TBI and PTSD are two of the signature injuries of Operation Enduring Freedom and Operation Iraqi Freedom, it is important to understand how any PTSD treatment used in the military might affect a patient who has also had a TBI. For example, many symptoms of TBIs, such as impaired cognitive functioning and amnesia or loss of consciousness during the trauma, could potentially interfere with PE. Bryant, Moulds, Guthrie, and Nixon (2003) investigated this hypothesis by conducting a small study comparing the effectiveness of CBT, including imaginal exposure, cognitive restructuring, and *in vivo* exposure) and that of a supportive counseling intervention in civilians with comorbid ASD and TBI within 2 weeks after injury. CBT was clearly superior to supportive counseling. In the CBT group, only 8% met PTSD criteria at posttreatment and 17% at 6-month follow-up, whereas 58% of the supportive counseling patients met PTSD criteria at posttreatment and follow-up. These results demonstrate that exposure-based techniques can be successfully implemented in a population with comorbid TBI. Overall, PE is a very effective and well-researched PTSD treatment that is easy to disseminate, well tolerated by patients, and versatile enough to use both in the deployment setting and in patients with comorbid TBI.

Limitations of PE with Military Personnel

Using PE with military personnel comes with a few challenges. PE (like other CBT protocols) requires a considerable time commitment on the part of the patient, who, according to the standard treatment protocol, should attend one or two 90-minute sessions per week for a total of 10–12 sessions. This can be particularly challenging for active-duty service members, who oftentimes have busy and tightly scheduled workdays. However, preliminary data indicate that similar improvements can be obtained with sessions of 60 minutes in duration (van Minnen & Foa, 2006).

Another concern for patients seeking PE for PTSD is the general stigma associated with seeking any type of mental health treatment in the military. Even if patients receive authorization to attend 90-minute PE sessions during the workday, they might then need to cope with social stigma when their coworkers discover the reason behind their absence. One potential solution is to allow behavioral health consultants to conduct PE in a primary care setting, because seeking primary care treatment is generally not as stigmatized as seeking mental health care.

There is some concern that PE is limited in its ability to address emotions often associated with PTSD, such as guilt, shame, and anger. These emotions are thought to be closely associated with negative trauma-related cognitions, such as "I am a horrible person" or "the world is a dangerous place." Emotional processing theory, which underlies and informs PE, hypothesizes that exposure, *in vivo* and in imagination, conducted during PE provides patients with experiences that disconfirm negative trauma-related cognitions. These cognitive changes lead to improvements in associated emotions such as guilt, shame, and anger. For example, a patient experiencing guilt resulting from the belief that "I should have been able to stop my buddy from dying" might come to realize that the death was not his fault after completing several imaginal exposure exercises. Some researchers hypothesize that treatments such as CPT lead to more improvement in emotions such as guilt, shame, and anger because they use the technique of cognitive restructuring to directly address maladaptive cognitions. Results from one study suggest that this might be the case. Resick et al. (2002) found that PE and CPT both significantly reduced global measures of guilt, but CPT was superior to PE on two out of the four guilt subscales. However, it should be noted that the feelings of guilt experienced by the sexual assault survivors in the Resick et al. (2002) study are likely to be different from the guilt experienced by combat veterans.

However, there are data that indicate that PE does address the negative cognitions related to PTSD. Foa and Rauch (2004) compared changes in trauma-related cognitions among patients treated with PE with those of a group treated with PE/CR. They found that both treatments equally improved negative trauma-related cognitions. Therefore, the addition of CR did not provide any further benefit to PE for improving negative trauma-related cognitions associated with guilt, shame, and anger. Moreover, Moser et al. (2010) found that the intensity of PTSD-related negative cognitions prior to treatment was more strongly correlated with good outcome when PE alone was used than when PE was combined with CR. Similarly, other studies have found that exposure-based therapies result in significant improvement in anger (Cahill, Rauch, Hembree, & Foa, 2003) and guilt (Taylor et al., 2003). It seems then that most existing studies do not support the view that the addition of CR is necessary for PE to modify negative cognitions such as guilt and shame.

Therapeutic Considerations

To implement PE, therapists should receive the recommended training and guidance. Training in PE typically includes attending an in-person workshop, during which PE experts describe the rationale and procedure for PE while offering opportunities to practice through role play. After attending a workshop, therapists can begin to use PE. However, therapists may find it helpful to obtain guidance as they treat their first few cases by attending weekly supervision meetings or teleconferences with experienced PE therapists. Several branches of the military are currently offering these workshops and weekly supervision teleconferences to their mental health providers.

Before beginning to implement PE, therapists should consider their level of tolerance for listening to detailed trauma stories. Oftentimes just listening to graphic accounts of a trauma during imaginal exposure can be an emotional experience for a PE therapist. However, the therapist should try to avoid expressing any extreme emotional reactions (e.g., horror or disgust) during the imaginal exposure exercise. The goal is to make patients feel comfortable retelling their trauma stories without worrying about the therapist's reaction or feeling that they should soften their stories. This said, if an imaginal exposure session is emotionally disturbing, the therapist should engage in self-care behaviors after the session, such as sharing cases with a colleague while maintaining the patient's anonymity. Anecdotally, therapists often experience these reactions when they first begin to practice prolonged exposure. However, as with PTSD patients, therapists usually habituate and cease to have extreme reactions to trauma stories after listening to several imaginal exposure exercises.

Case Vignette

John (not his actual name) is a 29-year-old Army sergeant. He is married and has three children, ages 9, 6, and 4. John was deployed twice to Iraq, once in 2003 and again in 2006, and returned from a deployment to Afghanistan about 5 months ago. He saw heavy combat during his initial tour in Iraq and was exposed to numerous blasts and other stressful events during his second tour. During his most recent deployment, John spent much of his time patrolling in areas of Afghanistan in which insurgent activity was high. His unit was exposed to a number of attacks and took heavy casualties; three members of the unit were killed, including one of John's best friends.

John presented reluctantly at the Behavioral Health Clinic seeking help for problems he had experienced since his return from Afghanistan. His complaints included disturbed sleep, angry outbursts, problems at work, and a sense that things were simply "not going well." He reported that he was at the clinic mostly because his wife was upset and had threatened to leave him if he didn't "get some help." A careful assessment indicated that John had PTSD with memories of several events from his deployments that flashed into his mind and about which he would often dream. He scored a 64 on the military version of the PTSD Checklist (PCL-M; Weathers, Huska,

& Keane, 1991), which ranges from a low of 17 to a high of 85, with scores higher than 50 indicating probable PTSD. In addition to PTSD, John was diagnosed with depression and an alcohol abuse problem, though he was not drinking to the extent to which he appeared dependent. After discussing the treatment with John, the therapist decided to initiate treatment with PE therapy.

During the first session of PE, the therapist described the rationale and procedures of PE and answered John's questions. John was reticent about initiating treatment and was particularly concerned with the prospect of having to relate the details of traumatic events during the imaginal exposure exercises. The therapist reassured John and told him that many veterans and trauma survivors had found this treatment to be difficult but ultimately healing. Having received assurance from John that he was willing to "give it a try," the therapist engaged John in a discussion about the events of his most recent deployment. Although a number of different events troubled John, the initial assessment had indicated one in particular, the death of his friend, as the most upsetting. Having confirmed this to be the case, the therapist went on to ask John a series of questions about the firefight during which his friend was killed. This interview provided the therapist with some details that had not been disclosed during the initial assessment and also allowed identification of the beginning and end points of the event. The therapist taught John how to help manage his arousal by controlling and slowing his breathing. At the end of session, John was instructed to practice this breathing exercise every day and listen to a recording of the session.

The second session began with the therapist answering any questions that John had about the treatment program or the last session and getting a report of how the breathing exercises had proceeded. Although John had not practiced the breathing exercise as often as he might, he had practiced some and reported that it was a little helpful. The therapist reinforced what John had done and encouraged him to continue to practice. The two then spent a portion of the session discussing common reactions to trauma and John's own reactions to his traumatic experiences. The therapist used this opportunity to reassure John that his responses did not indicate that he was crazy or weak and that many people who had had similar problems after returning from combat had been helped by PE treatment. After this conversation, the two worked to develop a hierarchy of items to be used during the *in vivo* exercises. Many of the items on John's hierarchy were common to those of other combat veterans, such as crowds, driving, the sound of gunfire, and news stories about the war. Other items were more specific to John's traumatic experience, such as places he used to go with his friend and images of blood or death. Working together, John and the therapist agreed on two items to be used for exercises during the ensuing week: shopping at the post exchange (PX) and driving alone on known roads without speeding. These items were selected because John reported that they would be arousing but not overwhelming.

At the beginning of the third session, John reported that he had successfully shopped at the PX twice but that he struggled to remain within the speed limit while driving. After discussing the homework and providing some encouragement, the therapist introduced the imaginal exposure exercise. Despite his reticence, John was able to relate the events of his trauma fairly well, and he repeated the story three times over the course of the exercise. Clearly upset by the memory, John appeared to actively fight to control his emotions, and throughout the exercise the therapist gently encouraged him to connect to his emotions. During the processing of the imaginal exercise the therapist helped John to explore the meaning of the event and his thoughts and feelings related to the loss of his friend. Homework for the week included *in vivo* exercises that were slightly more difficult than those of the previous week (also additional exercises focused on driving the speed limit) and repeatedly listening to the recording of the imaginal exercise.

At the start of Session 4, John scored a 51 on the PCL-M, indicating that his symptoms were decreasing. He was able to better engage with the memory during the imaginal exposure exercise and reported that he was able to complete his homework exercises the previous week. In session 5, John experienced a very strong emotional reaction as he related the details of his friend's death. Initially he became tearful and sad. After this, though, John became very angry and agitated. The therapist encouraged him to continue with the exercise despite the intense emotions and also to express all of his feelings and not to become focused only on his anger. With difficulty, John was able to continue with the exercise and process his reactions. Although this was a difficult session, John reported a sense of relief at having faced these feelings and "making it through." The therapist reinforced John's sense of accomplishment and encouraged him to keep working at the therapy to build on his progress.

Because session 5 was quite intense, the therapist decided to conduct the imaginal exposure exercise in session 6 using the full story rather than shifting to "hot spots." John, although still upset by the memory, was able to complete the exercise without the intense emotional reactions that occurred in session 5. In sessions 7 and 8 the imaginal exposure exercises focused on "hot spots" in the memory that John identified as particularly difficult: the point at which his friend was killed (session 7) and the beginning of the firefight (session 8). John continued to engage in the *in vivo* exercises, moving up the hierarchy at a steady pace and reported that he was feeling better and that his wife commented that she was noticing improvements as well.

In session 9 the therapist took some time to explore with John some of the other combat traumas that he experienced. Specifically, the therapist was trying to determine whether there were other memories that needed to be addressed through the imaginal exposure exercise. Based on the discussion, the fact that his PCL-M score had been reduced to a 34, and a review of John's report of reduced symptoms across sessions, it was decided that there was no need to address a different memory. The imaginal exposure exercise focused on a third "hot spot." This exercise went quickly and without incident, and following the exercise John and the therapist agreed that they would plan to end treatment with the next session.

In the final session, John retold the full memory and processed the experience of revisiting the memory and how that experience had changed over the course of treatment. The therapist reviewed John's *in vivo* hierarchy and had John re-rate the items on the hierarchy. From this exercise, it became clear that John had made substantial improvements but that a few items continued to bother him. The therapist helped John develop a plan to allow him to continue to work on these remaining items. Finally, the therapist confirmed that John's symptoms were largely reduced by conducting a symptom interview. The session ended with the therapist offering John encouragement and assuring him that should problems arise in the future, John could contact the therapist to get help if he wanted it.

References

Asukai, N., Saito, A., Tsuruta, N., Ogami, R., & Kishimoto, J. (2008). Pilot study on prolonged exposure of Japanese patients with posttraumatic stress disorder due to mixed traumatic events. *Journal of Traumatic Stress, 21,* 340–343.

Bradley, R., Greene, J., Russ, E., Dutra, L., & Westen, D. (2005). A multidimensional meta-analysis of psychotherapy for PTSD. *American Journal of Psychiatry, 162,* 214–227.

Bryant, R. A., Mastrodomenico, J., Felmingham, K. L., Hopwood, S., Kenny, L., Kandris, E., et al. (2008). Treatment of acute stress disorder: A randomized controlled trial. *Archives of General Psychiatry, 65,* 659–667.

Bryant, R. A., Moulds, M. L., Guthrie, R. M., Dang, S. T., Mastrodomenico, J., Nixon, R. D., et al. (2008). A randomized controlled trial of exposure therapy and cognitive restructuring for posttraumatic stress disorder. *Journal of Consulting and Clinical Psychology, 76,* 695–703.

Bryant, R. A., Moulds, M., Guthrie, R., & Nixon, R. D. (2003). Treating acute stress disorder following mild traumatic brain injury. *American Journal of Psychiatry, 160,* 585–587.

Cahill, S. P., Rauch, S. A., Hembree, E. A., & Foa, E. B. (2003). Effect of cognitive-behavioral treatments for PTSD on anger. *Journal of Cognitive Psychotherapy, 17,* 113–131.

Cigrang, J. A., Peterson, A. L., & Schobitz, R. P. (2005). Three American troops in Iraq: Evaluation of a brief exposure therapy treatment for the secondary prevention of combat-related PTSD. *Pragmatic Case Studies in Psychotherapy, 1,* 1–25.

Feeny, N. C., Zoellner, L. A., Mavissakalian, M. R., & Roy-Byrne, P. P. (2009). What would you choose?: Sertraline or prolonged exposure in community and PTSD treatment seeking women. *Depression and Anxiety, 26*, 724–731.

Feske, U. (2008). Treating low-income and minority women with posttraumatic stress disorder: A pilot study comparing prolonged exposure and treatment as usual conducted by community therapists. *Journal of Interpersonal Violence, 23*, 1027–1040.

Foa, E. B., Dancu, C. V., Hembree, E. A., Jaycox, L. H., Meadows, E. A., & Street, G. P. (1999). A comparison of exposure therapy, stress inoculation training, and their combination for reducing posttraumatic stress disorder in female assault victims. *Journal of Consulting and Clinical Psychology, 67*, 194–200.

Foa, E. B., Hembree, E. A., Cahill, S. P., Rauch, S. A. M., Riggs, D. S., Feeny, N. C., et al. (2005). Randomized trial of prolonged exposure for posttraumatic stress disorder with and without cognitive restructuring: Outcome at academic and community clinics. *Journal of Consulting and Clinical Psychology, 73*, 953–964.

Foa, E. B., Hembree, E. A., & Rothbaum, B. O. (2007). *Prolonged exposure therapy for PTSD: Emotional processing of traumatic experiences therapist guide.* New York: Oxford University Press.

Foa, E. B., & Kozak, M. J. (1986). Emotional processing of fear: Exposure to corrective information. *Psychological Bulletin, 99*, 20–35.

Foa, E. B., & Rauch, S. A. M. (2004). Cognitive changes during prolonged exposure versus prolonged exposure plus cognitive restructuring in female assault survivors with posttraumatic stress disorder. *Journal of Consulting and Clinical Psychology, 72*, 879–884.

Foa, E. B., Rothbaum, B. O., Riggs, D., & Murdock, T. (1991). Treatment of posttraumatic stress disorder in rape victims: A comparison between cognitive-behavioral procedures and counseling. *Journal of Consulting and Clinical Psychology, 59*, 715–723.

Foa, E. B., Zoellner, L. A., Feeny, N. C., Hembree, E. A., & Alvarez-Conrad, J. (2002). Does imaginal exposure exacerbate PTSD symptoms? *Journal of Consulting and Clinical Psychology, 70*, 1022–1028.

Galovski, T. E., Monson, C., Bruce, S. E., & Resick, P. A. (2009). Does cognitive-behavioral therapy for PTSD improve perceived health and sleep impairment? *Journal of Traumatic Stress, 22*, 197–204.

Hembree, E. A., Foa, E. B., Dorfan, N. M., Street, G. P., Kowalski, J., & Tu, X. (2003). Do patients drop out prematurely from exposure therapy for PTSD? *Journal of Traumatic Stress, 16*, 555–562.

Institute of Medicine. (2008). *Treatment of posttraumatic stress disorder: An assessment of the evidence.* Washington, DC: National Academies Press.

Keane, T. M., Fairbank, J. A., Caddell, J. M., & Zimering, R. T. (1989). Implosive (flooding) therapy reduces symptoms of PTSD in Vietnam combat veterans. *Behavior Therapy, 20*, 245–260.

Moser, J. S., Foa, E. B., & Cahill, S. (2010). Evidence for power outcome in patients with severe negative trauma-related cognitions: Implications for treatment making in posttraumatic stress disorder. *Journal of Nervous and Mental Disease, 198*, 72–75.

Nacasch, N., Foa, E. B., Fostick, L., Polliack, M., Dinstein, Y., Tzur, D., et al. (2007). Prolonged exposure therapy for chronic combat-related PTSD: A case report of five veterans. *CNS Spectrums, 12,* 690–695.

Nacasch, N., Foa, E. B., Huppert, J. D., Tzur, D., Fostick, L., Dinstein, Y., et al. (2010). Prolonged exposure therapy for combat- and terror-related PTSD: A randomized control comparison with treatment as usual. *Journal of Clinical Psychiatry.* Advance online publication. *doi:10.4088/JCP.09m05682blu*

Rauch, S. A., Defever, E., Favorite, T., Duroe, A., Garrity, C., Martis, B., et al. (2009). Prolonged exposure for PTSD in a Veterans Health Administration PTSD clinic. *Journal of Traumatic Stress, 22,* 60–64.

Resick, P. A., Nishith, P., Weaver, T. L., Astin, M. C., & Feuer, C. A. (2002). A comparison of cognitive-processing therapy with prolonged exposure and a waiting condition for the treatment of chronic posttraumatic stress disorder in female rape victims. *Journal of Consulting and Clinical Psychology, 70,* 867–879.

Schnurr, P. P., Friedman, M. J., Engel, C. C., Foa, E. B., Shea, M. T., Chow, B. K., et al. (2007). Cognitive-behavioral therapy for posttraumatic stress disorder in women: A randomized clinical trial. *Journal of the American Medical Association, 297,* 820–830.

Taylor S., Thordarson, D. S., Maxfield, L., Federoff, I. C., Lovell, K., & Ogrodniczuk, J. (2003). Efficacy, speed, and adverse effects of three PTSD treatments: Exposure therapy, relaxation training, and EMDR. *Journal of Consulting and Clinical Psychology, 71,* 330–338.

van Minnen, A., & Foa, E. B. (2006). The effect of imaginal exposure length on outcome of treatment for PTSD. *Journal of Traumatic Stress, 19,* 427–438.

Weathers, F., Huska, J., & Keane, T. (1991). *The PTSD Checklist Military Version (PCL-M).* Boston: National Center for PTSD.

CHAPTER 4

Cognitive Processing Therapy

Amy M. Williams
Tara E. Galovski
Karen A. Kattar
Patricia A. Resick

Cognitive processing therapy (CPT; Resick & Schnicke, 1992, 1993; Resick, Monson, & Chard, 2008) has been endorsed as a best-practice model in the International Society for Traumatic Stress Studies Practice Guideline (Foa, Keane, Friedman, & Cohen, 2008) and the Veterans Health Administration/Department of Defense clinical practice guideline (Veterans Health Administration, 2004). As one of the recommended treatments for posttraumatic stress disorder (PTSD), CPT is being increasingly employed in clinical settings with men and women in the armed forces. Although CPT was initially tested with samples consisting of survivors of sexual assault suffering from PTSD, its efficacy has since been demonstrated across a variety of types of trauma, including military-related traumatic events (Ahrens & Rexford, 2002; Chard, Schumm, Owens, & Cottingham, 2010; Galovski & Resick, 2008; Monson et al., 2006; Resick, Galovski, et al., 2008; Zappert & Westrup, 2008). Beginning in 2007, the National Center for PTSD began coordinating a systematic dissemination of CPT to clinicians in the Veterans Health Administration funded by the VA Office of Mental Health Services (McHugh & Barlow, 2010). Ongoing research continues to build the foundation of support for its effectiveness with a military population across modalities, including individual, group, and combined individual–group and cross-cultural applications, and across variations of the original manual (Falsetti, Resnick, Davis, & Gallagher, 2001; Otis, Keane, Kerns, Monson, & Scioli, 2009; Schulz, Huber, & Resick, 2006).

Theoretical Underpinnings of CPT

CPT is based on a social cognitive theory of PTSD that combines elements of information processing and social schema theories (Lang, 1977; McCann, Sakheim, & Abrahamson, 1988). The theory posits that all humans organize incoming information into schemas (i.e., stored bodies of knowledge). It is through these beliefs that individuals make sense of their world, interpret new information, and formulate expectations about future experiences. Trauma survivors, particularly those suffering from PTSD, commonly experience disruption in the areas of agency (reflecting the cause of the event), safety, trust, power, esteem, and intimacy (Janoff-Bulman, 1992; McCann et al., 1988).

In CPT, cognitive therapy techniques are utilized to focus on faulty thoughts or cognitions related to traumatic events. It is specifically theorized that individuals who develop PTSD following an exposure to a traumatic event experience significant disruptions in preexisting beliefs. CPT further posits that these disrupted beliefs are manifested in inaccurate self-statements that interrupt the normal recovery process. These inaccurate statements are termed "stuck points" because they tend to keep the individuals "stuck" in PTSD and prohibit the recovery to normal functioning. Stuck points essentially develop through the course of two cognitive processes. *Assimilation* is one such process that occurs when the new trauma memory can be incorporated without altering prior beliefs. If one's prior beliefs are already negative, then the trauma information would appear to confirm those beliefs ("I always knew that people in authority should not be trusted"). If one had prior positive beliefs, assimilation involves the alteration of the new trauma information to fit existing beliefs in a just world, in one's ability to control events, and so forth. Assimilated stuck points are past-oriented beliefs that often involve undoing, self-blame, and guilt. An example of an assimilated stuck point might include the statement, "It is my fault my buddy died. I should have shot sooner." The process of *over-accommodation* describes the extreme modification of entire existing belief systems in an effort to integrate trauma information and to resume an illusion of control over possible future events. An example of an over-accommodated stuck point might include the following statements: "The world is always dangerous" or "I cannot trust anyone." The goal of CPT is to assist the client in identifying stuck points and promoting the process of *accommodation*, balanced thinking that takes into account the reality of the traumatic event without going overboard. Through this process, the trauma survivor is able to generate alternative balanced beliefs such as, "Some places in the world are very dangerous, but there are many situations in which I am relatively safe."

CPT also addresses the emotions present in PTSD, including fear, anger, humiliation, shame, and sadness. Some emotions naturally occur in the face of a traumatic event (i.e., anger and loss in response to "an IED exploded next to my unit and killed my friend"). Others are manufactured in that they stem from appraisals and thoughts that may be distorted (i.e. guilt in response to "I should have known better than to take that road"). Clients are encouraged to feel their primary, natural emotions, elicited by writing a narrative of their traumatic experience at home and reading the trauma narrative aloud in session. Manufactured emotions (emanating from distorted thinking) are addressed at the cognitive level and spontaneously remit with more balanced, realistic thinking (i.e. "I did the best I could with the information I had at the time").

Format and Overview of CPT

CPT can be conducted in both individual and group settings or a combination of both. The course of treatment is typically 12 sessions, with a recommended follow-up session 1 month later. An additional optional traumatic bereavement session can be added when clinically indicated. Both individual and group treatment manuals for CPT have been revised with a focus on military trauma. The Veteran/Military versions of the CPT manuals offer detailed information regarding theory, suggestions for implementation, step-by-step descriptions of sessions, and reproducible worksheets (Chard, Resick, Monson, & Kattar, 2008; Resick, Monson, & Chard, 2008). Recent research (Resick, Galovski, et al., 2008) suggests that CPT can be equally effective without the inclusion of the written trauma account. This variation, CPT—Cognitive (CPT-C), is included in the manual. The course of CPT can be broadly conceptualized as including three phases, each with unique worksheets, goals, and tasks that are designed to be gradually mastered by the client as the client becomes his or her own therapist throughout the trauma recovery process.

Phase 1: Analyze, Gather Information, and Identify Feelings (Sessions 1–5)

In this phase, clinicians and clients embark on the process of understanding the meaning of the traumatic event. Clients are introduced to theory and treatment rationale in the first session of CPT. An impact statement is assigned in which clients are asked to describe why they think the event happened and the meaning of the event—the way in which the trauma has influenced their perspective on five belief systems: safety, trust, power/control, esteem, and intimacy. The clients are invited to look at how the traumas have affected or changed their belief systems and to identify stuck points that will be examined throughout the course of treatment. Assimilated stuck points are given special attention early in treatment because, if the clients are engaging in self-blame or are unable to accept the reality of the trauma, it is difficult to work on other issues. It is also easier to challenge the conclusions the clients have drawn about the traumatic event after the causes have been thoroughly examined. The relationships between thoughts and feelings are explored and discussed via an Events–Thoughts–Feelings worksheet (the A–B–C worksheet). The written account of the worst traumatic event occurs in this phase of treatment and is used to gather information about the trauma, including thoughts and feelings, as well as to provide clients with the opportunity to process natural emotions.

Phase 2: Challenge (Sessions 5–7)

Although some Socratic questioning and gentle cognitive challenging occurs in early sessions, phase 2 formally introduces the Socratic process to the clients. In this phase, the clinician introduces two worksheets that serve to guide the clients in independently beginning to challenge their own stuck points. The Challenging Questions and Patterns of Problematic Thinking worksheets encourage a client to begin acting as his or her own "scientist" in evaluating thoughts that have previously gone unquestioned. The overriding goal of this process is for clients to become their own therapists and develop more balanced ways of thinking and considering the world, an achievement that is essential in the maintenance of therapy gains and relapse prevention.

Phase 3: Change (Sessions 7–12)

In the final phase of CPT, clients are taught to use the Challenging Beliefs Worksheet (CBW), which is a compilation of all previous worksheets. The CBW uses multiple columns to (1) identify the event, thought, and feeling, (2) challenge the stuck point, and (3) modify maladaptive thoughts to experience a change in emotion. The last five sessions of CPT review each of the five schema areas often disrupted in those with PTSD (safety, trust, power/control, esteem, and intimacy). Modules about each schema are introduced that describe common symptoms related to having stuck points in that area. Possible thinking alternatives are suggested. Relevant stuck points are challenged, and alternative ways of thinking are generated by the client when using the CBW. In the final session of CPT, the client reads a new impact statement that includes current beliefs about the cause and meaning of the trauma. Treatment gains are consolidated, and goals are set for the future.

Research on CPT with Civilian Populations

Two decades of research involving CPT has supported its effectiveness with a variety of trauma groups. The first published study of CPT involved an open trial of a female sexual assault survivor sample and was administered in a group format (Resick & Schnicke, 1992). Following the promising outcomes of this original research, Resick, Nishith, Weaver, Astin, and Feuer (2002) compared CPT with prolonged exposure (PE; Foa, Rothbaum, Riggs, & Murdock, 1991) and a wait-list control group. Participants included women from a community sample who had been sexually assaulted. In addition to a decrease in PTSD symptoms, there was also a significant improvement in depression. For both guilt cognitions and health-related concerns, CPT showed a large pre- to posttreatment effect size that was significantly greater than the PE change (Resick et al., 2002; Galovski, Monson, Bruce, & Resick, 2009). Women with higher scores on a borderline characteristics scale were just as likely to demonstrate significant gains as those without borderline characteristics (Clarke, Rizvi, & Resick, 2009). An examination of complex PTSD symptoms comparing those with and without child sexual abuse histories demonstrated that CPT was effective for a wide range of symptoms in both groups, including dissociation, impaired self-reference, and tension reduction behaviors (Resick, Nishith, & Griffin, 2003).

Content analyses on the two impact statements completed for sessions 2 and 12 showed significant decreases in over-accommodated and assimilated clauses from the start to end of therapy. There was an increase in the number of accommodated clauses; accommodation clauses were significantly and negatively correlated with self-reported PTSD symptoms (Sobel, Resick, & Rabalais, 2009). A follow-up study revealed that participants maintained therapeutic changes 5–10 years posttreatment (Resick, Williams, Orazem, & Gutner, 2005).

The CPT protocol was extended in Chard's (2005) study with female adult survivors of childhood sexual abuse (CSA). Fifty-seven percent of participants reported more than 100 incidents of abuse. The treatment was conducted via a 17-week protocol that included a combination of group and individual sessions. The CPT—Sexual Abuse (CPT-SA) protocol added components of developmental theories, as well as information on assertiveness, sexual intimacy, and social support. CPT-SA was compared with a delayed-treatment condition, and a significant decrease in both PTSD and depression was documented.

In 2008, Resick and colleagues conducted a dismantling study with three conditions: CPT in its original format, CPT-C without a written account, and CPT-WA, which included only writing the account and reading it to the therapist and oneself. The community sample was composed of 150 women who had experienced a sexual trauma or physical assault.

Eighty-six percent of the participants had multiple traumatic events in their histories. Half of the participants also met criteria for major depressive disorder at pretreatment. Results suggested that all three formats produced large improvements, but overall, CPT-C was significantly more efficacious than CPT-WA and appeared to be the most efficient of the three conditions. In addition, clinically significant treatment effects were found for comorbid depression, general anxiety, and anger (Resick, Galovski, et al., 2008).

CPT has been effectively adapted and used in a variety of settings. There are published case and research studies using the CPT protocol with refugees (Schulz et al., 2006), survivors of motor vehicle accidents (Galovski & Resick, 2008), and incarcerated adolescents (Ahrens & Rexford, 2002). In addition, CPT has been used in combination with other therapies to address commonly comorbid psychiatric illnesses such as panic disorder (Falsetti et al., 2001).

Research on CPT with Military Populations

In 2006, Monson and colleagues conducted a treatment-as-usual control comparison study of CPT with 60 veterans (54 men, 6 women) who had chronic military-related PTSD. The mean age was somewhat older than previous civilian and community-based samples ($M = 54.9$ years). Although the majority of participants were Vietnam veterans (78%), this study also included veterans from Korean, post-Vietnam, and Gulf War periods of service. Forty percent of the intention-to-treat sample (i.e., including dropouts) receiving CPT did not meet criteria for a PTSD diagnosis at the end of treatment. Moreover, 50% had reliable improvement in their PTSD symptoms at posttreatment.

Chard, Schumm, Owens, and Cottingham (2010) examined cohort differences between recent veterans of the wars in Iraq and Afghanistan and Vietnam veterans before and after completing treatment for PTSD using CPT. Participants were treated on an outpatient basis and included 51 recent veterans and 50 Vietnam veterans. Anyone who attended at least one session was included in the study, and, in some cases, the treatment was extended beyond the protocol 12 sessions. Treatment dropouts did not differ on pretreatment assessment measures or demographics. Although all met criteria for PTSD diagnosis at the onset of treatment, only 41% of recent veterans and 60% of Vietnam veterans met posttreatment PTSD diagnostic criteria. When the authors controlled for PTSD severity pretreatment, findings emerged that recent veterans may have less severe PTSD symptoms following CPT than their Vietnam veteran counterparts.

Significant decreases in PTSD were also reported in a residential treatment setting that included CPT in the treatment approach (Owens, Chard

& Cox, 2005). Ninety-nine veterans received 7 weeks of treatment at a Veterans Administration (VA)-based PTSD residential rehabilitation program. The veterans were mixed gender (80% male, 20% female), and the majority included Vietnam War–era veterans. The mean age was 53 years. All patients received group and individual CPT in addition to other inpatient group programs. Although the effects cannot be attributed solely to CPT, significant decreases occurred from pre- to posttreatment on measures of PTSD, depression, and maladaptive cognitions. Owens et al. (2005) found no change in guilt, even though PTSD severity decreased. The authors note that previous findings regarding guilt came from sexual assault survivors and that the absence of a decrease in guilt, even with symptom improvement, may be unique to combat trauma samples (who may report having seen or been a part of events for which they later had feelings of guilt). In addition, the majority of participants were Vietnam-era veterans who were subjected to a great deal of social stigma following their return from war.

Zappert and Westrup (2008) published results from their implementation of CPT in a women's 60-day VA PTSD residential treatment program. The patients were admitted in cohorts, and CPT was provided in a group setting. Eighteen women completed treatment with CPT, and 15 of the 18 women had a statistically significant reduction in PTSD symptoms.

Similar to efforts in the civilian populations in which CPT has been combined with other treatments for comorbid dysfunction, results from a VA pilot study show promise for an integrated treatment for comorbid pain and PTSD (Otis et al., 2009). The 12-session protocol includes components of CPT and cognitive-behavioral interventions for pain. The authors note that a randomized controlled trial is being conducted and will compare CBT for pain, CPT for PTSD, integrated treatment, and a wait-list control condition.

Strengths of CPT with Military Personnel

Although part of the strength of CPT is that it is evidence based and manualized, it also offers a great deal of flexibility in its implementation. Because many service members may present with a variety of traumatic events beyond combat trauma, it is beneficial to have a treatment that can accommodate different types of life events in one treatment. As described before, CPT has been shown to be effective in treating PTSD arising from a number of different types of traumatic stressors. In addition, clients can address numerous personal traumatic incidents if necessary, all within the same course of treatment. For example, a client who presents with multiple traumatic events would first choose an "index trauma," which is identified as the trauma creating the worst symptoms for the client. After writing about this incident, the therapist and client could choose to write about an additional traumatic event. Or, instead of writing additional accounts, the client can simply use the CBW to identify and alter stuck points about additional traumatic events. Teaching a client to challenge his or her own thinking and modify extreme types of thinking (including overresponsibility and self-blame) may have a "ripple effect" on how the client views other traumatic events. Rather than having to begin a second, third, or fourth course of treatment for additional traumatic events, a goal of CPT is the resolution of stuck points related to the index trauma that can result in reduced disruption from other traumatic events.

In addition to being flexible within a single course of treatment, CPT is also flexible in its modality. It can be provided in various formats, including group, individual, or a combination of both. Delivering CPT in a group format allows service members to begin the process of trusting others in a social setting (decreasing isolation often found in traumatized individuals) while finding relief in learning that they are not alone. (For more information regarding group treatment approaches to PTSD, interested readers are referred to Foy et al., 2000). Group members in CPT provide support to each other via optional phone lists while learning how to receive support. This practice may translate to other relationships in their civilian lives, in which they are often disconnected from others.

Depending on the nature of the trauma, as well as the needs of the client, CPT can be conducted with or without completion of a written account (CPT-C). There are a number of reasons for a clinician to conduct CPT without a written account. First, CPT-C may result in a more rapid decline of symptoms at the onset of treatment (Resick, Galovski, et al., 2008). Providing quicker relief from PTSD symptoms may be important in situations involving an upcoming deployment, a move, or another leave of absence from treatment. Second, CPT-C may be beneficial if the client has no memory for the traumatic event for various reasons, including traumatic brain injury or drug-induced memory loss (i.e., Rohypnol, alcohol intoxication). Third, CPT-C can be used if the client absolutely refuses to write about the traumatic event.

In addition to treating past trauma, CPT may be a particularly effective treatment for those military personnel who plan to reenter combat zones in the future. Service members learn cognitive skills during the course of CPT that may be helpful when facing traumatic events in subsequent deployments. Many in the military often fear that treatment will reduce the survival skills necessary for combat, such as hypervigilance. One potential outcome of CPT is that clients learn to differentiate between dangerous (combat) and safe (civilian) situations. A goal of CPT is for service members to retain hypervigilance for dangerous situations but gain more mastery over when not to employ those skills.

Monson and colleagues (2006) noted that CPT may be well suited to a veteran population because of its "ability to address thoughts related to committing, witnessing and experiencing acts of violence, which often co-occur in the context of combat traumatization" (p. 904). The nature of war necessarily requires service members to be often in the position of not only being victimized but also having to commit acts of violence. Although this may be an expectation of war, it is still often a focus of treatment, especially when acts of violence were either intentionally or unintentionally directed toward members of society (e.g., civilian women and children). These acts may result in extreme cognitive and emotional distress, which may disrupt core beliefs about oneself and the world. CPT seeks to directly address related stuck points and help service members reconcile these internal conflicts.

A final potential strength of CPT that warrants further empirical investigation is its ability to be modified for clients struggling with literacy, cognitive impairment, and/or physical disability. Veterans returning from war may experience cognitive and physical impairments (e.g., traumatic brain injury, loss of limbs) that undermine their beliefs about themselves as productive members of society. In order to accommodate these impairments while targeting stuck points, clinicians have modified or selected worksheets according to user benefit. For instance, clinicians may opt to use A–B–C worksheets throughout the protocol for those whose cognitive impairments warrant less complex (and consequently less frustrating) worksheets. For service members who have physical impairments that may make CPT more difficult (such as writing difficulties), typing or audiotaping session content has been substituted on a case-by-case basis.

Limitations of CPT with Military Personnel

There is at this point no research published using CPT with active military, although several studies are ongoing. In addressing the limitations of CPT, clinicians are faced with some challenges specific to military personnel and others more general in nature. The inherent nature of military training requires that a combatant contain emotions in order to "get the job done." Although this is a necessary skill in the heat of battle, this learned style of coping with great distress often hinders recovery of trauma-related symptoms. Service members learn to avoid experiencing emotions and traumatic memories. Military culture can send the message that feeling emotions equates to weakness and inadequacy. Needing treatment may be interpreted to mean that one is incapable of handling situations. There can be a fear of being "found out as weak" if one is seen by other service members in a treatment program. Because CPT involves feeling emotions, this can be a challenge for military personnel.

Any treatment requires attendance and participation to be successful. CPT is significantly enhanced with active participation in weekly practice assignments. Although most are not overly time-consuming, the addition of practice assignments can present a challenge for some clients. Time constraints may also pose a treatment barrier. Avoidant behavior common in PTSD may be exhibited in CPT by incomplete practice assignments and/ or missing session(s) altogether. These therapy-interfering behaviors can be targeted therapeutically and may be addressed throughout a course of CPT using the worksheets explained earlier. Attention early in treatment to avoidance or lack of compliance with assignments can be very helpful in successfully implementing CPT.

Therapeutic Considerations

As a result of efforts to implement evidence-based treatments in the VA and the Department of Defense, CPT has enjoyed increased visibility, and there have been numerous opportunities for clinicians in these settings to attend training. The current VA training recommendations include attending a 2-day workshop to learn individual CPT and a third day for group CPT training. Following workshop attendance, clinicians begin to implement the treatment, with opportunities for weekly group phone consultation with expert CPT clinicians. Advanced lectures and discussions are offered on a regular basis by the VA.

For additional review and training, interested clinicians may also access online materials through the Medical University of South Carolina National Crime Victims Research and Treatment Center at *cpt.musc.edu*. The online course provides Web-based learning in nine modules and was developed to complement use of the manual and/or attending a workshop. The National Center for PTSD is also in the process of developing a Web-based course in CPT. It is important to note that completion of a Web-based course is not considered sufficient to deliver CPT. Opportunities for consultation and supervision in developing the necessary skills for implementation are an important part of the learning process.

Case Vignette

Bill (not his actual name) is a 28-year-old battlefield corpsman who recently completed a tour of duty in Iraq. During his tour, he was stationed with the Marines and rendered emergency medical care following numerous combat situations. Through the course of this service, he was often in harm's way and witnessed significant injuries, burns, and death, as well as surviving heavy fire himself. He identified his index trauma as the first time that he was not able to save a young soldier's life due to the extent of the injuries suffered. Bill presented to the PTSD clinic after being diagnosed with PTSD (his score on the PTSD Checklist was a 78 out of a possible 85) and major depressive disorder (MDD; his score on the Beck Depression Inventory—2 was a 47 out of a possible 66). He had initially been referred to the local VA for services for substance dependence because his family and friends encouraged him to seek help following a conviction for driving while intoxicated and several fights in bars as well as his inability to hold down a job. Although Bill had heard of PTSD before, he was largely unfamiliar with the symptom picture, had avoided talking about his experiences in Iraq at all, and described himself as no longer able to experience emotions—except possibly when under the influence of some substance, and then he only felt rage.

Bill and his therapist decided to engage in trauma-focused therapy to resolve PTSD and agreed to begin a course of CPT. The initial session of the therapy provided significant psychoeducation regarding PTSD, specifically highlighting the idea that the normal recovery process had been interrupted in a number of ways (less than accurate interpretations of the event, the subsequent engagement in avoidance strategies, etc.). The therapist and Bill began discussions about identifying stuck points and continued this process when reading the impact statement in session 2. Assimilated stuck points that became evident in this early stage of therapy seemed to focus primarily around Bill's belief that he "had not done enough to save these guys." Through the process of Socratic dialogue, it was furthered discovered that Bill felt ashamed of the fear and horror that he felt during his first encounters with wounded soldiers in the very beginning of his tour. He felt that his fear was so great that it must have prevented him from applying his medical interventions adequately. He concluded that lives were lost due to his incompetence. The Socratic process in this early stage of the therapy allowed Bill the latitude to recount his experiences, particularly his identified index event, more completely. Through this process, he was able to realize that it was normal to feel fear in the face of danger, and he came to acknowledge that the men who lost their lives on the battlefield that day died because of the extent of their injuries, not due to his incompetence. He was able to start feeling sadness about these deaths, rather than the overwhelming guilt and shame that he had been experiencing.

Experiencing natural emotions such as sadness was, at first, significantly distressing to Bill. He reported that he was feeling worse and that this therapy was not working. His PCL scores had decreased only slightly and were holding at 71. He told his therapist that he had "stopped feeling entirely" after this index event and was not going to ever find himself in that position (of feeling fear, helplessness, vulnerability) again. This threat of imminent dropout occurred at session 7 and coincided with the introduction of the CBW.

At this point in therapy, Bill had become very familiar with the concept of identifying his stuck points, those self-statements that were preventing his recovery. In examining what he was telling himself at this point in therapy, Bill identified the stuck point concerning "feeling his emotions" as the following: "If I begin to feel again, I will be vulnerable to losing control." The following includes the Socratic dialogue that ensued in session 7.

THERAPIST: OK—let's spend a little time with this. "If I begin to feel again, I will be vulnerable to losing control." Losing control? Hmmmm, what do you mean by that?

BILL: You know–going crazy. Losing control.

THERAPIST: What kinds of things might you do if you were to "go crazy"?

BILL: I might punch a wall or punch people. You know how many fights I got into—that's what got me in here to begin with.

THERAPIST: So if you started to feel sad about all of the soldiers that were hurt or killed over in Iraq, you would punch walls? Is this what happened when you got into fights after you returned stateside?

BILL: No, those fights happened when I was drinking and when I got really pissed off, usually for no reason at all, like someone was looking at me wrong. I would just start thinking about Iraq and couldn't take it and needed to stop, so I drank and got ugly.

THERAPIST: So, it sounds like you would work pretty hard *not* to think and feel about everything that happened in Iraq. Part of working hard was drinking to forget? Blowing off steam in another way by picking fights?

BILL: (*Stares at therapist.*) Yeah—I did, and do, everything I could ... to turn off Iraq in my head.

THERAPIST: How do you think that helped?

BILL: (*Stares at his hands.*) It didn't. Here I am.

THERAPIST: From the way that you describe this, it almost sounds like you haven't tried feeling your feelings in a long time. In fact, you've done everything that you can *not* to feel any feelings. It may be difficult to say, then, that you would lose control if you were to feel your feelings. It may be that working so hard *not* to feel your feelings is actually resulting in some of these out-of-control behaviors. What might happen if, say today, you were to feel very, very sad over the loss of life in Iraq?

BILL: (*Looks therapist right in the eye.*) I might cry, and that is unacceptable. Crying shows weakness and, where I've been, weakness can get you dead. Becoming emotional is a distraction and makes you vulnerable. If you're distracted, you can lose focus, and in the work I did, that means someone might die.

THERAPIST: It sounds like you needed to stay very tightly controlled over in Iraq in order to perform your duties. A lot was riding on it?

BILL: What was I supposed to do? Take a piss and moan break while people were dying around me? Tie up a tourniquet while bawling over the soldier whose leg was blown off?

THERAPIST: You're right, a lot was riding on it. A lot depended on you staying focused. Those guys are lucky they had you. What about now? Do the same rules apply?

BILL: I didn't think about it like that. I keep feeling like I had to hold it together for these guys, and I guess I just keep holding it together.

THERAPIST: That makes a lot of sense to me. Choosing safe, appropriate times and ways to mourn the losses that you've experienced. Tell you what—why don't you spend a little time thinking about this? Maybe do a worksheet on it between sessions?

BILL: Yeah—I can do that.... Hey—thanks.

References

Ahrens, J., & Rexford, L. (2002). Cognitive processing therapy for incarcerated adolescents with PTSD. *Journal of Aggression, Maltreatment and Trauma, 6,* 201–216.

Chard, K. M. (2005). An evaluation of cognitive processing therapy for the treatment of posttraumatic stress disorder related to childhood sexual abuse. *Journal of Consulting and Clinical Psychology, 73,* 965–971.

Chard, K. M., Resick, P. A., Monson, C. M., & Kattar, K. A. (2008). *Cognitive processing therapy therapist group manual: Veteran/military version.* Washington, DC: Department of Veterans Affairs.

Chard, K. M., Schumm, J. A., Owens, G.P., & Cottingham, S.M. (2010). A comparison of OEF and OIF veterans and Vietnam veterans receiving cognitive processing therapy. *Journal of Traumatic Stress, 23*(1), 25–32.

Clarke, S. B., Rizvi, S. L., & Resick, P. A. (2009). Borderline personality characteristics and treatment outcome in cognitive-behavioral treatments for PTSD in female rape victims. *Behavior Therapy, 39*(1), 72–78.

Falsetti, S. A., Resnick, H. A., Davis, J. A., & Gallagher, N. G. (2001). Treatment of posttraumatic stress disorder with comorbid panic attacks: Combining cognitive processing therapy with panic control treatment techniques. *Group Dynamics: Theory, Research, and Practice, 5*(4), 252–260.

Foa, E. B., Keane, T. M., Friedman, M. J., & Cohen, J. A. (Eds.). (2008). *Effective treatments for PTSD: Practice guidelines from the International Society for Traumatic Stress Studies* (2nd ed.). New York: Guilford Press.

Foa, E. B., Rothbaum, B. O., Riggs, D. S., & Murdock, T. B. (1991). Treatment of posttraumatic stress disorder in rape victims: A comparison between cognitive-behavioral procedures and counseling. *Journal of Consulting and Clinical Psychology, 59*, 715–723.

Foy, D. W., Glynn, S. M., Schnurr, P. P., Jankowski, M. K., Wattenberg, M. S., Weiss, D. S., et al. (2000). Group therapy. In E. B. Foa, T. M. Keane, M. J. Friedman, & J. A. Cohen (Eds.), *Effective treatments for PTSD: Practice guidelines from the International Society for Traumatic Stress Studies* (pp. 155–175). New York: Guilford Press.

Galovski, T. E., Monson, C., Bruce, S. T., & Resick, P. A. (2009) Does cognitive-behavioral therapy for PTSD improve perceived health and sleep impairment? *Journal of Traumatic Stress, 22*, 197–204.

Galovski, T. E., & Resick, P. A. (2008). Cognitive processing therapy for posttraumatic stress disorder secondary to a motor vehicle accident: A single-subject report. *Cognitive and Behavioral Practice, 15*, 287–295.

Janoff-Bulman, R. (1992). *Shattered assumptions: Towards a new psychology of trauma*. New York: Free Press.

Lang, P. J. (1977). Imagery in therapy: An information processing analysis of fear. *Behavior Therapy, 8*, 862–886.

McCann, I. L., Sakheim, D. K., & Abrahamson, D. J. (1988). Trauma and victimization: A model of psychological adaptation. *Counseling Psychologist, 16*, 531–594.

McHugh, R. K., & Barlow, D. H. (2010). The dissemination and implementation of evidence-based psychological treatments: A review of current efforts. *American Psychologist, 65*(2), 73–84.

Monson, C. M., Schnurr, P. P., Resick, P. A., Friedman, M. J., Young-Xu, Y., Stevens, S. S. (2006). Cognitive processing therapy for veterans with military-related posttraumatic stress disorder. *Journal of Consulting and Clinical Psychology, 74*(5), 898–907.

Otis, J. D., Keane, T. M., Kerns, R. D., Monson, C., & Scioli, E. (2009). The development of an integrated treatment for veterans with comorbid chronic pain and posttraumatic stress disorder. *Pain Medicine, 10*(7), 1300–1311.

Owens, G. P., Chard, K. A., & Cox, T. A. (2005). The relationship between maladaptive cognitions, anger expression and posttraumatic stress disorder among veterans in residential treatment. *Journal of Aggression, Maltreatment and Trauma, 17*(4), 439–452.

Resick, P. A., Galovski, T. E., Uhlmansiek, M. O., Scher, C. D., Clum, G. A., & Young-Xu, Y. (2008). A randomized clinical trial to dismantle components of cognitive processing therapy for posttraumatic stress disorder in female victims of interpersonal violence. *Journal of Consulting and Clinical Psychology, 76*, 243–258.

Resick, P. A., Monson, C. M., & Chard, K. M. (2008). *Cognitive processing therapy: Veteran/military version*. Washington, DC: Department of Veterans Affairs.

Resick, P. A., Nishith, P., & Griffin, M. G. (2003). How well does cognitive-behavioral therapy treat symptoms of complex PTSD?: An examination of child sexual abuse survivors within a clinical trial. *CNS Spectrums, 8*, 340–355.

Resick, P. A., Nishith, P., Weaver, T. L., Astin, M. C., & Feuer, C. A. (2002). A comparison of cognitive processing therapy with prolonged exposure and a waiting condition for the treatment of chronic posttraumatic stress disorder in female rape victims. *Journal of Consulting and Clinical Psychology, 70,* 867–879.

Resick, P. A., & Schnicke, M. K. (1992). Cognitive processing therapy for sexual assault victims. *Journal of Consulting and Clinical Psychology, 60,* 748–756.

Resick, P. A., & Schnicke, M. K. (1993). *Cognitive processing therapy for rape victims: A treatment manual.* Newbury Park, CA: Sage.

Resick, P. A., Williams, L., Orazem, R., & Gutner, C. (2005, November). *Can we cure PTSD?: Five-year follow-up of a clinical trial comparing CPT and PE.* Paper presented at the annual meeting of the Association for Behavioral and Cognitive Therapies, Washington, DC.

Schulz, P. M., Huber, L. C., & Resick, P. A. (2006). Practical adaptations of cognitive processing therapy with Bosnian refugees: Implications for adapting practice to a multicultural clientele. *Cognitive and Behavioral Practice, 13*(4), 310–321.

Sobel, A. A., Resick, P. A., & Rabalais, A. E. (2009). The effect of cognitive processing therapy on cognitions: Impact statement coding. *Journal of Traumatic Stress, 22,* 205–211.

Veterans Health Administration. (2004). *VA/DoD clinical practice guideline for the management of posttraumatic stress (Version 1.0).* Washington, DC: Department of Defense, Veterans Health Administration.

Zappert, L. N., & Westrup, D. (2008). Cognitive processing therapy for posttraumatic stress disorder in a residential treatment setting. *Psychotherapy Theory, Research, Practice, Training, 45*(3), 361–376.

CHAPTER 5

Eye Movement Desensitization and Reprocessing

Mark C. Russell
Howard Lipke
Charles Figley

Developed by Francine Shapiro in 1987, "eye movement desensitization" (EMD) was introduced primarily as a counterconditioning technique, informed by behavioral theory, that utilized patients' eye movements tracking the therapist's rapid back-and-forth hand gestures to elicit desensitization. Shapiro's (1989) inaugural study with 22 trauma survivors, including several Vietnam War veterans, revealed the potential for significant reduction of posttraumatic stress disorders (PTSD) symptoms after a single EMD session, maintained at 3-month follow-up. Although skepticism over EMD's nontraditional methodology and single-session effects reigned, positive multiple-case studies (e.g. Lipke & Botkin, 1992; Marquis, 1991) spurred randomized clinical trials (RCTs) discussed later.

In 1990, Shapiro added "reprocessing" (R) to EMD to better account for broad and often rapid information processing changes believed to exceed mainstream CBT theoretical explanations (Shapiro, 2001). Her rejection of an established paradigm for an untested, "accelerated" information processing theory coupled with restrictive training requirements led to a two-decade-long controversy with profound implications for military populations (Russell, 2008a).

Amid a long and often acrimonious debate over EMDR theory, sufficient RCTs and meta-analyses established the efficacy of EMDR and its recognition as an evidence-based treatment (EBT) for PTSD by the International Society for Traumatic Stress Studies (Foa, Keane, Friedman, & Cohen, 2009), the Department of Veterans Administration (DVA) and Department of Defense (DoD) *Practice Guidelines for Management of Traumatic Stress Disorders* (2004), the American Psychiatric Association (2004), and nearly every other major domestic and international trauma guideline (Russell, 2008a).

Overview of EMDR

EMDR Theory

In short, Shapiro's (2001) current theory of EMDR, "adaptive information processing" (AIP), posits that psychopathology reflects dysfunctional stored information in memory (neural) networks often "derived from earlier life experiences that set in motion a continued pattern of affect, behavior, cognitions, and consequent identity structures" (p. 16) that both influences and is triggered by present experience. Pathological or maladaptive patterns of behavior signify the brain's natural self-healing. Therefore, identifying and targeting past, present, and future (anticipated) pathogenic experiential contributors, whether conventional "traumatic" events (i.e., combat) or less conventional traumatic events (e.g., divorce), that have far-reaching impact is essential for adaptive processing or healing to occur. According to the AIP model, maintaining "dual focused" or conscious attention to internal stimuli (i.e., image, thought, emotion, sensation) while also attending to alternating (left–right) rhythmic external stimuli (i.e., eye movements, auditory tones, kinesthetic vibrations), often referred to as "bilateral stimulation" (BLS), activates at least one of the brain–body's natural processing mechanisms that assimilates or accommodates information into more adaptive memory networks. Conceptually, this tendency of humans to process information to adaptive resolution is consistent with basic assumptions of humanistic psychology. And the view that memory storage underlies trauma-based psychopathology is consistent with some psychodynamic theory (e.g., Horowitz, 1976). Shapiro (2001) readily admits that her model is a "working hypothesis," given the status of neuroscience.

Description of EMDR Therapy

EMDR is an integrative psychotherapy that focuses on all aspects of the traumatic memory, including visual imagery, cognition, emotion, and sensation, as well as preferred modes of functioning, to provide the desensitization and reprocessing that provides relief of traumatic stress symptoms.

EMDR consists of the following eight phases, although there may be variation depending on many clinical factors, especially in treating clients not yet ready for intensive trauma-focused work.

Phase I: Client History

Phase I comprises standard history taking, rapport building, mental status, safety screening, and informed consent.

Phase II: Client Preparation

Phase I comprises rapport building, explaining the theory, testing eye movements [EM], teaching coping skills (i.e., "safe place" stress management exercises), and addressing client fears. As with most effective treatments, there is considerable discussion with the client about preferences, comfort, skill building, self-regulation and self-care, and establishing expectancy of relief provided by the method.

Phase III: Assessment

In Phase III, the clinician identifies target memories and components by asking clients to bring the trauma to awareness and then selecting an image and/or other sensory stimuli, as well as a present negative cognition (NC), emotion(s), physical sensation(s) and body location; obtaining baseline subjective distress (SUDS) rating, from 0, "no distress," to 10, "worst ever." He or she also solicits a preferred positive cognition (PC)—an adaptive self-statement related to target memory—and a baseline rating on the Validity of Cognitions scale (VoC), with 1 standing for "completely untrue" and 7 for "completely true." Over the course of treatment, components of each target memory, as well as anticipated problem situations, are assessed in this manner, though such thorough treatment may not be practical in some situations, such as operational or deployed settings.

Phase IV: Desensitization

In Phase IV, called "desensitization," the traumatic memory is chiefly expected to be adaptively "reprocessed." Clients are instructed to start by focusing on the target memory image, NC, emotions, and body sensations and to track the BLS (i.e., therapist's hand movements) for approximately 24 back-and-forth movements (10 seconds). Afterward the clinician asks open-ended questions (e.g., "what are you aware of now?"). If the response reflects change or movement, the therapist will typically initiate further BLS sets with the client's free associations until no further change in self-report or desensitization occurs (e.g., a SUDS of 0–1). If processing seems to be blocked, the therapist will use a variety of brief interventions, such as a change in direction of EM, directing attention to a specific aspect of the trauma experience, or a brief cognitive therapy-type intervention, as the content of awareness as the next set of BLS begins.

Phase V: Installation

After desensitization–reprocessing appears complete, in Phase V the new adaptive PCs associated with the target memory are paired with BLS sets until a VoC of 6–7 is achieved. Client progress is clinically assessed in light of the initially established cognitive goal, and reprocessing is extended if it was not completed previously. It should be noted that the target SUDS and VoC numbers are only guidelines and that other clinical indicators of progress are also employed.

Phase VI: Body Scan

In Phase VI, the client focuses on the target memory and scans his or her body for negative physical sensations that, if present, are processed with BLS sets until absent. In this phase the progress apparently made in the desensitization phase is checked for aspects of the traumatic memory that were not fully processed. These aspects are often associated with memories linked with a particular body sensation and perhaps not significantly different from the experience of phantom limb syndrome among amputees (e.g., Russell, 2008b).

Phase VII: Closure

Activity in Phase VII is determined by several factors, especially whether or not reprocessing appears complete. When it appears that processing will be incomplete, the therapist in debriefing the client before the end of session may utilize relaxation techniques to "seal over" disturbing material that may have surfaced and prepare the client for possible after-effects. When processing appears complete, there can be more extensive therapeutic discussion.

Phase VIII: Reevaluation

In Phase VIII clinician reevaluates status of target memory at the beginning of the next session and follow-up. If all past memories are processed, the clinician can proceed to present triggers, then future template (if practical).

Research on EMDR with Civilian Populations

The research previously noted that involves EMDR treatment of civilians establishes EMDR as a possible frontline treatment for PTSD. Meta-analyses of RCTs with head-to-head comparisons between EMDR and trauma-focused cognitive-behavioral therapy (CBT) found both to be comparably effective (Bisson & Andrew, 2007), with EMDR effects reported as more rapid and efficient as it does not require extensive homework (Seidler & Wagner, 2006). In addition, a blind RCT sponsored by the National Institute of Mental Health (NIMH) compared EMDR with placebo and Prozac in treating adults with childhood-onset PTSD and adult-onset PTSD, finding EMDR superior to both other conditions (van der Kolk et al., 2007). Other notable civilian research of relevance to the military includes at least five neuroimaging EMDR treatment case studies revealing functional pre- and posttreatment brain changes, coinciding with self-reported symptom improvement (see Russell, 2008a).

Since the comparisons of EMDR with other methods have now established its general effectiveness, other research questions become worth considering, for example, the role of EM or a substitute activity in EMDR. Although clinical dismantling studies have not had the power to definitively address this issue, analogue research, even by critics of EMDR, has found that EM reduces the intensity of visual images and emotion related to memories with a strong emotional component (see Maxfield, Melny, & Hayman, 2008).

On the subject of methodology, in one of the few reviews of PTSD treatment that has not shown evidence for EMDR, the Institute of Medicine (IOM, 2007), while failing to accurately read the outcome data on some of the EMDR studies being reviewed (Lee & Schubert, 2009), also criticized the research on all methods as being potentially tainted by allegiance effects. Contrary to the IOM statement, three strong studies supporting the value of EMDR have been conducted by principal investigators who were allied with other methods of treatment (Carlson, Chemtob, Rusnak, Hedlund, & Muraoka, 1998; Rothbaum, Astin, & Marsteller, 2006; Rothbaum, 1997).

The controversy around EMDR has extended beyond just the reading of studies. Corrigan (2001), in criticizing recently developed methods of treatment, including EMDR, acceptance and commitment therapy (ACT), and dialectical behavior therapy (DBT), for "getting ahead of the data," posits that there is not enough research to support their promotion.

Research on EMDR with Military Populations

A review of DoD and DVA research on EMDR revealed that, despite its being designated as an EBT by DVA/DoD (2004) and despite pressing mental health needs, inexplicably no EMDR RCTs have been conducted in DoD nor within DVA since the beginning of Operation Iraqi Freedom and Operation Enduring Freedom (Russell & Friedberg, 2009). Prior to 2000, EMDR RCTs by DVA with Vietnam War vets were inconclusive, ranging from minimal (i.e., Boudewyns, Stwertka, Hyer, Albrecht, & Sperr, 1993) to significant (Carlson, Chemtob, Rusnak, Hedlund, & Muraoka, 1998) benefit.

Carlson et al. (1998) found that 77% of 35 combat veterans no longer met criteria for PTSD, with results maintained at 9-month follow-up as a result of demonstrating adequate treatment fidelity periods targeting multiple memories. In addition, a small nonrandomized study of multiple memories of combat veterans with chronic combat PTSD found EMDR to be superior to biofeedback and relaxation training on seven of eight measures (Silver, Brooks, & Obenchain, 1995).

Military clinicians have published small and large EMDR case studies with active-duty patients treated in an array of actual clinical and operational/deployed settings, deemed essential to establish external validity of EBT. Subsequently, EMDR's potential effectiveness has been demonstrated at a U.S. Navy field hospital at which four Iraqi War medical evacuees were successfully treated for acute stress disorder (ASD) or acute PTSD (Russell, 2006), and a U.K. soldier with acute stress reaction was treated at a field mental health unit with sustained improvement at 18 months (Wesson & Gould, 2009). In addition, single-case studies of EMDR treatment in military outpatient clinics involving phantom-limb pain from traumatic amputation (Russell, 2008b), combat-related medically unexplained conditions (Russell, 2008c; Silver, Rogers, & Russell, 2008), and inpatient treatment of non-combat PTSD with 40 German soldiers (Zimmermann, Biesold, Barre, & Lanczik, 2007) were all positive, signifying EMDR's utility "in the trenches." Furthermore, a grassroots joint DoD/VA EMDR training program monitored training efficacy by nonrandomized archival chart review of 63 military outpatient treatment cases, including 48 with combat PTSD, submitted by nine military therapists and reported significant symptom reduction on average of four EMDR sessions (eight if wounded in action; Russell, Silver, Rogers, & Darnell, 2007).

Treatment of postmilitary combat trauma in veterans has ranged from significantly effective to minimally beneficial. The most notable study has been an RCT comparing EMDR with biofeedback and routine clinical care in 35 veterans (Carlson et al., 1998). The authors concluded, "Compared to the other conditions, significant treatment effects were obtained at posttreatment on a number of self-report, psychometric and standardized treatment measures. Relative to other treatment groups, these effects were generally maintained at 3-month follow-up" (p. 3). At the other end of the range, in a study of veterans designed to clarify the role of eye movement, Pitman et al. (1996) found minimal treatment effects that were not sustained (Macklin et al., 2000), echoing previous results of minimal effects in this treatment team's findings on "imaginal flooding" (Pitman et al., 1996). Although a direct comparison of the studies is not possible, it can be noted that Pitman et al. (1991) reported the presence of "under-recognized complications occurring during flooding therapy for post-traumatic stress disorder " (p. 17) in 6 of the first 20 subjects treated. No such problems were reported in the EMDR study. These and other RCTs with combat veterans are reviewed by Maxfield and Hyer (2002).

Strengths of EMDR with Military Personnel

In regard to psychotherapies with military personnel, a premium is placed on practicality, flexibility, efficiency, rapidity, and effectiveness within a believable therapeutic framework that is respectful of warrior culture and ethos. To that end, EMDR therapy appears uniquely suited.

Practicality

Unlike CBT, the effectiveness of EMDR is not dependent on clients' compliance with 40–60 hours of daily or weekly homework assignments (e.g., listening to exposure sessions) in the privacy of their homes, luxuries that military personnel residing in crowded barracks, tents, or ships do not enjoy. Competing military demands can also interfere with homework compliance. Generally speaking, extensive homework requirements are often impractical in the military, a problem EMDR avoids altogether, except for, perhaps, noting issues that the client would like to bring up at a next meeting.

Additionally, EMDR does not require expensive computerized equipment or virtual reality software, nor mass reproduction or purchase of workbooks, homework sheets, and daily self-rating forms, which may be inaccessible during deployment. The DVA/DoD (2004) PTSD guidelines cite EMDR's potential for rapid therapeutic gains in fewer sessions than conventional talk therapies, a critical factor for time-sensitive dispositions. Generalization of EMDR treatment effects with heterogeneous, complicated, and comorbid presentations, delivered by actual military clinicians "in the trenches" (i.e., Russell, 2006), is another important consideration.

Flexibility

Whether at frontline combat-stress clinics (Wesson & Gould, 2009), field evacuation hospitals (Russell, 2006), military outpatient clinics (Silver et al., 2008; Russell, 2008b, 2008c; Russell, Silver, & Rogers, 2007), or military inpatient hospitals (Zimmerman et al., 2007), EMDR has been demonstrated to be a low-cost, low-tech, and highly adaptable therapeutic tool. Material requirements are a secluded area with a therapist capable of generating back-and-forth hand movements.

Another aspect of EMDR's unique flexibility is its application of exposure. In typical EMDR desensitization sessions, patients are instructed to "just be aware of" their free associations and the BLS. Unlike in prolonged exposure, EMDR clinicians avoid redirecting the client's attention repetitively to the initially targeted traumatic memory and actively encourage free associations, tantamount to positively reinforcing escape behaviors. However, EMDR's client-centered approach sets it apart from directive CBT methods, an approach that is likely responsible for the DVA/DoD's (2004) conclusion that "EMDR may be more easily tolerated for patients who have difficulties engaging in prolonged exposure therapy" (p. 2)—thereby providing military clinicians and patients an invaluable alternative to exposure-based therapies.

Efficiency

Comprehensive treatment of war trauma goes beyond PTSD diagnosis, including diverse DSM diagnoses (e.g., depression), and/or medically unexplained conditions (MUC), sometimes referred to as "war syndromes" (e.g., chronic pain). In addition, high rates of PTSD and comorbidity (e.g., mood disorder) are prevalent in wounded service members. A multitude of CBT packages have been developed to specifically target individual DSM and MUC diagnoses. That said, reports of using EMDR to "simultaneously" treat military patients (including those wounded in action and diagnosed with ASD/PTSD and depression; i.e., Russell et al., 2007)—that is, a Marine with PTSD, depression, and phantom limb pain (Russell, 2008b); a soldier with PTSD, depression, and suicidal ideation (Silver et al., 2008); and a Marine with PTSD and atypical cardiac pain (Russell, 2008c)—illustrate its comprehensive capacity. These findings are consistent with civilian studies that have shown significant decreases in depression scale scores when PTSD subjects were treated with EMDR (e.g., Rothbaum, 1997). Moreover, published accounts of EMDR's effectiveness as an acute trauma intervention both within (i.e., Wesson & Gould, 2009) and outside (i.e., Shapiro, 2009) military circles, further suggests therapeutic efficiency.

Last, a high prevalence of childhood traumatic events and military sexual trauma has been reported in PTSD research with veterans, implicating early trauma exposure as a risk factor for adult PTSD. In terms of efficiency, EMDR has been identified as an EBT for childhood trauma and sexual assault, supported by an RCT comparison with Prozac (van der Kolk et al., 2007). As opposed to making already overstretched clinicians learn multiple CBT protocols to effectively treat common comorbidities found in traumatized patients—whether acute or chronic, early childhood or adult onset—EMDR presents a single, modifiable platform delivering comprehensive treatment.

Rapidity

In a highly mobile, time-sensitive, and often restrictive treatment environment such as the military, there is an inherent need for brief interventions that produce rapid, enduring outcomes. As noted in the DVA/DoD guidelines (2004, p. 127), "the possibility of obtaining significant clinical improvements in PTSD in a few sessions presents this treatment [EMDR] method as an attractive modality worthy of consideration." Military reports of significant symptom improvement after a single EMDR session (Russell, 2006), four consecutive sessions (Wesson & Gould, 2009), and an average of four sessions (eight if wounded in action) in 63 military patients, including 48 with combat PTSD (Russell et al., 2007), are noteworthy. Moreover, experiencing tolerable, rapid symptom relief in a single or a few sessions can foster treatment confidence and prevent premature termination.

Credible Therapeutic Frame

EMDR theory lends itself to scientifically framed, credible explanations, including the role of hemispheric lateralization, neural networks, REM sleep, and emotional processing in PTSD, explanations tacitly supported by EMDR neuroimaging studies, that can shape client expectations that EMDR will be different from talk therapy. Furthermore, the clinician's belief in treatment efficacy can also influence outcome. Seventy-four percent of a DVA-sponsored survey of EMDR-trained clinicians reported EMDR as having more beneficial treatment effects than other methods, whereas only 4% indicated less benefit (Lipke, 1995). A recent RCT examined 255 trauma experts about their preferences for exposure therapy for nonmilitary PTSD patients and found that clinicians rated EMDR as significantly more credible than supportive counseling or exposure therapy that was rarely used in actual clinical settings, especially with multiple or childhood traumas (van Minnen, Hendriks, & Olff, 2010).

Culturally Sensitive to Warrior Ethos

Unlike CBT or prolonged-exposure (PE) approaches, EMDR does not compel repetitive, detailed, and often painful retelling of traumatic experiences to be effective. Nor does EMDR require disputing irrational cognitions, frequently challenging dysfunctional beliefs, or intrusive sharing of undesirable, guilt-laden, embarrassing, or shameful self-disclosures. Thus EMDR offers a unique advantage when working with military populations, as reiterated by the DVA/DoD (2004) guidelines that "EMDR processing is internal to the patient, who does not have to reveal the traumatic event" (p. 1). At the outset, EMDR clients are informed that they are in control of the process, including the amount of exposure, when to stop, and how much or how little they choose to disclose. Explicitly assigning locus of control to clients may serve to enhance trust and rapport. Just as important, it may reduce the common fears associated with mental health care that are prevalent in military culture and run counter to the warrior ethos. These involve sanctions against self-revelation, displaying weakness and admitting vulnerability, as well as the fear of risking short- or long-term loss of emotional control, all of which may interfere with one's ability to function or stay in the military.

Respecting client versus therapist control over the therapeutic process to the degree seen in EMDR is also in keeping with traditional military expectations of senior enlisted and officers.

Limitations of EMDR with Military Personnel

Several potential limitations of EMDR therapy exist with military populations. These include their feelings about the treatment's credibility (e.g., therapist's hand movements); premature termination or dropout; barriers to care and stigma regarding mental health treatment; frequent missed sessions due to military duties; unwillingness to self-disclose even to the modest degree EMDR requires; survivor guilt response, in which some individuals may feel unjustified in seeking relief; guilt over having killed nonenemy combatants, either accidentally (i.e., friendly fire) or intentionally (i.e., fog of war); ambivalence toward treatment and/or return to duty; traumatic grief and fear of losing the memory of fallen friends; and/or secondary gain (i.e., escaping military duty, pursuing VA disability). Of course, none of the above limitations is unique to EMDR, and clinicians should anticipate and be proactive and open to dealing with such issues as they arise. In the case of EMDR, the military patient's ambivalence, beliefs that he or she deserves to suffer, and so forth, can be proactively solicited by the clinician and become the focus of EMDR before trauma work (Lipke, 2000; Silver & Rogers, 2001).

With regard to specific EMDR limitations, military patients with seizures or complicated pregnancies, and those acutely suicidal, actively psychotic, or intoxicated, may not be suited for EMDR until appropriate safety and mental status concerns are cleared. Moreover, although no two clients are identical in their responses to EMDR, changes in perceptual detail, cognitions, and emotional response to traumatic experiences is common (Shapiro, 2001). Therefore, clinicians should be wary of using EMDR in courts-martial cases without prior consultation with the Judge Advocate General if preservation of unaltered, vivid recollections of witnesses is essential.

In addition, military patients may be averse to the possibility of recalling certain premilitary or other military-related distressing or traumatic experiences. Thus appropriate informed consent stating that the patient understands that EMDR effects may generalize beyond the present incident must be obtained (Shapiro, 2001). Similarly, service members (and their treating clinicians) experiencing acute stress reactions within operational/deployed settings may find EMDR's potential to process memories beyond the immediate precipitant to be counterproductive of goals aimed at rapid symptom stabilization, reduction, and return to duty. However, military clinicians have demonstrated effective EMDR modifications in operational/deployed settings (i.e., Wesson & Gould, 2009) by redirecting the client's focused attention to the current incident, instead of freely associating to other memories.

Therapeutic Considerations

In 1995, the EMDR International Association (EMDRIA), an independent professional association, emerged as the authoritative voice for EMDR training standards and now accepts applications from prospective EMDR trainers. EMDRIA training standards include 20 hours of didactic work, 20 hours of supervised practicum, and 10 hours of consultation. Separate training criteria exists for certified EMDR therapists, consultants, facilitators, and trainers (www.emdria.org). However, the expansion of empirically untested EMDR training requirements and accretion of requirements to establish and maintain levels of status within EMDRIA can fuel speculations of proprietary intentions that reinforces resistance by mainstream academia and researchers (i.e., Russell, 2008a).

Nonetheless, while empirical validation of EMDRIA training standards (as well as all psychotherapy approaches) is pending, at least one requirement appears essential: the need for supervised practice (Lipke, 1995). Unique aspects of EMDR are difficult to learn from a journal article or treatment manual, regardless of clinical expertise. For instance, nuances of target memory assessment, when to start and stop EM, dealing with processing difficulties, and adherence to EMDR's client-centered, free-associative approach may appear exceptionally simple ("just have the patient imagine the trauma and track back-and-forth hand movements with their eyes"), but novices often discover EMDR to be more challenging to learn and to run counterintuitively to prior clinical training.

Case Vignette

A 29-year-old married Asian American male Navy Corpsman Petty Officer (E-5) with 8 years' continuous active-duty service was referred to a Navy mental health clinic by his senior chief for uncharacteristic anger outbursts, social withdrawal, apathy, and decrease in work performance since returning from deployment to Iraq over 8 months ago. The primary target memory was his role as first responder to a suicide bombing of a dining facility.

The following dialogue is taken from the "desensitization" phase of his first EMDR session. The letters "EM" indicate when eye movements have been initiated.

Near the beginning of this phase the client describes this content of his awareness: "I'm looking at all the bodies and body parts all over the place ... it's hard to see because of the smoke, but I can see some people crawling on the floor, and hear them yelling for me to help them ... but there's just too many...." (stops talking, staring ahead and eyes tearing up). As the session unfolded he expressed considerable anger, and then came the following exchange:

PETTY OFFICER: I was just thinking that all the deaths did not have to happen that day ... if I hadn't froze .. maybe the Gunny or others would have lived?

THERAPIST: Think of that [EM] ... what do you notice?

PETTY OFFICER: But there were so many people, so many bodies, I don't know what anyone could do?

THERAPIST: Stay with that [EM] ... what do you get now?

PETTY OFFICER: The whole thing was a nightmare, even one of our best docs, Doc B, was overwhelmed, I saw him breaking down outside

THERAPIST: Notice that [EM].... What are you aware of now?

[Much information required to fully consider this client's situation is omitted because of space limitations (based on actual treatment case after altering personal identifiers).]

PETTY OFFICER: Hmmm.... I guess we all did the best we could ... it was so freakin' chaotic.

THERAPIST: Think of that [EM] ... what do you notice now?

PETTY OFFICER: I don't know what I would or could have done differently, but I can't stop thinking that maybe there was some way to save Gunny.

[It appears that the client's processing might be stuck, so the therapist gently reminds the client of information that might be useful, then allows the process to unfold.]

THERAPIST: Earlier, you described being surprised that he survived as long as he did given the nature of his wounds?

PETTY OFFICER: Yeah, ... that's true

THERAPIST: Stay with that [EM].... What are you aware of now?

PETTY OFFICER: Yeah ... that's what Doc B told me, too.

THERAPIST: By the way, do you know whether any of the people you helped that day survived?

PETTY OFFICER: (*pause*) ... I haven't ever thought about that ... but when you asked me ... I remember, I think it was Doc B telling me a few days later ... that a couple of the Marines I had worked on, did survive ... in fact, he even told me that I had saved their lives ... that's weird ... I completely blocked that out....

THERAPIST: Okay, well just stay with that [EM] ... what do you get now?

PETTY OFFICER: Huh, that was really cool when Doc told me that.

THERAPIST: Stay with that [EM].... What do you notice now?

PETTY OFFICER: Hmmm ... I still feel bad that Gunny did not survive, but that wasn't something that I could control, it does feel good to know that I at least was able to help others.

THERAPIST: Good, focus on that [EM] ... what do you get now?

PETTY OFFICER: I don't know, I guess I did the best I could under the circumstances.

THERAPIST: Stay with that [EM] ... what are you aware of now?

PETTY OFFICER: Nothing, really, it's something that I'll never forget.

THERAPIST: All right, let's go back to the initial tent bombing memory we started with, bring up the picture and thoughts "I can't handle this." Do you got it?

PETTY OFFICER: Yes.

THERAPIST: What do you notice right now?

PETTY OFFICER: Huh ... I can still see the scene, but the picture seems to be faded some, it's not as overwhelming now ... when I think about it now ... it's still an ugly picture, the fact that so many people were killed ... it's not something I'll ever forget ... but I don't feel as tense ... or overwhelmed now.

THERAPIST: Using that scale of 0 to 10, 0 meaning completely relaxed, not upset at all, and 10, the most upset you've ever been, how would you rate how you feel right now when you bring up the mess tent memory?

PETTY OFFICER: Hmmm ... maybe a 3 or 2½ ... I don't know....

The session continued and was wrapped up with consolidation of these gains and preparation for the rest of the day and the next session.

References

American Psychiatric Association. (2004). *Practice guidelines for the treatment of patients with acute stress disorder and posttraumatic stress disorder.* Arlington, VA: Author.

Bisson, J., & Andrew, M. (2007). Psychological treatment of posttraumatic stress disorder (PTSD). *Cochrane Database of Systematic Reviews, 3* (Article No. CD003388).

Boudewyns, P. A., Stwertka, S. A., Hyer, L. A., Albrecht, J. W., & Sperr, E. V. (1993). Eye movement desensitization and reprocessing: A pilot study. *Behavior Therapist, 16,* 30–33

Carlson, J. G., Chemtob, C. M., Rusnak, K., Hedlund, N. L., & Muraoka, M. Y. (1998). Eye movement desensitization and reprocessing for combat-related posttraumatic stress disorder. *Journal of Traumatic Stress, 11,* 3–24.

Corrigan, P. W. (2001) Getting ahead of the data: A threat to some behavior therapies. *Behavior Therapist, 24,* 189–193.

Department of Veterans Affairs and Department of Defense. (2004). *VA/DoD clinical practice guideline for the management of post-traumatic stress.* Washington, DC: Department of Defense, Department of Veterans Affairs and Health Affairs, Veterans Health Administration (Office of Quality and Performance Publication No. 10Q-CPG/PTSD-04).

Foa, E. B., Keane, T. M., Friedman, M. J., & Cohen, J. A. (2009). *Effective treatments for PTSD: Practice guidelines of the International Society for Traumatic Stress Studies.* New York: Guilford Press.

Horowitz, M. (1976). *Stress response syndromes.* New York: Aronson.

Institute of Medicine. (2007). *Treatment of posttraumatic stress disorder: An assessment of the evidence.* Washington, DC: National Academies Press.

Lee, C. W., & Schubert, S. (2009). Omissions and errors in the Institute of Medicine's Report on Scientific Evidence of treatment for posttraumatic stress disorder. *Journal of EMDR Practice and Research, 3,* 32–38.

Lipke, H. (2000). *EMDR and psychotherapy integration.* Boca Raton, FL: CRC Press.

Lipke, H. J. (1995). EMDR clinicians survey In F. Shapiro (Ed.), *Eye movement desensitization and reprocessing (EMDR): Basic principles, protocols and procedures.* New York: Guilford Press.

Lipke, H. J., & Botkin, A. (1992). Case studies of eye movement desensitization and reprocessing (EMDR) with chronic posttraumatic stress disorder. *Psychotherapy, 29,* 591–595.

Macklin, M. L., Metzger, L. J., Lsako, N. B., Berry, N. J., Orr, S. P., & Pitman, R. K. (2000). Five-year follow-up study of eye movement desensitization and reprocessing therapy for combat-related posttraumatic stress disorder. *Comprehensive Psychiatry, 41,* 24–27.

Marquis, J. N. (1991). A report on seventy-eight cases treated by eye movement desensitization. *Journal of Behavior Therapy and Experimental Psychiatry, 22,* 187–192.

Maxfield, L., & Hyer, L. (2002). The relationship between efficacy and methodology in studies investigating EMDR treatment of PTSD. *Journal of Clinical Psychology, 58,* 23–42.

Maxfield, L., Melnyk, W. T., & Hayman, C. A. G. (2008). A working memory explanation for the effects of eye movement in EMDR. *Journal of EMDR Practice and Research, 2,* 247–268.

Pitman, R. K., Orr, S. P., Altman, B., Greenwald, E., Longpre, R., Poiré, R. E., et al. (1991). Psychiatric complications during flooding therapy for posttraumatic stress disorder. *Journal of Clinical Psychiatry, 52,* 17–20.

Pitman, R. K., Orr, S. P., Altman, B., Longpre, R., Poiré, R. E., & Macklin, M. L. (1996). Emotional processing during eye movement desensitization and reprocessing therapy of Vietnam veterans with chronic posttraumatic stress disorder. *Comprehensive Psychiatry, 37,* 419–429.

Rothbaum, B., Astin, M., & Marsteller, F. (2006). Prolonged exposure versus eye movement desensitization and reprocessing (EMDR) for PTSD rape victims. *Journal of Traumatic Stress, 18,* 607–616.

Rothbaum, B. O. (1997). A controlled study of eye movement desensitization and reprocessing in the treatment of posttraumatic stress disordered victims. *Bulletin of the Menninger Clinic, 61,* 317–334.

Russell, M. C. (2006). Treating combat-related stress disorders: A multiple case study utilizing eye movement desensitization and reprocessing (EMDR) with battlefield casualties from the Iraqi war. *Military Psychology, 18,* 1–18.

Russell, M. C. (2008a). Scientific resistance to research, training, and utilization of EMDR therapy in treating post-war disorders. *Social Science and Medicine, 67*(11), 1737–1746.

Russell, M. C. (2008b). Treating traumatic amputation-related phantom limb pain: A case study utilizing eye movement desensitization and reprocessing (EMDR) within the Armed Services. *Clinical Case Studies, 7,* 136–153.

Russell, M. C. (2008c). War-related medically unexplained symptoms, prevalence and treatment: Utilizing EMDR within the armed services. *Journal of EMDR Practice and Research, 2*(2), 212–225.

Russell, M. C., & Friedberg, F. (2009). Training, treatment access and research on trauma intervention in the armed services. *Journal of EMDR Practice and Research, 3,* 24–31.

Russell, M. C., Silver, S. M., Rogers, S., & Darnell, J. N. (2007). Responding to an identified need: A joint DoD-DVA training program in EMDR for clinicians providing trauma services. *International Journal of Stress Management, 14*(1), 61–71.

Seidler, G. H., & Wagner, F. E. (2006). Comparing the efficacy of EMDR and trauma-focused cognitive-behavioral therapy in the treatment of PTSD: A meta-analytic study. *Psychological Medicine, 36*(11), 1515–1522.

Shapiro, E. (2009). EMDR treatment of recent trauma. *Journal of EMDR Practice and Research, 3*(3), 141–151.

Shapiro, F. (1989). Efficacy of the eye movement desensitization procedure in the treatment of traumatic memories. *Journal of Traumatic Stress, 2,* 199–223.

Shapiro, F. (2001). *Eye movement desensitization and reprocessing (EMDR): Basic principles, protocols, and procedures* (2nd ed.). New York: Guilford Press.

Silver, S., & Rogers, S. (2001). *Light in the heart of darkness: EMDR and the treatment of war and terrorism survivors.* New York: Norton.

Silver, S. M., Brooks, A., & Obenchain, J. (1995). Treatment of Vietnam War veterans with PTSD: A comparison of eye movement desensitization and reprocessing, biofeedback, and relaxation training. *Journal of Traumatic Stress, 8,* 337–342.

Silver, S. M., Rogers, S., & Russell, M. (2008). Eye movement desensitization and reprocessing (EMDR) in the treatment of war veterans. *Journal of Clinical Psychology: In Session, 64*(8), 947–957.

van der Kolk, B. A., Spinazzola, J., Blaustein, M. E., Hopper, J. W., Hopper, E. K., Korn D. L., et al. (2007). A randomized clinical trial of eye movement desensitization and reprocessing (EMDR), fluoxetine, and pill placebo in the treatment of posttraumatic stress disorder: Treatment effects and long-term maintenance. *Journal of Clinical Psychiatry, 68*(1), 37–46.

van Minnen, A., Hendriks, L., & Olff, M. (2010). When do trauma experts choose exposure therapy for PTSD patients?: A controlled study of therapist and patient factors. *Behavioral Research and Therapy, 48*(4), 312–320.

Wesson, M., & Gould, M. (2009). Intervening early with EMDR on military operations. *Journal of EMDR Practice and Research, 3*(2), 91–97.

Zimmerman, P., Biesold, K. H., Barre, K., & Lanczik, M. (2007). Long-term course of posttraumatic stress disorder (PTSD) in German soldiers: Effects of inpatient eye movement desensitization and reprocessing therapy and specific trauma characteristics in patients with non-combat-related PTSD. *Military Medicine, 172*(5), 456–460.

CHAPTER 6

Virtual Reality Exposure Therapy

Greg M. Reger
Kevin M. Holloway

Innovative approaches to treatment are receiving increased attention because of the growing number of service members and veterans with posttraumatic stress disorder (PTSD). In the general population, lifetime prevalence rates of PTSD are 10.4% for women and 5% for men (Kessler, Sonnega, Bromet, Hughes, & Nelson, 1995). However, individuals exposed to combat are at increased risk. Estimates of lifetime prevalence of PTSD for Vietnam veterans are 26.9% and 30.9% for female and male veterans, respectively (Kulka et al., 1988). When these data were reanalyzed with a conservative correction to require functional impairment and documentation of exposure to combat-related trauma, the lifetime prevalence rate of PTSD for Vietnam veterans was 18.7% (Dohrenwend et al., 2006).

Recent studies confirm that veterans of the current combat operations in Iraq and Afghanistan are also at increased risk. Hoge et al. (2004) conducted cross-sectional research involving an anonymous survey to U.S. service members before and after deployments to Iraq and Afghanistan. Results suggested that service members deployed to Iraq screened positive for PTSD at rates of 18 to 19.9%. Of those deployed to Afghanistan, 11.5% screened positive for PTSD. An analysis of responses to the Post-Deployment Health Assessment (PDHA) of soldiers and marines after deployment to Iraq and Afghanistan (Hoge, Auchterlonie, & Milliken, 2006) found that 9.8% of those deployed to Iraq and 4.7% of those deployed to Afghanistan screened positive for PTSD. A follow-up population-based study (Milliken, Auchter-lonie, & Hoge, 2007) screened soldiers approximately 6 months after returning from deployment to Iraq. Nearly 17% of those soldiers screened positive for PTSD. A recent large study of soldiers 12 months after deploy-ment (Thomas et al., 2010) found that 7.3% of active component and 11.3% of National Guard SMs met a strict screening definition of PTSD. Veterans also face similar difficulties. A large study of veterans of Opera-tion Iraqi Freedom (OIF) and Operation Enduring Freedom (OEF) (Seal, Bertenthal, Miner, Sen, & Marmar, 2007) found that 16% of veterans who sought treatment at Veterans Affairs (VA) facilities within a 4-year window met criteria for PTSD.

Overview of Virtual Reality Exposure Therapy

These studies underscore the need for effective treatments for combat-related PTSD. Exposure therapy is one effective treatment, and it presents the context within which virtual reality exposure therapy (VRE) is under-stood. Exposure therapy is a cognitive-behavioral therapy (CBT) based on behavioral and cognitive models of human learning. Mowrer's (1960) clas-sic two-factor theory is often used to explain the development and mainte-nance of PTSD. However, due to the limitations of this theory to adequately explain all of the symptoms observed in PTSD (Foa, Steketee, & Rothbaum, 1989; Foa & Hearst-Ikeda, 1996), emotional processing theory was pro-posed (Foa & Kozak, 1986). This theory modified the purely behavioral rationale of exposure therapy to incorporate information processing compo-nents. Specifically, PTSD is thought to be the continuation of a pathological fear structure, which consists of associations among stimuli (e.g., exploding vehicle), responses (e.g., racing heart), and the meaning (e.g., threat to one's life). This fear structure is broadly generalized so that it is accessed eas-ily. Behavioral and cognitive avoidance prevent the learning of information that would be inconsistent with this fear structure and thus prevents recov-ery. According to this model, recovery requires activating the fear structure (i.e., encountering stimuli represented in the fear structure) and learning new information that is disconfirming. The closer the match is between the stimuli encountered and those present in the fear structure, the greater is the activation of the memory (Foa, Huppert, & Cahill, 2006). Prolonged exposure therapy (PE; Foa, Hembree, & Rothbaum, 2007) is a manual-ized exposure therapy protocol grounded in emotional processing theory. Based on this theoretical rationale, patients in exposure therapy are asked to approach feared memories or anxiety-provoking situations, activities, places, or people for prolonged periods of time until anxiety decreases. The two most common forms of exposure are imaginal exposure, which requires the patient to repeatedly imagine or revisit the memory of the trauma, and *in vivo* exposure, which involves repeatedly confronting safe situations or objects that are anxiety provoking because they remind the individual of the trauma (Foa et al., 2007).

VRET Treatment Protocol

There are a few minor variants of VRE (Rothbaum, Difede, & Rizzo, 2008), but many of them are based on exposure therapy and often exposure therapy protocols (e.g., Foa et al., 2007). The major components of PE are often present in the VRE protocols, including psychoeducation regarding PTSD and trauma reactions, relaxation training usually in the form of breathing retraining, data collection, homework exercises, *in vivo* exposure, and imaginal exposure. The major difference between standard PE and VRE is that during the imaginal exposure segment of treatment, the client does not close his or her eyes to imagine the index trauma but rather experiences an immersive, interactive computer simulation of the index trauma while he or she tells the story of the event in as much detail as possible. The therapist manipulates various elements of the virtual environment to match as closely as possible the details of the event as they are told by the client.

The structure of VRE sessions typically consists of approximately eight to twelve 90-minute therapy sessions conducted once or twice a week. The first two sessions are generally psychoeducational in nature and include discussions of the rationale of exposure therapy, expectations for treatment, common reactions to trauma, and breathing retraining. Session 2 may include a brief orientation to the virtual reality equipment using a neutral virtual environment. The intent of this orientation is to familiarize the client with the use and function of the virtual reality equipment to be used during VRE beginning in session 3, but in an environment that is unlikely to activate distress (e.g., a city park, a professional office scene).

Session 3 begins with a review of homework followed by a review of the rationale for the use of virtual reality in exposure therapy. The client then dons the virtual reality equipment and is instructed to tell the story of his or her index trauma in the present tense, including as much detail as possible, repeating the story enough times to fill 40–45 minutes. While the client tells the story, the therapist attempts to match the details of the event as closely as possible by activating relevant stimuli in the virtual environment. This may include settings such as time of day, type of scenario (e.g., mounted versus dismounted), position in the vehicle (if relevant), presence of other service members, presence of civilians, and ambient noise. The therapist also activates events in real time to match the client's story, such as an improvised explosive device (IED) detonation, vehicle-borne IED detonation, weapons fire, incoming rocket-propelled grenades (RPGs), aircraft flyovers, smoke, or injuries to virtual characters. The therapist titrates the intensity of the stimuli activated in the virtual environment according to the client's response, keeping the intensity of sufficient strength to facilitate habituation and accommodation of corrective information. Following VRE, the client and therapist engage in processing the experience, which may include highlighting the experience of habituation during exposure, reinforcing the courage to complete the exposure, identifying unhelpful interpretations of events or views of oneself, generating alternative ways to understand the event, identifying emotions and cognitions related to the exposure, and processing unrealistic guilt or responsibility taking. Homework includes continued *in vivo* exposure exercises and daily listening to an audio recording of the VRE session.

Sessions 4 through the end of treatment continue as session 3, with minor alterations. The rationale for VRE is reviewed as needed throughout treatment, though it may not be discussed explicitly at each session. Consistent with other exposure therapy protocols, the focus of VRE shifts in session 5 or 6 to "hot spots," which are segments of the overall index trauma that are especially distressing to the client. Throughout therapy, the therapist's role is to support and encourage the client to fully engage in therapeutic exposure, which is often difficult and distressing, reminding him or her of the rationale for exposure, and celebrating all successes, including minor approximations of success. VRE also requires that the therapist be actively engaged in the VRE process, matching the virtual environment to the client's descriptions and titrating the intensity of exposure.

Virtual Reality Equipment

The most common hardware configurations for VRE include a computer running a virtual Iraq or Afghanistan simulation, often using a head-mounted display (HMD) with head orientation tracking to present the visual components of the simulation. Headphones provide the audio components, and a game controller allows for client-controlled navigation. The use of an HMD with head tracking is thought to increase the psychological sense of participating in the virtual environment as compared with a flat panel computer monitor, though use of flat panel monitors may achieve adequate "presence" for some clients. Presence may be enhanced by including other peripherals. For example, some virtual reality systems include a "rumble platform," a raised platform to which bass-shaker speakers are attached, which respond to low-frequency sound effects by vibrating beneath the client. Some systems incorporate a scent machine, which releases relevant premanufactured scents into the therapy room. Each hardware component aims to help activate the trauma memory through the presentation of stimuli relevant to the index trauma.

Research on VRE with Civilian Populations

VRE has been used to treat fear of heights, public speaking, spiders, fly-ing, and close spaces since the early 1990s (Parsons & Rizzo, 2008). More recently it has been applied to the treatment of PTSD. Existing research pro-vides initial support for this emerging tool in exposure therapy. However, clinical research to date has included small samples and methodologically limited designs. Additional quality research is needed.

A small study explored the effectiveness of VRE in treating a case series of six patients with PTSD or subsyndromal PTSD from motor vehicle accidents (Beck, Palyo, Winer, Schwagler, & Ang, 2007). Participants were treated with 10 sessions of VRE using a 3D driving simulator. Statistically and clinically significant reductions in PTSD symptoms were found post-treatment relative to the pretreatment baseline. There were no significant reductions in self-reported depression or general anxiety.

Research has also explored the effectiveness of a virtual environment in treating survivors of 9/11. The first report was a case study of PTSD that resulted from the attack on the World Trade Center (Difede & Hoff-man, 2002). A positive treatment outcome was reported using VRE with a patient who had failed to improve with traditional exposure therapy. A quasi-experimental wait-list controlled study followed, which used the same World Trade Center virtual reality application (Difede et al., 2007). Ten virtual reality participants received 6–13 VRE sessions. Results indicated statistically and clinically significant decreases on the Clinician-Adminis-tered PTSD Scale (CAPS). These changes were significant relative both to pretreatment symptoms and to the 8 wait-list control participants. Five of the 10 virtual reality patients were treated with imaginal exposure therapy prior to the study, with limited benefit. These findings suggested promise for VRE, even for patients who had not improved from other evidence-based treatments.

A case report presented the effective treatment of a survivor of a ter-rorist bus attack in Israel using a virtual environment known as BusWorld (Freedman et al., 2010). The patient received 10 sessions of VRE, and treat-ment resulted in large reductions in PTSD and depression.

Research on VRE with Military Populations

The first applications of VRE to treat combat-related PTSD explored its potential as an exposure tool to treat Vietnam veterans. A case report described the treatment outcomes of VRE with a male veteran who was a former helicopter pilot in Vietnam (Rothbaum et al., 1999). He received 14 treatment sessions that used a Virtual Vietnam as part of the exposure therapy. His symptoms fell in the "severe" range at pretreatment but were in the "moderate" range at posttreatment. His improvements were maintained at 3 and 6 months posttreatment.

This pilot study was followed by a small open clinical trial (Rothbaum, Hodges, Ready, Graap, & Alarcon, 2001). In this study, nine veterans with PTSD completed an average of 13 exposure therapy sessions. Treatment included exposure to two virtual environments. One included a virtual jungle clearing with a range of combat-related stimuli such as gunfire, mines, and helicopters, and so forth. Stimuli could be customized in terms of intensity. The second environment was a virtual helicopter ride. Treatment resulted in an appreciable decrease in PTSD symptoms, which reached statistical significance at the 3-month and 6-month follow-ups.

The military operations associated with OIF and OEF have resulted in significant interest in the potential of VRE to address the growing treatment needs of this military population. At least three groups have built virtual Iraq or Afghanistan environments (Koffman & Wood, 2009; Miyahira, Folen, Hoffman, & Garcia-Palacios, 2009; Rizzo, Reger, Gahm, Difede, & Rothbaum, 2009), and VRE has also been used clinically in the combat theater (McLay, McBrien, Wiederhold, & Wiederhold, 2010). Some early questions surrounded the willingness of service members to use virtual reality as part of their mental health treatment. A survey research study of 352 active-duty soldiers (Wilson, Onorati, Mishkind, Reger, & Gahm, 2008) found that 58% of the sample reported a willingness to use virtual reality as a part of mental health treatment. Of those reporting that they would not be willing to use traditional talk psychotherapy, 19% reported that they were neutral to very willing to receive virtual-reality-based mental health care.

Regarding initial evidence of effectiveness, two published case studies report positive treatment outcomes with veterans of OIF. One case report (Gerardi, Rothbaum, Ressler, & Heekin, 2008) used virtual reality exposure therapy with a 29-year-old National Guardsman who was treated approximately 6 months postdeployment. He received four treatment sessions over 4 weeks and reported clinically and statistically significant reductions in PTSD. Another case report of an active-duty soldier (Reger & Gahm, 2008) reported treatment outcomes following six sessions of VRE using a simulated tactical convoy. Results indicated a substantial reduction in PTSD symptoms posttreatment relative to baseline. Posttreatment self-reported symptoms for this patient were well below the recommended cut point for a positive screening for PTSD.

A recent study described the effectiveness of VRE for active-duty soldiers treated in a military behavioral health clinic (Reger et al., 2011). Patients included 24 active-duty soldiers who were treated with an average of seven treatment sessions. Relative to their pretreatment PTSD symptoms, soldiers reported a significant decrease at posttreatment. VRE resulted in clinically meaningful change for 62% of patients.

A number of studies of VRE for combat-related PTSD are currently under way. Much more will be known about the effectiveness of this exposure tool when these studies are complete. For example, we are aware of two ongoing open clinical trials. One that was conducted at the Naval Medical Center, San Diego, and Camp Pendleton is evaluating the effectiveness of VRE with veterans of OIF with PTSD. Preliminary results from 20 treatment completers found a statistically significant decrease in self-reported symptoms of PTSD and a 50% reduction in symptoms for 16 of 20 participants (Rizzo et al., 2009).

A second open clinical trial is being planned at the Baltimore VA. This study plans to study the effectiveness of VRE for PTSD among 15 OEF/OIF veterans. The study will also investigate the impact of VRE on experiential avoidance, barriers to care, and quality of life. Participants will be recruited from the Trauma Recovery and Returning Veterans Outreach and Education Programs at the Perry Point and Baltimore VA medical centers (E. Romero, personal communication, March 2, 2010).

An open clinical trial evaluating an anxiety management approach to using VR is being conducted by the Virtual Reality Medical Center (Koffman & Wood, 2009). This treatment protocol deviates significantly from traditional exposure therapy, as it does not require the patient to revisit a specific trauma during each exposure but aims to train anxiety management techniques (i.e., meditation) with rehearsal of these skills in virtual reality combat environments. This treatment protocol was supported by a published case study that reported mild but clinically meaningful reductions in PTSD symptoms after 10 sessions (Wood et al., 2007). There were no meaningful changes in posttreatment self-reported depression or general anxiety. A second case study using this protocol treated a 26-year-old active-duty Navy woman with PTSD (Wood et al., 2009). After 20 treatment sessions, substantial reductions in self-reported PTSD symptoms, depression, and anxiety were reported. In addition, preliminary results from the first 12 treatment completers of an open clinical trial suggested a mild but clinically meaningful reduction in self-reported PTSD symptoms and depression (Koffman & Wood, 2009).

More important, at least three randomized clinical trials (RCTs) are under way to evaluate the efficacy of VRE for treating service members with PTSD. Our organization, the National Center for Telehealth and Technology (T2), is collaborating with Madigan Army Medical Center in an RCT comparing PE with VRE with a wait-list control group. This clinical trial has randomized 81 patients to date but the study is blind and still ongoing. Accordingly, preliminary results are not available. In the second RCT at

Walter Reed Army Medical Center, preliminary results for the first four VR treatment completers suggested a mild but clinically meaningful reduction in PTSD symptoms for two of four patients (Roy, 2009). The third RCT is evaluating VR exposure relative to a minimal-attention control group at Tripler Army Medical Center (Miyahira et al., 2009). Preliminary results are not currently available.

Finally, an additional study is examining the combination of VRE with medications that may affect the learning that takes place during exposure. Preliminary results from the first 14 treatment completers of an Emory University study testing virtual reality-based exposure therapy combined with Xanax, d-cycloserine, or placebo found a mean drop in scores on the CAPS from a baseline of 83 to 60. Medication treatment groups remain blind, so these symptom reductions are best accounted for by the VRE (Rothbaum, 2008).

Strengths of VRE with Military Personnel

Within the cognitive-behavioral research literature on treating PTSD, exposure therapies, including PE, have received significant empirical support. Exposure therapy has been studied in randomized clinical trials for a wide range of trauma populations, including female sexual and nonsexual assault survivors (Resick, Nishith, Weaver, Astin, & Feuer, 2002; Foa et al., 1999; Foa et al., 2005), survivors of motor vehicle accidents (Maercker, Zollner, Menning, Rabe, & Karl, 2006), male Vietnam War veterans (Keane, Fairbank, Caddell, & Zimering, 1989), female Vietnam veterans (Schnurr et al., 2007) and mixed trauma groups (Marks, Lovell, Noshirvani, Livanou, & Thrasher, 1998). Based on this body of research, the Institute of Medicine (OM; 2008), the International Society for Traumatic Stress Studies Clinical Practice Guidelines (Foa, Keane, Friedman, & Cohen, 2009), and the VA/ DoD Clinical Practice Guideline Working Group (Department of Veterans Affairs and Department of Defense, 2004) unanimously recommend exposure therapy as an effective treatment for PTSD.

However, there are potential barriers to using exposure therapies with service members. First, treatment stigma may interfere with individuals' willingness to seek care. A study of 708 U.S. military service members returning from a peacekeeping mission in Bosnia (Britt, 2000) found that 61% agreed that admitting a psychological problem would harm their careers. Similarly, 45% agreed that admitting a psychological problem would cause their coworkers to spend less time around them. Admitting a psychological problem was associated with significantly greater perceived stigma than admitting a medical problem. Given the fears associated with admitting a psychological problem, it is possible that service members may be hesitant to engage in treatment that may put them at risk of having such problems identified. Indeed, previously deployed OIF/OEF service members reported significant treatment stigma, which was greatest among service members reporting the most difficulties (Hoge et al., 2004). Only 38 to 45% of those who screened positive for a mental health problem reported an interest in accessing care.

A second challenge in treating soldiers with PTSD is the difficulty in achieving the degree of emotional engagement required for effective exposure therapy. The activation of affect during exposure has been proposed to be related to treatment outcome for decades (Lang, 1977). Consistent with this finding, one study found that facial expressions of fear during the first PTSD exposure treatment session were related to greater reductions on treatment outcome measures (Foa, Riggs, Massie, & Yarczower, 1995). Furthermore, a second study found that a high level of emotional engagement, based on self-reported subjective units of distress, was key to positive treatment outcomes. Accordingly, the authors recommend that when problems with emotional engagement are observed during treatment, techniques to increase engagement should be employed (Jaycox, Foa, & Morral, 1998). For example, the PE treatment protocol (Foa et al., 2007) suggests that increased activation can be encouraged by asking for more details and emotion-producing stimuli.

Problems with emotional engagement may be of particular concern for military service members with combat-related trauma. A meta-analytic review of PTSD treatment studies (Bradley, Greene, Russ, Dutra, & Westen, 2005) found that patients with combat-related traumas benefited significantly less from PTSD treatments than did patients with other trauma types. One potential explanation is poor emotional engagement during exposure. Long, stressful combat deployments with multiple exposures to potentially traumatic events may result in adaptive emotional disengagement that assists soldiers in getting through a difficult deployment. Upon redeployment, however, this adaptive emotional disengagement may interfere with the activation of the trauma memory for PTSD patients during exposure therapy.

The stigma associated with traditional "talk therapies" and the challenges associated with emotional engagement suggests that new treatment approaches are needed to reduce stigma and facilitate emotional engagement during exposure therapy. VRE may present new tools for modulating emotional engagement during exposure and may provide a form of treatment that is more appealing to some service members than other types of psychotherapy. If correct, VRE may increase the willingness of some military personnel to seek care and provide a new clinical tool to improve treatment outcome.

Limitations of VRE with Military Personnel

Virtual reality therapies are still relatively new. Although it is assumed that VRE is effective because it is based heavily on the procedures and theoretical underpinnings of exposure protocols, there is still limited research supporting this treatment in a military population, especially among active-duty service members. The development of virtual environments for use in VRE can be a long, expensive process requiring a significant investment of time and resources. Despite a number of virtual environments available for use in VRE that are designed to cover the most commonly reported combat-related index traumas, not every index trauma can be represented in a virtual environment. It is likely that virtual environments need not be a perfect match to a client's index trauma to effectively augment imaginal exposure. However, perhaps the most potent limitation of VRE is the possibility that the introduction of extraneous stimuli in a virtual environment may dilute the effectiveness of VRE for some patients. This issue deserves more research in the future.

Because VRE requires the patient to don electronic hardware, patients with certain injuries may be unable to engage in VRE. For example, patients with head or neck injuries may experience discomfort wearing the HMD unit. Additionally, some patients may experience "cyber sickness," which McCauley and Sharkey (1992, as cited in Lawson, Graeber, Mead, and Muth, 2002) described as "the motion-sickness-like symptoms associated with [virtual environments]." Although many patients may experience some mild cyber sickness symptoms, such as dizziness, disorientation, nausea, and headache, while using VRE, approximately 5% of patients will experience these symptoms to such severity that they cannot tolerate prolonged use of virtual environments (Lawson et al., 2002). However, it is sometimes difficult to differentiate cyber sickness symptoms from physiological anxiety reactions common during exposure therapy.

Therapeutic Considerations

Many therapeutic considerations for VRE are similar to those related to other exposure therapies. For example, a strong commitment to exposure therapy theory and rationale is important to successfully implementing VRE. It is important that VRE, like other exposure therapies, be considered a tool to be used by a skilled, trained clinician, not as a self-help solution or a replacement for a qualified, trained therapist.

Most, if not all, exposure therapies for PTSD focus primarily on PTSD symptoms and their reduction and therefore should be used when PTSD symptoms are the primary clinical concern. Some PTSD patients may have complex clinical presentations that may include additional or related symptoms, such as severe risk of harm to self or others, that require direct attention and amelioration prior to the initiation of exposure therapy.

The technological aspects of VRE require therapists to be comfortable with the use of computer systems and to have some troubleshooting skills in case the computer systems malfunction mid-session. Additionally, therapists need to be able to effectively divide their attention between the patient's story, affect, and distress and the need to control the events in the virtual environment so that the simulation matches the patient's narration and is of appropriate intensity.

Not all therapists are cut out to be exposure therapists. Therapists need to make honest assessments of themselves regarding their ability to help their patients engage in uncomfortable and distressing experiences, to tolerate significant patient emoting, and to hear their patients' darkest experiences. However, exposure therapy can be very rewarding for therapists, as they often see significant improvements in patient symptoms and functioning in a relatively short time frame.

Case Vignette

Joe (not his actual name) was a 26-year-old Army sergeant with two prior deployments to Iraq. In the final month of his most recent deployment, he and a good friend were in the same vehicle during a combat patrol. About halfway through the mission, they switched positions, and Joe drove while his friend took the turret. Later that evening, they were driving down a quiet, narrow road when an IED struck their vehicle, which nearly turned over from the blast. Joe was shook up and shocked but uninjured. The personnel on site responded well, and security was quickly established. No enemy combatants were identified, and no one returned any fire. Joe was with his injured friend immediately, and he was horrified by the injuries he saw. Nonetheless, he was well trained, and he responded according to his training. Attempts to render first aid did not appear to be successful, and as the medical evacuation helicopter took off, Joe correctly feared that his friend was dead.

In the month that followed, Joe changed dramatically. He found a reason to avoid driving in theater for the remainder of the deployment. He couldn't seem to get any rest, and about three times a week he had terrifying nightmares of the IED blast or of his friend's horrifying injuries. Accordingly, he began to fear sleep, and he found himself playing video games during downtime, when he should have been sleeping. He was irritable with everyone, kept his conversations with his family very brief, and, except for his daughter, he felt very little concern for much of anything. Following his return home, he expected things would improve, but they did not. His previous interest in socializing was gone, and he and his wife had little to talk about. He found driving too uncomfortable, and he spent most of his time in his home. His wife took him to work most days, and he avoided any destination that required driving down narrow lanes or in congested traffic. The demands at work were minimal in the first month, but as things picked up, he had significant difficulty focusing on the task at hand. His thoughts frequently drifted off, and despite his best attempts not to think about the traumatic episode, his mind often went back to that horrible day in Iraq.

In VRE treatment, Joe responded well to the first two sessions. He was willing to help the therapist understand the event in which his friend died, and he actively engaged in a discussion of exposure therapy. Although he was not looking forward to facing his memory, he readily understood that uncomfortable things got easier with repetition; his military training had already taught him this. He tried the breathing retraining but confessed that he felt self-conscious and stated that he would not likely try it again. During the second session, Joe appeared happy to learn that he wasn't going crazy; he was relieved to hear that his reactions were common among combat-trauma survivors. He was not so sure that he wanted to tell the story at the next session, but his life was a self-described "wreck," and he was willing to try anything. He was interested in the VR equipment and seemed to get mild enjoyment out of trying the HMD and navigating around a computer-generated peaceful park. Joe also made a long list of things that he avoided because they reminded him of his friend's death. He returned for session 3 pleased to find that he had actually enjoyed one aspect of his *in vivo* home-work—a dinner with his wife at a very quiet restaurant.

During session 3, he tried to listen to a brief description of the rationale for using virtual reality in exposure, but he was distracted, as he was antici-pating having to recall his friend's death. When Joe put on the HMD, he worked with the therapist to find a stretch of road that most closely resem-bled the area where his friend was killed. During this first session of using virtual reality to revisit the memory, the therapist customized the scenario to match the environmental conditions of the memory without including the simulated combat. The therapist adjusted the time of day of the scenario and placed Joe in the virtual turret of the vehicle. Joe began to revisit the memory and told the therapist what happened in the first person, present tense. When he remembered the vehicle moving, Joe drove the vehicle in the virtual environment. The seat he sat on rumbled with the idle of the vehicle. When Joe reached the point of the story at which he traded roles with his friend, the clinician customized the scenario and put him in the driver's seat of the computer-generated vehicle. Joe cried as he described the events lead-ing up to his friend's death, but he courageously continued; when he reached the end of the story, he began again at the beginning, and the environment was customized in real time to correspond to the part of the event he was telling.

During session 4, his therapist talked with Joe about incorporating the simulated IED attack, and they collaboratively agreed to include all relevant stimuli. Joe revisited the memory with the environment customized to the same state as the previous session. When Joe recalled the IED blast, the clinician triggered a simulated IED blast that gently shook the chair in which Joe sat. A simulated Blackhawk was added to correspond to the memory of the air evacuation of his buddy. At the end of the story, he started again and repeated the event in virtual reality three times, over approximately 40 minutes.

Consistent with reports of patients in other exposure therapy protocols, Joe reported a slight increase in symptoms after his initial VR exposure. This was expected; he had stopped avoiding the memory, and intentionally confronting it resulted in a brief increase in distress. However, he stuck with the protocol, and by session 8 he was reporting significant habituation to the memory. His self-reported discomfort during VRE in session had dropped significantly. After 10 sessions, his self-reported PTSD symptoms were significantly reduced relative to his pretreatment reports. His functioning in his job and at home were similarly improved, and he and his therapist collaboratively agreed to terminate treatment.

Conclusion

VRE is an innovative treatment approach that may represent a more appealing form of treatment to service members than other PTSD treatment approaches. Theoretically, the use of multisensory stimuli presents an opportunity to increase activation of the trauma memory and improve emotional engagement during exposure. By customizing computer-generated stimuli to resemble aspects of the individual's traumatic event, clinicians can leverage a tool that may fit with the clinical needs of the PTSD patient population in general and military personnel with PTSD in particular. Preliminary research provides initial support for VRE. If ongoing RCTs find that VRE is efficacious, this exciting new treatment option may help address the needs of a growing number of service members with combat-related PTSD.

Acknowledgment

The authors would like to thank Joe Edwards for his manuscript review and editing.

References

Beck, J. G., Palyo, S. A., Winer, E. H., Schwagler, B. E., & Ang, E. J. (2007). Virtual reality exposure therapy for PTSD symptoms after a road accident: An uncontrolled case series. *Behavior Therapy, 38,* 39–48.

Bradley, R., Greene, J., Russ, E., Dutra, L., & Westen, D. (2005). A multidimensional meta-analysis of psychotherapy for PTSD. *American Journal of Psychiatry, 162,* 214–227.

Britt, T. W. (2000). The stigma of psychological problems in a work environment: Evidence from the screening of service members returning from Bosnia. *Journal of Applied Psychology, 30*(8), 1599–1618.

Department of Veterans Affairs and Department of Defense. (2004). *VA/DoD clinical practice guideline for the management of posttraumatic stress, Version 1.0.* Washington, DC: Department of Defense, Department of Veterans Affairs and Health Affairs, Veterans Health Administration.

Difede, J., Cukor, J., Jayasinghe, N., Patt, I., Jedel, S., Spielman, L., et al. (2007). Virtual reality exposure therapy for the treatment of posttraumatic stress disorder following September 11, 2001. *Journal of Clinical Psychiatry, 68,* 1639–1647.

Difede, J., & Hoffman, H. G. (2002). Virtual reality exposure therapy for World Trade Center posttraumatic stress disorder: A case report. *CyberPsychology & Behavior, 5,* 529–535.

Dohrenwend, B. P., Turner, J. B., Turse, N. A., Adams, B. G., Koenen, K. C., & Marshall, R. (2006). The psychological risks of Vietnam for U.S. veterans: A revision with new data and methods. *Science, 313,* 979–982.

Foa, E. B., Dancu, C. V., Hembree, E. A., Jaycox, L. H., Meadows, E. A., & Street, G. P. (1999). The efficacy of exposure therapy, stress inoculation training, and their combination in ameliorating PTSD for female victims of assault. *Journal of Consulting and Clinical Psychology, 67,* 194–200.

Foa, E. B., & Hearst-Ikeda, D. (1996). Emotional dissociation in response to trauma: An information-processing approach. In L. K. Michelson & W. J. Ray (Eds.), *Handbook of dissociation: Theoretical and clinical perspectives* (pp. 207–222). New York: Plenum Press.

Foa, E. B., Hembree, E. A., Cahill, S. P., Rauch, S. A., Riggs, D. S., Feeny, N. C., et al. (2005). Randomized trial of prolonged exposure for PTSD with and without cognitive restructuring: Outcome at academic and community clinics. *Journal of Consulting and Clinical Psychology, 73,* 953–964.

Foa, E. B., Hembree, E. A., & Rothbaum, B.O. (2007). *Prolonged exposure therapy for PTSD: Emotional processing of traumatic experiences: Therapist guide.* New York: Oxford University Press.

Foa, E. B., Huppert, J. D., & Cahill, S. P. (2006). Emotional processing theory: An update. In B. O. Rothbaum (Ed.), *Pathological anxiety: Emotional processing in etiology and treatment* (pp. 3–24). New York: Guilford Press.

Foa, E. B., Keane, T. M., Friedman, M. J., & Cohen, J. A. (Eds.). (2009). *Effective treatments for PTSD: Practice guidelines from the International Society for Traumatic Stress Studies* (2nd ed.). New York: Guilford Press.

Foa, E. B., & Kozak, M. J. (1986). Emotional processing of fear: Exposure to corrective information. *Psychological Bulletin, 99*(1), 20–35.

Foa, E. B., Riggs, D. S., Massie, E. D., & Yarczower, M. (1995). The impact of fear activation and anger on the efficacy of exposure treatment for posttraumatic stress disorder. *Behavior Therapy, 26*, 487–499.

Foa, E. B., Steketee, G., & Rothbaum, B. O. (1989). Behavioral/cognitive conceptualizations of posttraumatic stress disorder. *Behavior Therapy, 20*, 155–176.

Freedman, S. A., Hoffman, H. G., Garcia-Palacios, A., Weiss, P. L., Avitzour, S., & Josman, N. (2010). Prolonged exposure and virtual reality-enhanced imaginal exposure for PTSD following a terrorist bulldozer attack: A case study. *Cyberpsychology, Behavior, and Social Networking, 13*(1), 95–101.

Gerardi, M., Rothbaum, B. O., Ressler, K., & Heekin, M. (2008). Virtual reality exposure therapy using a virtual Iraq: Case report. *Journal of Traumatic Stress, 21*, 209–213.

Hoge, C. W., Auchterlonie, J. L., & Milliken, C. S. (2006). Mental health problems, use of mental health services, and attrition from military service after returning from deployment to Iraq or Afghanistan. *Journal of the American Medical Association, 295*(9), 1023–1032.

Hoge, C. W., Castro, C. A., Messer, S. C., McGurk, D., Cotting, D. I., & Koffman, R. L. (2004). Combat duty in Iraq and Afghanistan, mental health problems, and barriers to care. *The New England Journal of Medicine, 351*(1), 13–22.

Institute of Medicine. (2008). *Treatment of posttraumatic stress disorder: An assessment of the evidence.* Washington, DC: National Academies Press.

Jaycox, L. H., Foa, E. B., & Morral, A. R. (1998). Influence of emotional engagement and habituation on exposure therapy for PTSD. *Journal of Consulting and Clinical Psychology, 66*(1), 185–192.

Keane, T. M., Fairbank, J. A., Caddell, J. M., & Zimering, R.T. (1989). Implosive (flooding) therapy reduces symptoms of PTSD in Vietnam combat veterans. *Behavior Therapy, 20*, 245–260.

Kessler, R. C., Sonnega, A., Bromet, E., Hughes, M., & Nelson, C. B. (1995). Posttraumatic stress disorder in the National Comorbidity Survey. *Archives of General Psychiatry, 52*(12), 1048–1060.

Koffman, R., & Wood, D. P. (2009, June). *Virtual reality exposure therapy with arousal control for the treatment of combat-related posttraumatic stress disorder.* Paper presented at the annual Cybertherapy Meeting, Lago Maggiore, Verbania, Italy.

Kulka, R. A., Schlenger, W. E., Fairbank, J. A., Hough, R. L., Jordan, B. K., Marmar, C. R., et al. (1988). *National Vietnam Veterans Readjustment Study (NVVRS): Description, current status, and initial PTSD prevalence estimates.* Washington, DC: Veterans Administration.

Lang, P. J. (1977). Imagery in therapy: An information processing analysis of fear. *Behavior Therapy, 8*(5), 862–886.

Lawson, B. D., Graeber, D. A., Mead, A. M., & Muth, E. R. (2002). Signs and symptoms of human syndromes associated with synthetic experiences. In K. M. Stanney (Ed.), *Handbook of virtual environments* (pp. 589–618). Mahwah, NJ: Erlbaum.

Maercker, A., Zollner, T., Menning, H., Rabe, S., & Karl, A. (2006). Dresden PTSD treatment study: Randomized controlled trial of motor vehicle accident survivors. *BioMed Central Psychiatry, 6,* 1–8.

Marks, I., Lovell, K., Noshirvani, H., Livanou, M., & Thrasher, S. (1998). Treatment of posttraumatic stress disorder by exposure and/or cognitive restructuring: A controlled study. *Archives of General Psychiatry, 55,* 317–325.

McLay, R. N., McBrien, C., Wiederhold, M., & Wiederhold, B. (2010). Exposure therapy with and without virtual reality to treat PTSD while in the combat theater: A parallel case series. *Cyberpsychology, Behavior, and Social Networking, 13*(1), 37–42.

Milliken, C. S., Auchterlonie, J. L., & Hoge, C. W. (2007). Longitudinal assessment of mental health problems among active and reserve component soldiers returning from the Iraq war. *Journal of the American Medical Association, 298*(18), 2141–2148.

Miyahira, S., Folen, R. A., Hoffman, H. G., & Garcia-Palacios, A. (2009, June). *Treating combat PTSD with virtual reality exposure therapy.* Paper presented at the annual CyberTherapy and CyberPsychology Conference, Villa Caramora, Italy.

Mowrer, O. H. (1960). *Learning theory and behavior.* New York: Wiley

Parsons, T. D., & Rizzo, A. A. (2008). Affective outcomes of virtual reality exposure therapy for anxiety and specific phobias: A meta-analysis. *Journal of Behavior Therapy and Experimental Psychiatry, 39,* 250–261.

Reger, G. M., & Gahm, G. A. (2008). Virtual reality exposure therapy for active-duty soldiers. *Journal of Clinical Psychology, 64*(8), 940–946.

Reger, G. M., Holloway, K. M., Candy, C., Rothbaum, B. O., Difede, J., Rizzo, A. A., et al. (2011). Effectiveness of virtual reality exposure therapy for active-duty soldiers in a military mental health clinic. *Journal of Traumatic Stress, 24,* 93–96.

Resick, P. A., Nishith, P., Weaver, T. L., Astin, M. C., & Feuer, C. A. (2002). A comparison of cognitive-processing therapy with prolonged exposure and a waiting condition for the treatment of chronic posttraumatic stress disorder in female rape victims. *Journal of Consulting and Clinical Psychology, 70*(4), 867–879.

Rizzo, A. A., Reger, G. M., Gahm, G. A., Difede, J., & Rothbaum, B. O. (2009). Virtual reality exposure therapy for combat-related PTSD. In P. Shiromani, T. Keane, & J. LeDoux (Eds.), *Posttraumatic stress disorder: Basic science and clinical practice* (pp. 375–400). New York: Humana Press.

Rothbaum, B. O. (2008, May). *Virtual reality therapy for post-traumatic stress disorder in Iraq war Veterans.* Paper presented at the 161st Annual Meeting of the American Psychiatric Association, Washington, DC.

Rothbaum, B. O., Difede, J., & Rizzo, A. A. (2008). *Therapist treatment manual for virtual reality exposure therapy: Posttraumatic stress disorder in Iraq combat Veterans.* Lakewood, WA: Geneva Foundation.

Rothbaum, B. O., Hodges, L., F., Alarcon, R., Ready, D., Shahar, F., Graap, K., et al. (1999). Virtual reality exposure therapy for PTSD Vietnam veterans: A case study. *Journal of Traumatic Stress, 12,* 263–271.

Rothbaum, B. O., Hodges, L. F., Ready, D., Graap, K., & Alarcon, R. D. (2001).

Virtual reality exposure therapy for Vietnam veterans with posttraumatic stress disorder. *Journal of Clinical Psychiatry, 62,* 617–22.

Roy, M. J. (2009, August). *An update on the ViRTICo (Virtual Reality Therapy and Imaging in Combat Veterans) trial.* Paper presented at the annual World Congress of IBMISPS Brain Mapping and Image Guided Therapy, Boston, MA.

Schnurr, P. P., Friedman, M. J., Engell, C. C., Foa, E. B., Shea, M. T., Resick, P. A., et al. (2007). Cognitive behavioral therapy for posttraumatic stress disorder in women: A randomized controlled trial. *Journal of the American Medical Association, 297,* 820–830.

Seal, K. H., Bertenthal, D., Miner, C. R., Sen, S., & Marmar, C. (2007). Bringing the war back home: Mental health disorders among 103,788 U.S. Veterans returning from Iraq and Afghanistan seen at Department of Veterans Affairs facilities. *Archives of Internal Medicine, 167*(5), 476–482.

Thomas, J. L., Wilk, J. E., Riviere, L. A., McGurk, D., Castro, C. A., & Hoge, C. W. (2010). Prevalence of mental health problems and functional impairment among active component and National Guard Soldiers 3 and 12 months following combat in Iraq. *Archives of General Psychiatry, 67,* 614–623.

Wilson, J. A. B., Onorati, K., Mishkind, M., Reger, M. A., & Gahm, G. A. (2008). Soldier attitudes about technology-based approaches to mental healthcare. *CyberPsychology & Behavior, 11*(6), 767–769.

Wood, D. P., Murphy, J., Center, K., McLay, R., Reeves, D., Pyne, J., et al. (2007). Combat-related posttraumatic stress disorder: A case report using virtual reality exposure therapy with physiological monitoring. *CyberPsychology & Behavior, 2,* 309–315.

Wood, P. D., Webb-Murphy, J., Center, K., McLay, R., Koffman, R., Johnston, S., et al. (2009). Combat-related posttraumatic stress disorder: A case report using virtual reality graded exposure therapy with physiological monitoring with a female Seabee. *Military Medicine, 174,* 1215–1222.

CHAPTER 7

Psychodynamic Psychotherapy

Harold Kudler

Background and Overview
of Psychodynamic Psychotherapy

The history of psychodynamic treatment for posttraumatic stress disorder (PTSD) and its application to military personnel abounds in ironies. Psychoanalytic theory and practice date back to the late 19th century, but the principles on which they are based are as old as human nature and have likely played a role in society's response to the needs of warriors, their families, and their communities for as long as there have been wars.

As Jonathan Shay demonstrates in *Achilles in Vietnam* (1994) and *Odysseus in America* (2002), Homeric epics have served two key purposes over the past three millennia by providing (1) words for the often unspeakable experiences of war and (2) a forum in which the warrior's experience may be "communalized" as an essential component of homecoming. Modern readers think of the *Iliad* and the *Odyssey* as great books to be read privately, but these epics were developed and employed as community events through which warriors, their families, and their fellow citizens could share a common narrative that was sung in a public setting (an ancient form of the rap videos currently being produced by service members in Iraq and Afghanistan).

Four hundred years after Homer, Sophocles, a seasoned general, wrote plays specifically for the Greek soldiers who attended them. Athenian soldiers sat in the theater by division and rank to watch plays drawn from classic myths and Homeric epic but that had been crafted to evoke images and concerns relevant to their most recent campaigns. Sophocles' works were not entertainment in the modern sense. They were meant to evoke a spiritual "mystery." Through theater, Greek society sanctioned community-based expression of combat experiences within which combatants, their families, and their fellow citizens could confront and process stressors of war from the safer distance of metaphor. Then as now, theater provides a unique opportunity to toggle between past and present, reality and fantasy, self and other, relief and grief, wish and fear in an effort to confront psychological dissonance and, hopefully, spur its resolution. Greek theater, like the Homeric epics that preceded and informed it, was deliberately constructed as a cathartic experience meant to assist war fighters, their families, and their communities in processing their experiences and subsequent readjustment problems as they transitioned from warriors to citizens.

A century after Sophocles, Aristotle tutored one of history's most celebrated warriors, Alexander the Great. Tradition holds that Alexander slept with a copy of the *Iliad*, personally annotated by Aristotle, under his pillow because it embodied, as Dryden framed it in his translation of Plutarch's *Life of Alexander,* "a perfect portable treasure of all military virtue and knowledge." Perhaps Alexander believed that Homer's narrative, coupled with Aristotle's philosophy, enhanced his strategy and his resilience in the face of war.

In contemplating the nature of Greek poetry and drama, Aristotle defined catharsis in his *Poetics* as the release of pent-up emotion that would overcome a character in a play and/or the audience watching that play. Catharsis was to be understood as an emotional cleansing and/or spiritual purification of the characters in a play and/or of its audience. The literary critic F. L. Lucas pointed out that Aristotle had already defined catharsis in purely medical terms (as a purgative of excessive bodily substances) in writings prior to *The Poetics* so the literary use of the term should be understood as a medical metaphor connoting "the human soul that is purged of its excessive passions" (Lucas, 1928, p. 24).

Trauma and catharsis came together again more than 2,000 years later in Breuer and Freud's 1895 *Studies on Hysteria*, which marks the beginning of psychoanalysis and modern psychotherapy. For the purposes of this chapter, the terms *psychoanalytic* and *psychodynamic* will be used interchangeably. *Studies* broke with the contemporary view that hysterical symptoms, including anxiety, dissociation, or conversion, even if triggered by a traumatic event, were primarily a reflection of a biological defect usually summarized as "degeneracy." Modern usage associates degeneracy with moral failure, but, in the late 19th century, the term referred to biological degeneration of the central nervous system *and* the intellectual and moral corruption associated with it. *Hysteria*, a term derived from the ancient

Greek medical literature, was assumed to represent the impaired workings of a biologically degenerate brain.

Breuer and Freud famously asserted that "hysterics suffer mainly from reminiscences" (p. 7), meaning that traumatic memories and the survivor's thoughts and feelings in response to them were, in themselves, the cause of hysteria. Breuer and Freud described the use of hypnosis to enable repressed traumatic memories and the ideas and feelings associated with them to be brought into consciousness and shared with the therapist. They pointed out that simply remembering and sharing the traumatic narrative was insufficient; the memory had to be brought forward, along with the pent-up affect that accompanied it, if symptoms were to be relieved. This was a rediscovery and medical application of the ancient Greek principle, and *catharsis* was precisely the term Breuer and Freud used to describe their new therapy.

Breuer and Freud went on to consider that "instead of a single, major trauma ... a number of partial traumas [may form] a *group* of provoking causes" (p. 6), thus anticipating the modern concept of cumulative trauma by a century and pointing the way toward an understanding of complex trauma (a concept still hotly debated today). They concluded that "the psychical trauma—or more precisely the memory of the trauma—acts like a foreign body which long after its entry must continue to be regarded as an agent that is still at work" (p. 6). Hypnosis was the first psychodynamic means of plucking that foreign body out of the psyche, much as one might remove a festering splinter or eradicate a germ from within its host.

Psychoanalysis has been evolving steadily since 1895. Even in his first case in *Studies*, Freud tried to move beyond hypnotic suggestion and simply talk with his patient about her problems. Over time, he came to realize that, although many sequelae of traumatic experiences were responsive to catharsis, most of the problems in living with which his patients presented were more complex and required a more thoroughgoing technique. Freud came to distrust hypnosis as "a mystical ally" (Freud, 1910, p. 22) that, although often helpful in eradicating specific symptoms, could distract both patient and therapist from more fundamental issues. Whereas Breuer held that traumatic memories haunted people through hysterical symptoms because they were simply unable to remember them, Freud wondered whether survivors defended themselves against remembering them (repression). Thus Freud understood repression as a defense and came to understand posttraumatic symptoms as a set of compromises between what the survivor could neither entirely forget nor allow him- or herself to remember.

In order to help the patient understand and overcome hysterical symptoms, Freud developed the strategic use of free association, which remains essential to psychodynamic psychotherapy. Rather than being induced to remember under hypnosis, the patient is asked to speak openly about whatever is on his or her mind even if what comes forth seems irrelevant, embarrassing, banal, rude, or even shocking. Based on the belief that "no mortal can keep a secret" (Freud, 1905, p. 215), free association helps the patient become increasingly aware of the content and process of his or her own thoughts and feelings, including his or her own rules about what is acceptable and his or her characteristic defenses against what is unacceptable. This effort requires honesty, insight, trust, and no small amount of courage on the part of the patient, along with the steady facilitation of the therapist. Many of these psychological contents and rules predominantly function outside conscious awareness. Through free association, psychoanalysis moved beyond pure catharsis to become the analysis of unconscious mental contents and operations.

The idea that a significant component of what drives a person's behavior resides in the unconscious was one of the most radical innovations of psychoanalytic theory. Freud (1933) once described the relationship between the personified, known aspects of a person (the "me" or, as his classically inclined translator, James Strachey, dubbed it, the "ego") and the unconscious, often disowned "not me" or "it" aspects of the self (as per Strachey, the "id") within the following metaphor:

> One might compare the relation of the ego to the id with that between a rider and his horse. The horse provides the locomotor energy, and the rider has the prerogative of determining the goal and of guiding the movements of his powerful mount towards it. But all too often in the relations between the ego and the id we find a picture of the less ideal situation in which the rider is obliged to guide his horse in the direction in which it itself wants to go. (1933, p. 77)

Freud recognized dreams as compromise formations arising out of the same conflicts that underlie hysterical symptoms. For Freud dreams were the "royal road to the unconscious" (Freud, 1900) because the psychological system operates differently during sleep than while awake. When a patient brings forward a dream within waking associations, it becomes possible to juxtapose waking and dream thoughts in ways that triangulate on the concerns and defenses common to both. Further, the patient's realization that the dream is surely his or her own creation confronts the patient with the strong possibility that the dream has something useful to say about his or her own thoughts and feelings.

After abandoning hypnosis, Freud enjoined his patients to collaborate with him on the analysis of their thoughts, feelings, dreams, and patterns of behavior, conscious and unconscious, but was surprised to encounter a paradox: The more intensively he worked with them, the more likely his patients were to become sidetracked by the eruption of inaccurate yet compelling attitudes toward the therapist. Although each patient had his or her own characteristic set of concerns about the therapist, these fit a common pattern in that they were predictably intense and inappropriate and in that, whether positive or negative in character, they consistently obstructed the progress of therapy. Through systematic exploration of these unexpected resistances, Freud realized that they were *transferences* of the patient's past relationships onto the therapeutic relationship.

At first, Freud saw transference as the patient's self-defensive efforts against the therapy itself that had to be overcome (often by assertion of the therapist's authority) in order to continue the work. In time, he came to appreciate that transference offers a unique opportunity for patient and therapist to learn something that might not otherwise have been apparent or even available to either of them. Because transference literally reinserts the past into the present, it provides invaluable clues about developmental problems that brought the patient into treatment in the first place. Those issues are alive in the transference (a demonstration of Freud's hypothesis that the unconscious has no sense of time). It is one thing for the patient to come to therapy and talk about past developmental experiences and quite another thing to reexperience the past in real time with the therapist. The patient's progressive appreciation of his or her transference responses helps drive the analysis by bringing the intensity, character, and enduring impact of earlier life experiences to present-day interactions in therapy and in the outside world. For these reasons, psychoanalysis has evolved into the analysis of transference.

The realignment of psychoanalysis on transference required certain technical innovations. Freud urged therapists to limit self-disclosure in order to provide the patient with a blank screen upon which to project transference distortions. Frequent meetings (classical psychoanalysis usually requires four–five sessions per week of 45–50 minutes each) and the patient's position on the couch looking away from the analyst are deliberate efforts to precipitate more intense transference. The therapist then works with the patient to confront and decipher what has been projected. In this way, psychoanalysis became a systematic method of working through old problems rather than simply reliving them. It is interesting to speculate that the same processes of reliving, confronting, and moving beyond past experiences and current compromises are at play in psychoanalysis as in catharsis but that psychoanalytic treatment harnesses these elements such that they are less mystical, more fully articulated, more clearly within the grasp of both subject and therapist, and more reliably effective.

It is important to note that, unlike classical psychoanalysis (which remains widely practiced), not all psychodynamic psychotherapies focus on the analysis of transference. As a rule of thumb, the more a psychodynamic psychotherapy centers on expressive elements (free association, insight, interpretation), the more it focuses on transference. Psychoanalytic psychotherapy usually refers to transference-based therapy conducted face-to-face with sessions of 45–50 minutes that are held one to three times per week. Contrary to popular opinion, more frequent sessions are indicated not because the patient is "sicker" but rather because they provide the patient a greater opportunity to confront and work through transference. Less frequent psychodynamic sessions may be indicated when a patient is more likely to feel overwhelmed by transference feelings. Often this feeling correlates with the patient's ability to form a positive therapeutic relationship. Psychoanalytic psychotherapists distinguish between the "real relationship" with the therapist (Greenson, 1967) and the transference relationship in order to describe the interplay between two enduring, coherent, but often opposing, constructions on the part of the patient. As an example, clinical experience shows that patients with borderline personality disorder tend to have more difficulty distinguishing their real relationship with the therapist from their transference relationship with the therapist. Therefore, patient–therapist relationships tend to be very rocky and sometimes even intolerable for patients with borderline personality disorders. In such cases, it is often wise to decrease the frequency of sessions or, sometimes, the length of sessions in order to titrate the level of transference to more tolerable levels. Psychodynamic psychotherapy is effective in work with borderline patients when technical applications are applied to meet their specific problems and needs (Clarkin, Levy, Lenzenweger & Kernberg, 2007).

Psychodynamic psychotherapy usually involves a higher level of therapist activity than classical psychoanalysis, but the therapist retains relative abstinence from self-disclosure in order not to muddy the waters as transference coalesces and expresses itself. Without the development of transference, insight-oriented psychodynamic psychotherapy would lack its central focus. On the other hand, the closer psychodynamic psychotherapy comes to the supportive end of the therapeutic spectrum (typified by reassurance, help with self-esteem and self-reliance, and greater activity and more self-disclosure on the part of the therapist), the less it centers on transference interpretation. For example, in more supportive modes of psychodynamic psychotherapy, the therapist's hypotheses may be informed by the patient's transference, but his or her therapeutic interventions are designed to strengthen the patient's coping abilities, not to help interpret transference distortions. As is demonstrated by other forms of psychotherapy, it is not always necessary to analyze a problem down to its fundamental components in order to achieve a meaningful and lasting therapeutic result. Supportive psychodynamic psychotherapy "supports the ego" in order to assist the patient in mobilizing his or her own strengths and adaptive strategies to reach a better compromise with current problems so that life can be managed with less pain, greater freedom, and higher levels of effectiveness. There is no evidence that clinical outcomes achieved through supportive psychotherapy are any less profound or enduring than those achieved by more insight-oriented psychoanalytic treatment (Werman, 1984). As in any form of treatment, the form of psychodynamic therapy employed should reflect the patient's wants, needs, and abilities at the time of therapy rather than the therapist's theoretical principles or routine practices.

Cognitive-behavioral therapy, which derives from psychoanalytic therapy, also holds that psychopathology may reflect unconscious patterns of thought and behavior but assumes that such problems arise from simple misunderstandings that can be corrected by the therapist. The patient then works to incorporate the corrected knowledge through thought and practice until it is fully integrated into a new, more adaptive schema. The essential difference between cognitive therapy and psychoanalytic therapy is that psychoanalytic theory holds that such "mistakes" are not simply failures to understand reality or perform effectively but rather are "bargains" made as part of a purposeful if often unconscious effort to sidestep reality and avoid still more painful issues. The fact that both therapies can be successful does not prove one or disprove the other. It may simply be that many patients can make progress by working with a trusted therapist in a structured effort to confront and correct problematic behaviors at the level of thought or behavior, whereas other patients either prefer or need to work at other levels of conflict before they can grasp and overcome maladaptive patterns. A third group of patients may not be able to employ either method of therapy because they lack the capacity to form the trusting therapeutic relationship essential to both.

Another distinctive attribute of psychodynamic psychotherapy is the role it assigns to countertransference. Whereas teachers and clinical supervisors of other psychotherapies may warn about potential boundary crossings and other problems associated with the therapist's countertransference, psychoanalytic clinicians emphasize the important ways in which countertransference can inform the therapy. Originally conceived of as the therapist's inappropriate response to the patient based on his or her own past relationships and characteristic psychological responses (and therefore a good reason for psychotherapists to pursue their own analysis in order to become aware of potentially troublesome tendencies and blind spots), psychoanalytic clinicians also understand countertransference to include the therapist's conscious and unconscious response to the patient's transference. As the therapist works to sort out which of his or her responses to the patient are primarily idiosyncratic and which reflect responses reciprocal to the patient's attitudes and behaviors, transferential and otherwise, the therapist forms hypotheses about what the patient is doing, to paraphrase Sullivan (1970), *with* the therapist and *to* the therapist (p. 55). By working to either confirm or disconfirm those hypotheses, the therapist becomes increasingly aware of important patterns that this particular patient brings to the therapeutic relationship. Some of these patterns are too subtle to be observed directly but become apparent when viewed through the lens of the therapist's countertransference (*if* the therapist is attuned to his or her own responses). Disciplined attention to countertransference informs the therapist's efforts to help the patient become aware of those patterns as well.

Transference and countertransference are unique aspects of the therapeutic relationship that psychodynamic psychotherapists exploit for the benefit of the patient. They provide powerful tools for exploring aspects of the patient's development that have crystallized as persistent unconscious representations expressed in recurring maladaptive patterns. Such problems are particularly suitable for psychoanalytic approaches so long as the patient is open to this approach and prepared to undertake it. Among the qualities that a patient should bring to psychoanalytic psychotherapy are a strong motivation to understand, a tolerance for frustration, the capacity for insight, good reality testing, the ability to sustain a relationship despite stress, and a history of significant suffering (Gabbard, 2005).

Psychodynamic psychotherapy can be conducted individually, in groups, or in family therapy on either an inpatient or an outpatient basis. No one form of psychodynamic psychotherapy is intrinsically superior to others. The choice of therapy will reflect patient needs, wishes, attributes, and practical concerns, as well as the judgment, training, and experience of the therapist. The goal is to match the treatment to the specific patient within a specific clinical situation.

Research on Psychodynamic Psychotherapy with Civilian Populations

Despite more than a century of clinical experience and research, psychodynamic psychotherapy receives, at best, a second-tier recommendation in clinical practice guidelines for PTSD (Forbes et al., 2010). The reason is that randomized clinical trials (RCTs) are the gold standard for designating a treatment as an "evidence-based therapy," and controlled investigations of the efficacy of psychodynamic therapies are few. Beyond noting that lack of evidence is not evidence of nonefficacy, it is important to point out two key reasons for the paucity of research on psychoanalytic treatment. The first was summarized by Shedler (2010):

> There is a belief in some quarters that psychodynamic concepts and treatments lack empirical support, or that scientific evidence shows that other forms of treatment are more effective. The belief appears to have taken on a life of its own. Academicians repeat it to one another, as do healthcare administrators, as do healthcare policy makers. With each repetition, its

apparent credibility grows. At some point, there seems little need to question or revisit it because—everyone knows it to be so. (p. 98)

But if the larger scientific community sees little point in pursuing research on psychoanalytic concepts and treatments, why haven't psychoanalysts taken the lead in producing the needed body of research? Unfortunately, many leaders in the psychoanalytic community question the relevance, the probity, or even the possibility of such research. They argue that RCTs focus on the symptoms of a disorder, whereas psychodynamic treatment applies a highly individualized perspective that looks beyond symptom reduction to focus on the growth and potential of a specific person. They add that psychodynamic research must always focus on the individual rather than on the treatment of a specific disorder across a broad range of patients. They conclude that RCT research inherently compromises psychoanalytic practices and treatment goals to the point at which their findings no longer reflect psychoanalytic ideas at all. Unfortunately, by limiting their focus to the individual patient, psychodynamic researchers run the risk of depriving the many of the potential benefits of psychoanalytic treatment for PTSD. Fonagy, Roth, and Higgit (2005) end their exhaustive review of the psychotherapy outcomes literature with a set of recommendations including that researchers "end the splendid isolation of psychoanalysis by undertaking active collaboration with other scientific and clinical disciplines" (p. 45).

Although individual case reports make up the bulk of the psychodynamic literature on the treatment of psychological trauma, a small and growing group of empirical investigations and case series with controlled variables and validated outcome measures support psychodynamic therapy as a treatment option for PTSD (Kudler, Blank, Krupnick, Herman, & Horowitz, 2008). Brom, Kleber, and Defares (1989) conducted an RCT comparing a manualized brief psychodynamic psychotherapy with an exposure-based hypnotherapy, a desensitization therapy, and a wait-list control group in the treatment of patients with PTSD. Symptoms of intrusion and avoidance improved significantly in each of the treatment groups, but not in the control group. Psychodynamic psychotherapy was the most effective in improving coping ability and self-esteem. The psychodynamic psychotherapy group showed more improvement in the posttermination phase than did others. Participants in all three treatment conditions improved more than those in the wait-list group.

Schottenbauer, Glass, Arnkoff, and Gray (2008) recently reviewed the literature on empirically supported psychodynamic approaches for PTSD. They argued for psychodynamic treatment on the basis that it may address crucial areas in the clinical presentation of PTSD and the sequelae of trauma not targeted by other therapies and that it may be particularly helpful when treating complex PTSD. They point to empirical and clinical evidence suggesting that psychodynamic approaches may result in increased ability to resolve reactions to trauma through improved reflective functioning, increased reliance on mature as opposed to immature defenses, internalization of more secure working models of relationships, and improved social functioning. They also note a trend across studies that patients in psychodynamic psychotherapy continue to improve after treatment ends (as was observed in Brom et al.'s [1989] PTSD study).

By definition, RCTs are not representative of clinical practice because they do not reflect the true complexity of most patients. For example, PTSD is rarely found without comorbid disorders such as major depression and/or substance abuse, but comorbidity is not usually studied in RCTs. Randomization, although essential in RCTs, is not representative of clinical conditions in which patients themselves tend to seek out the type of treatment they prefer for highly personal reasons. Effectiveness studies, which test the success of treatment under real-world conditions, offer a new lens that may help inform clinicians about the value of psychodynamic psychotherapy and other psychotherapies for PTSD in real-world settings. It will, however, be necessary to develop standards for incorporating effectiveness research findings into clinical practice guideline recommendations before such studies have a significant impact on what is generally considered "evidence-based" treatment of PTSD or other disorders.

Research on Psychodynamic Psychotherapy with Military Populations

Psychoanalytic psychotherapy began with trauma survivors, and its growth has been spurred by the challenges presented in caring for combat veterans. Shell shock, the signature injury of World War I, was originally conceptualized as a purely physical injury resulting from the effect of exploding artillery shells on the structure of the central nervous system (Mott, 1916; Jones, Fear, & Wessely, 2007). By the war's end, psychoanalytic ideas were already being applied to shell shock and other psychiatric problems of combat veterans. W. H. R. Rivers, whose work at the Craiglockhart War Hospital with British neuropsychiatric casualties was famously portrayed in Pat Barker's historical novel, *Regeneration* (1991), wrote an influential 1918 paper on the role of repression in the development and maintenance of war neuroses. Freud's observations on the nightmares of World War I veterans led him to write *Beyond the Pleasure Principle* (1920), in which he reconsidered his theory of dreams in light of an apparent compulsion to repeat traumatic memories that later became a core component of the PTSD diagnosis. Grinker and Spiegel's 1945 *Men Under Stress* summarized their experience treating hundreds of combat veterans with cathartic treatments utilizing either hypnosis or sodium amytal. Their approach, based on the psychoanalytic view that the conversion and dissociative symptoms of combat veterans (then termed "battle fatigue") were caused by repression of traumatic memories, was remarkably effective. The success of psychoanalytic principles in military medicine led to the growth of psychoanalysis and of psychiatry itself in the postwar years.

Despite its excellent service record, there have been no large-scale studies on the psychoanalytic treatment of combat veterans since World War II.

Strengths of Psychodynamic Psychotherapy with Military Personnel

As noted previously, psychodynamic theory proved of immense help in resolving conversion, dissociative, and anxiety disorders from past wars. The use of hypnosis or sodium amytal to overcome pathological repression of psychological trauma would likely be as effective today in the treatment of conversion and dissociation—especially in acute cases—but it is important to note that these suggestive techniques require expert application. Clinicians practicing these approaches would need to be certified in hypnotherapy and possess expertise in conscious sedation.

Deployment-related psychological problems may be more likely among individuals who have suffered trauma in earlier life, including sexual abuse, physical abuse, or profound neglect (Breslau, Chilcoat, Kessler, & Davis, 1999). Survivors of early life trauma are sometimes described as having complex PTSD (Herman, 1992). Because of its focus on basic problems in interpersonal relationships, psychodynamic psychotherapy may be particularly useful in treating patients with complex PTSD (Courtois, 1999; Roth & Batson, 1997; Shengold, 1989), although studies have not been conducted in military populations. Psychodynamic psychotherapy may also be useful in treating patients suffering complex PTSD stemming from other prolonged and/or mixed stressors as might be experienced during multiple deployments or as prisoners of war but there is, as yet, little research evidence to support this recommendation.

Limitations of Psychodynamic Psychotherapy with Military Personnel

The greatest limitation to the use of psychoanalytic psychotherapy with military personnel is the lack of a strong evidence base in military settings. On the other hand, the available evidence suggests that brief psychodynamic psychotherapy such as was applied in the Brom et al. (1989) study mentioned earlier may be of value in treating military-related PTSD.

Psychodynamic ideas have, in some instances, been misapplied in clinical work with survivors of childhood trauma, giving rise to concern about the creation or elaboration of so-called *false memories* (Roth & Friedman, 1998). It may be that trauma survivors are particularly prone to this phenomenon given their tendency toward dissociation. It is not clear that this same concern applies to work with combat veterans, but it is important that clinicians be properly trained before undertaking psychodynamic treatment of trauma survivors.

Therapeutic Considerations

At the time of this writing, an unforeseen consequence of reliance on RCTs and the clinical practice guidelines based on them is playing out within the U.S. Department of Veterans Affairs (VA) as it ramps up efforts to meet the clinical needs of over 100,000 veterans of the wars in Iraq and Afghanistan who have already been diagnosed with PTSD. Thousands of VA clinicians are being trained and supervised in at least one of two first-tier psychotherapies for PTSD (prolonged exposure [PE] and cognitive processing therapy [CPT]). No such investment is being made to train clinicians to provide psychodynamic treatment for PTSD. Because VA is a major employer of mental health professionals nationally and the country's largest training system for mental health professionals, its decision to deemphasize psychodynamic psychotherapy reverberates within every American community and across the nation.

Clinical leaders often argue that there are insufficient research data to recommend a greater investment in psychoanalytic psychotherapy at this time. Unfortunately, doubt about the standing of psychodynamic psychotherapy for PTSD seems to have only increased the stigma associated with researching a treatment that, as Shedler notes, "everyone knows" does not work. Investigators tend to design studies on therapies that reviewers consider "more scientific" and more fundable. There seems to be a vicious cycle that bodes poorly for the future of psychodynamic psychotherapy unless clinicians, researchers, and funding agencies begin to work together to expand the evidence base for psychoanalytic psychotherapy for PTSD. Hopefully, competition among rivals can be reformulated as collaboration among colleagues.

Training in psychoanalytic psychotherapy has never been more widely available. Psychoanalytic institutes that prepare candidates to become eligible for certification by the American Psychoanalytic Association exist in major populations centers across the nation. In addition, there is a growing number of psychoanalytic psychotherapy training programs that provide clinicians with a firm grounding in psychoanalytic principles and techniques without requiring a commitment to undertake the extra years of training and practice necessary to become a certified psychoanalyst. Some of these are aligned with psychoanalytic institutes, whereas others are based in universities or in association with large clinical institutions. Distance-learning options are also proliferating. Although once largely a medical enterprise, psychoanalytic trainees now typically include psychologists, social workers, pastoral counselors, and lay people. Most psychoanalytic training is based on a "tripartite system" that integrates coursework with supervised practice and personal psychotherapy.

Psychoanalytic training is experiencing a renaissance just as research and funding in psychoanalytic psychotherapy are at a nadir. Perhaps renewed interest in psychodynamic training reflects a perceived need for the listening skills, clinical strategies, and clinical supervision associated with psychoanalytic practice as a complement to what is offered in the training and practice of other psychotherapies. Psychoanalysis is unique among the psychotherapies in its emphasis on the importance of self-care and introspection on the part of the therapist in order to prevent countertransferential obstacles from arising and to better inform the therapist about the patient. As new generations of clinicians struggle with their patients' trauma narratives and associated problems in living, they may be reaching for the profound conceptualizations, sophisticated technical skills, and thoughtful supervision that inform and enrich psychoanalytic psychotherapy. Hopefully, a new generation of psychoanalytic researchers will not be far behind.

This brief description of psychodynamic psychotherapy is obviously incomplete but has hopefully provided a practical scaffold for this introductory chapter. Although psychodynamic psychotherapy is the oldest psychotherapy for the treatment of traumatic stress, it remains among the most controversial. A final irony may be found in one of the U.S. Department of Defense Centers of Excellence for Psychological Health and Traumatic Brain Injury's (DCoE) newest therapeutic programs for the new veterans of Operation Enduring Freedom in Afghanistan and Operation Iraqi Freedom. The DCoE's Theater of War program (*www.theater-of-war.com*) employs public readings of Sophocles' plays *Ajax* and *Philoctetes* to military audiences to destigmatize deployment-related psychological injuries and to create a safe space for dialogue about the challenges faced by service members and veterans and their families in the course of the deployment cycle. Under contract with DCoE, Theater of War is being performed for military audiences at military bases, suicide prevention conferences, service academies, war colleges, and medical schools. Available in three formats (military, military member and family, and female veteran), Theater of War builds on ancient Greek theater (and the thousands of years of human experience and wisdom that Greek theater incorporates) to create a cathartic community experience for the benefit of modern service members and veterans and their families. In doing so, it provides a psychodynamically informed intervention of significant power and depth. The more things change, the more they stay the same.

Case Vignette

A 23-year-old male Army National Guard member who had served three tours in Iraq was referred from the gastrointestinal clinic where he had been worked up for severe episodic vomiting. After extensive evaluation, no physical cause for his vomiting could be found, and consultation was requested "to screen for psychogenic causes." The patient had no prior psychiatric diagnoses but, on evaluation, did meet criteria for PTSD. He also noted "temper problems" at work but was keeping his anger under control and was not judged imminently dangerous to himself or others. He had a history of multiple head traumas, some associated with brief loss of consciousness (never longer than a few seconds), but workup for traumatic brain injury was unrevealing. His medical and psychiatric history were otherwise unremarkable except for his having been seen by a counselor at age 7 for "signs of depression" (social and emotional withdrawal, trouble sleeping, new onset of enuresis) after his mother died in a car accident. His father remarried, and the patient reported excellent relations with both parents.

The mental health team recommended a course of cognitive processing therapy for PTSD, but the patient dropped out of treatment after four sessions, saying that he preferred a treatment in which he could "talk out" his problems. The team assigned him to brief (12–20 sessions) psychodynamic psychotherapy.

Upon beginning psychodynamic psychotherapy, the patient focused on an incident that had occurred during his third tour. As a squad leader for a convoy security team, he prided himself on his ability to keep his soldiers safe even if it meant plotting special routes and taking some heat from his officers. His squad was known for exceptional performance and a low casualty rate. At the time of the incident, they were just back from the road and sitting down to their first meal in a secure area in several days when a mortar scored a direct hit on their mess hall. Three of his team were killed outright and two were critically injured. The patient escaped with minor injuries. It was, in his words, "a slaughterhouse."

The patient seemed to be making a good adjustment in the days after the incident until the vomiting began during his first trip outside the wire. At first, he chalked it up to food poisoning ("there had been some bad bologna and a lot of people had stomach problems then"), but the problem became more intense and more frequent over time—especially when he was on the road. He did not seek medical attention while in the country but, instead, chose to skip meals "in order to keep an empty stomach." As his tour came to an end, he hoped his vomiting would go away but, instead, the problem worsened to the point at which he wasn't sure he could keep his civilian job as a truck driver.

His therapist noted a possible link between the mortar attack, the act of eating, and his vomiting, but the patient insisted that "worse things happened to other people" and denied any possibility of a connection there. Although the patient had requested "a chance to talk openly," his therapist began to feel increasingly frustrated by a sense that the patient, although open to talking about events in considerable detail, seemed determined to gloss over any feelings connected to those events. Further, the patient seemed determined to negate any helpful effort that the therapist made, often with a dismissive statement such as "if you knew what it was like over there, Doc, you wouldn't say that." The therapist began to dread seeing this patient. As he thought about why, he realized that he had come to doubt whether he was "good enough" to help this patient and that he was feeling guilty for having "let him down."

When the therapist brought these issues up in supervision, his supervisor noted that it was unusual for this therapist to lack reasonable confidence. She wondered if the therapist's concerns about not being "good enough" and having "let down" someone who depended on him might be a countertransferential response. She suggested that the therapist's feelings reflected the patient's own feelings, which he, himself, did not want to be aware of but which he could bring into therapy by making the therapist feel them instead. They agreed that the therapist should listen closely for any concerns about guilt within the patient and follow up with questions should they arise.

At the next session, the patient reported a dream: "I was driving down the road with my wife and we were arguing about seatbelts. She wouldn't put hers on and I was getting angrier and angrier. Suddenly there was a bear in the road and we hit it. We both got out of the car and it turned out that the bear wasn't really dead. It jumped up and swallowed my wife—just like the wolf swallowed the grandmother in the Red Riding Hood story. I woke up screaming and ran to the bathroom where I vomited. Then I was up all night after. I feel queasy again just telling you about it."

As they discussed the dream, the patient found it strange that he had been so angry at his wife in it. Although he still got angry at work, he rarely felt anger toward his family. He then recalled that, earlier that evening before the dream, his wife had criticized him for being too harsh with their 2-year-old son. The patient had yelled at the boy for playing too close to their space heater. He denied being angry and insisted that he was simply teaching his son an important lesson that he had learned "the hard way" in Iraq: "If you're not careful, somebody will die."

The therapist agreed that this was an important lesson but also noted the wife's objection that the child was only 2 years old. When the patient admitted that he might have been too hard on the boy, the therapist asked him if he could also be very hard on himself. The patient became quiet for the moment (which was unusual for him) and then spoke about how angry he got when he remembered that the soldiers who died in the mortar attack would never come home to *their* families. Over the next few sessions, he made a series of connections between his sense of guilt for having survived that attack and the anger he was feeling toward other people. He spoke of how hard it was to "swallow my anger" so he wouldn't have to feel like "a bad person." He had always taken great pride in his successful efforts to keep his soldiers safe. To him, this was the mark of a good soldier and a good person. After the mortar attack, he had begun to wonder if the shelling was "the Universe's confirmation that I was never really any good to begin with." With the therapist's support, he was able to recall his initial relief that he had survived when his buddies had not. He considered this "the most shameful confession of my life." He wondered if his anger at other people might not be an expression of anger he harbored against himself.

In the course of these sessions, the presenting symptom of vomiting became less and less frequent such that it no longer impaired him at work and rarely surfaced at home. His PTSD symptoms had also lessened; he felt he had "a longer fuse." He was proud to report that his wife had recently been complimenting him about how nice he was to be around and what a good father he was.

During his 12th session, he described having narrowly avoided a car accident the afternoon before. The other driver appeared to be drunk. The patient pulled over and jumped out of his truck just in time to vomit on the roadside. The therapist worried to himself that the patient had suffered a setback but was then surprised and impressed by the patient's explanation of the sequence of events: "I guess I learned that there is just so much anger I can swallow, Doc. All that anger had to go somewhere so I guess I just threw it up!" That was the last episode of vomiting that the patient ever reported. He completed his course of psychotherapy 1 month later and, as his primary care physician has documented, continues to do well at work and home with no significant medical problems in the 2 years since his last treatment session.

References

Barker, P. (1991). *Regeneration*. New York: Plume.

Breuer, J., & Freud, S. (1895). Studies on hysteria. In *The standard edition of the complete psychological works of Sigmund Freud* (Vol. 2, pp. 1–319). London: Hogarth Press

Breslau, N., Chilcoat, H. D., Kessler, R. C., & Davis, G. C. (1999). Previous exposure to trauma and PTSD effects of subsequent trauma: Results from the Detroit Area Survey of Trauma. *American Journal of Psychiatry, 156*, 902–907.

Brom, D., Kleber, R. J., & Defares, P. B. (1989). Brief psychotherapy for posttraumatic stress disorders. *Journal of Consulting and Clinical Psychology, 57*, 607—612.

Clarkin, J. F., Levy, K. N., Lenzenweger, M. F., & Kernberg, O. F. (2007). Evaluating three treatments for borderline personality disorder: A multiwave study. *American Journal of Psychiatry, 164*, 922–928.

Courtois, C. A. (1999). *Recollections of sexual abuse: Treatment principles and guidelines*. New York: Norton.

Fonagy, P., Roth, A., & Higgitt, A. (2005). Psychodynamic psychotherapies: Evidence-based practice and clinical wisdom. *Bulletin of the Menninger Clinic, 69*(1), 1–58.

Forbes, D., Creamer, M., Bisson, J., Cohen, J., Crow, B., Foa, E., et al. (2010). A guide to guidelines for the treatment of PTSD and related conditions. *Journal of Traumatic Stress, 23*(5), 537–552.

Freud, S. (1900). The interpretation of dreams. In *The standard edition of the complete psychological works of Sigmund Freud* (Vol. 4, pp. 1–338). London: Hogarth Press.

Freud, S. (1905). Fragment of an analysis of a case of hysteria. In *The standard edition of the complete psychological works of Sigmund Freud* (Vol. 7, pp. 1–122). London: Hogarth Press.

Freud, S. (1910). Five lectures on psycho-analysis. In *The standard edition of the complete psychological works of Sigmund Freud* (Vol. 11, pp. 1–56). London: Hogarth Press.

Freud, S. (1920). Beyond the pleasure principle. In *The standard edition of the complete psychological works of Sigmund Freud* (Vol. 18, pp. 1–64). London: Hogarth Press

Freud, S. (1933). New introductory lectures on psychoanalysis. In *The standard edition of the complete psychological works of Sigmund Freud* (Vol. 22, pp. 1–182). London: Hogarth Press.

Gabbard, G. O. (2005). *Psychodynamic psychotherapy in clinical practice* (4th ed.). Arlington, VA: American Psychiatric Publishing.

Greenson, R. R. (1967). *The technique and practice of psychoanalysis*. New York: International Universities Press.

Grinker, R. R., & Spiegel, J. P. (1945). *Men under stress*. Philadelphia: Blakiston.

Herman, J. L. (1992). Complex PTSD: A syndrome in survivors of prolonged and repeated trauma. *Journal of Traumatic Stress, 5*(3), 377–391.

Jones, E., Fear, N. T., & Wessely, S. (2007). Shell shock and mild traumatic brain injury: A historical review. *American Journal of Psychiatry, 164*, 1641–1645.

Kudler, H. S., Krupnick, J. L., Blank, A. S., Herman, J. L., & Horowitz, M. J. (2008). Psychodynamic therapy for adults. In E. B. Foa, T. M. Keane, M. J. Friedman, & J. A. Cohen (Eds.), *Effective treatments for PTSD: Practice guidelines from the International Society for Traumatic Stress Studies* (pp. 346–369). New York: Guilford Press.

Lucas, F. L. (1928). *Tragedy in relation to Aristotle's Poetics.* London: Hogarth Press.

Mott, F. W. (1916). Special discussion on shell shock without visible signs of injury. *Proceedings of the Royal Society of Medicine, 9,* i–xxiv.

Plutarch. *The life of Alexander* (J. Dryden, trans.). *classics.mit.edu/Plutarch/alexandr.html.*

Rivers, W. H. R. (1918). The repression of war experience. *Lancet, 96,* 513–533.

Roth, S., & Batson, R. (1997). *Naming the shadows: A new approach to individual and group psychotherapy for adult survivors of childhood incest.* New York: Free Press.

Roth, S., & Friedman, M. J. (1998). Childhood trauma remembered: A report on the current scientific knowledge base and its applications. *Journal of Child Sexual Abuse, 7,* 83–109.

Schottenbauer, M. A., Glass, C. R., Arnkoff, D. B., & Gray, S. H. (2008). Contributions of psychodynamic approaches to treatment of PTSD and trauma: A review of the empirical treatment and psychopathology literature. *Psychiatry, 71,* 13–34.

Shay, J. (1994). *Achilles in Vietnam: Combat trauma and the undoing of character.* New York: Atheneum.

Shay, J. (2002). *Odysseus in America: Combat trauma and the trials of homecoming.* New York: Scribner.

Shedler, J. (2010). The efficacy of psychodynamic psychotherapy. *American Psychologist, 65*(2), 98–109.

Shengold, L. (1989). *Soul murder: The effects of childhood abuse and deprivation.* New Haven, CT: Yale University Press.

Sullivan, H. S. (1970). *The psychiatric interview.* New York: Norton.

Werman, D. S. (1984). *The practice of supportive psychotherapy.* New York: Brunner/Mazel.

CHAPTER 8

Group Therapy

David W. Foy
Kent D. Drescher
Patricia J. Watson
Iya Ritchie

In this chapter we present a review of recent studies on group therapy for combat-related posttraumatic stress disorder (PTSD), followed by a brief overview of four different group approaches for treating PTSD and related issues: (1) prevention and early intervention; (2) reducing core PTSD symptoms; (3) dual-diagnosis groups; and (4) groups to address auxiliary issues. The emphasis is on their usefulness for current (active-duty) and former (veteran) military personnel. Two empirically based forms of group therapy for direct treatment of core PTSD symptoms—trauma-focused group therapy (TFGT) and present-centered group therapy (PCGT)—are described. Additionally, we present a group approach that addresses a frequent auxiliary issue with combat-related PTSD—that is, negative changes in key dimensions of spirituality, such as forgiveness and meaning making. Finally, a recent group adaptation of combat operational stress first aid (GCOSFA) for prevention of and early intervention for PTSD is presented. Particular strengths and limitations of group therapy for use with active duty members and veterans are discussed. Finally, issues related to group leader key competencies, fidelity to group therapy guidelines or manualized instructions, and necessary supervision of group leaders are addressed.

Overview and Rationale for Group Therapy with Military Personnel

Using group approaches for combat-related trauma benefits individuals by providing a group context in which to improve their coping with trauma consequences such as isolation, alienation, shame, and restricted or diminished feelings. Combat-related trauma groups are especially appropriate because many former combatants feel ostracized from society and have not shared their combat experiences, and they may even perceive judgment or blame from others for their distress. Other advantages of a group approach include acknowledgment and validation of members' combat experiences, normalization of their trauma-related responses, and validation of behaviors required for survival during combat-related traumas (Foy, Drescher, & Watson, in press).

Group interventions for combat-related trauma were first used following World War II with veterans struggling with the psychological consequences of their war experiences. The first groups were supportive in nature and were conducted months or years after the war's end (e.g., Dynes, 1945). The readjustment needs of Vietnam veterans also stimulated the development of combat-related group interventions. In 1979 the Veterans Administration (VA) established a nationwide network of community-based vet centers to serve these veterans in other than traditional hospital settings. "Rap groups," led by counselors who themselves were Vietnam veterans, were featured in these centers (Sipprelle, 1992). Within VA hospital-based PTSD treatment programs, a multimodal approach, featuring a combination of individual and group therapies, was widely adopted (e.g., Seidel, Gusman, & Abueg, 1994; Gusman, et al., 1996). Groups were also developed to meet a wide range of rehabilitation needs among veterans with chronic combat-related PTSD. More recently, timely group interventions have been developed so that single-session groups are now often used to provide psychoeducation and support within the first few days or weeks after a destabilizing event or upon exiting the war zone.

Research on Group Therapy for PTSD among Military Personnel

Table 8.1 displays 12 studies published over the past 15 years that deal with PTSD and related issues among veterans (10 studies) or active-duty service members (2 studies). Among these studies four different group types are represented. Five studies (Nos. 5, 8, 10, 11, and 12) represent group approaches aimed directly at reducing core symptoms of combat-related

TABLE 8.1. Studies of Group Interventions for Active-Duty Military or Veterans

Study	Treatment group (N)	Comparison group (N)	Number of sessions	Population	Major findings
1. Adler et al. (2008)	Critical incident stress debriefing group (CISD) (312)	Stress management (SM) (359); survey only (SO) (281)	Single session, 50–150 minutes' duration	U.S. soldiers serving as peacekeepers; 96% male	No significant differences between groups in PTSD symptom reduction at two postdeployment assessments.
2. Adler, Bliese, McGurk, Hoge, & Castro (2009)	Battlemind debriefing (BD) (586), battlemind training (BT) in small (565) and large (618) groups	Usual postdeployment stress education (SE) (528)	Single session, 30–50 minutes' duration	U.S. soldiers after 12-month Iraq combat deployment; 95% male	BD and training in BT in small or large groups more effective than SE for participants with high combat exposure on measures of PTSD and other symptoms at 4-month follow-up.
3. Bolton et al. (2004)	CBT in succession: understanding PTSD (105), stress (62), and anger management groups (30)	N/A	Series of three consecutive groups, each 12 weeks' duration	Male veterans in VA outpatient treatment for PTSD and related concerns	Pre–post results indicated modest reduction in distress levels and high participant satisfaction; results favorable for behavior-specific group interventions
4. Cook, Walser, Kane, Ruzek, & Woody (2006)	CBT seeking safety (18)	N/A	25 sessions	Male veterans in VA treatment for PTSD, substance-use disorders	Significant improvements in PTSD and quality of life
5. Creamer, Elliott, Forbes, Biddle, & Hawthorne (2006)	Predominantly CBT group-based program, plus limited individual therapy sessions (2,223)	N/A	12 weeks, six member cohorts	Male Australian Vietnam veterans	Significant improvements in PTSD, anxiety, depression, anger at 6 months; smaller gains through 24-month follow-up

(continued)

TABLE 8.1. (continued)

Study	Treatment group (N)	Comparison group (N)	Number of sessions	Population	Major findings
6. Donovan, Padin-Rivera, & Kowaliw (2001)	Group CBT skills training, trauma processing, and peer support (46)	N/A	12 weeks, 10 hrs of group treatment per week	Male veterans with PTSD, substance-use disorders	Significant reductions in PTSD symptoms and addiction severity; maintained at 6- and 12-month follow-ups
7 Dunn et al. (2007)	Self-management therapy (SMT) (51)	Active-control therapy (ACT) (50)	14 weekly sessions	Male veterans in VA treatment for combat PTSD	SMT group demonstrated lower depression scores than ACT at posttreatment, but no differences in PTSD or depression at 3-, 6-, or 12-month follow-ups
8. Frueh, Turner, Beidel, Mirabella, & Jones (1996)	Multicomponent behavioral treatment, trauma management therapy (TMT) (15)	N/A	14 group sessions (1–3 per week); 15 individual sessions	Male Vietnam Veterans in VA treatment for combat PTSD, with comorbidity	Significant improvement for trauma-related symptoms, sexual problems, self-esteem, and general distress
9. Murphy, Thompson, Murray, Rainey, & Uddo (2009)	PTSD motivation enhancement group (PME) (60)	Psychoeducational group (PE) (54)	Four weekly sessions	Male veterans in VA outpatient treatment for PTSD	Compared to PE, PME group showed significantly more readiness for change, higher ratings for treatment relevance, and higher attendance rates

Study	Treatment (n)	Comparison (n)	Population	Dosage	Outcomes
10. Rademaker, Vermetten, & Kleber (2009)	Multimodal exposure-based group therapy (22)	N/A	Male Dutch U.N. peacekeeping veterans	Day treatment, 1 day/week, 18 months' duration	Pre–post reductions in PTSD symptoms, depression, anxiety and work-related difficulties; improvements in coping strategies and self-esteem
11. Ready et al. (2008)	Group-based exposure therapy (GBET), including stress management (102)	N/A	Male veterans in VA treatment for PTSD	16–18 sessions, biweekly	Clinically significant symptomatology reduction in most patients, maintained at 6-month follow-up; low dropout rate
12. Schnurr et al. (2003)	CBT trauma-focused group therapy (TFGT) (162)	Present-centered group therapy (PCGT) (165)	Male veterans in VA treatment for PTSD	30 weekly, followed by 5 monthly, booster sessions	Significant pre–post test improvements in PTSD for both treatment groups; no overall difference between treatment types; improvements maintained at 12 months' follow-up

PTSD; three reports (Nos. 4, 6, and 7) are "dual diagnosis" in nature, focusing on PTSD and either substance use disorder or depression; two most recent studies (Nos. 1 and 2) evaluate different group approaches to early intervention and prevention among active duty soldiers; and two studies (Nos. 3 and 9) address auxiliary issues such as motivation to participate in PTSD treatment, stress control, and anger management. Thus group therapy developers have addressed a broad range of combat-related PTSD issues, both direct and indirect. Cognitive-behavioral group approaches in a multimodal context have been used most often. Seven of the studies presented are limited in their experimental designs by the absence of control groups. However, it is encouraging that the remaining five studies are randomized controlled trials (Nos. 1, 2, 7, 9, and 12), and these offer rigorous empirical support for several group methods.

In the next section we present brief descriptions of four selected group modalities that may be particularly useful, either for active-duty members or veterans, or for both groups. Two of these formats have strong empirical support for their clinical use, whereas the others are promising but still need further field testing.

Overview of Two Empirically Based Group Therapy Methods for Core PTSD Symptoms

Trauma-Focused Group Therapy

TFGT emphasizes two cognitive-behavioral methods, systematic prolonged exposure and cognitive restructuring, to process each group member's selected combat experience. Each group member has the opportunity to recount his or her story as others listen. Therefore, group members take part in trauma processing through direct experience of their own trauma event, as well as vicariously through the experiences of others. The TFGT group model encourages both the strength of personal narrative and the power of group support; members "stand together" and bear witness to the trauma experiences of one another without judgment. Psychoeducational material regarding normal reactions to trauma and use of key coping skills bolsters group members' resources for response to current and future trauma-related reminders and symptoms (Foy, Ruzek, Glynn, Riney, & Gusman, 2002). Early-stage TFGT sessions include education about PTSD, coping resource assessment, and information about self-management of symptoms. Middle-stage sessions involve premilitary autobiographies, war zone scene identification, exposure, and cognitive restructuring. Final sessions focus on termination and relapse prevention (Schnurr et al., 2003).

Present-Centered Group Therapy

PCGT is a form of supportive group therapy that is problem oriented, providing members with additional social support in the group to improve current coping. PCGT groups avoid actual details of members' traumatic experiences, although personal consequences of trauma are acknowledged and validated. Groups are managed so that members engage emotionally with their own middle-range affects (e.g., frustration, sadness, happiness, hurt), whereas rage and terror are diffused. These groups infrequently use structured materials, and expectations for members' participation rarely involve homework or testing for mastery of material. Unlike other types of experiential groups, PCGT groups attempt to maintain a sense of interpersonal comfort and to keep transference at a low to moderate level. Other features include an active, facilitative leadership style, emphasis on members' strengths, process-encouraging interventions, combination of pragmatic and "here and now" focus, low to moderate structure, and view of change as gradual and incremental. Level of confrontation is kept in the low to moderate range (Schnurr et al., 2003).

In PCGT, early sessions focus on initiation of rapport, education about PTSD symptoms and associated features, and the connection between PTSD symptoms and difficulties in relationships and problem solving. Middle-stage sessions are aimed at identification and clarification of individual members' specific issues and the development of plans for dealing with these issues, relying heavily on interaction of group members for input and feedback. Final-stage PCGT sessions review experiences and progress in the group and other termination issues.

Overview of Two Promising Group Therapy Methods for Auxiliary Issues

Spirituality and Trauma Group Module

The spirituality and trauma group module (ST) was developed to meet the needs of veterans in residential treatment for combat-related PTSD. It is a manualized eight-session group treatment in clinical use with combat veterans since 2001. It was designed as an adjunct to other empirically supported PTSD treatments, not as a primary PTSD treatment. It utilizes brief didactic presentations by facilitators, member-to-member interactions, and large and small group discussion. Detailed descriptions of the group's development and of the module's potential for application to additional trauma populations have been provided previously (Drescher et al., 2004; Drescher, Smith, & Foy, 2007).

The ST group module has several overarching goals. One is to encourage members to consider the role that healthy spirituality might play as a healing resource in coping with traumatic events. Members' responses may include strengthening and deepening personal spiritual understandings and practices and reconnecting with their own religious or spiritual roots and traditions from childhood. Members may also explore new avenues of spiritual experience and expression that are more immediately relevant to their recent experiences. Group activities are selected to honor diversity and the inherent value of a wide variety of spiritual experiences. A second ST goal is to facilitate cognitive processing of the meanings associated with traumatic events and the personal significance members attach to them. This includes identifying cognitive distortions (e.g., inappropriate survivor guilt, including self-blame) and helping members to restructure their understandings in ways that are more adaptive. It may also include finding personal answers to the difficult existential questions of "why" and "how" these events have occurred. Group sessions include sharing feedback and reflections from other group members about the meanings they associate with these questions.

It may be that some service members return with their units from combat deployment to communities honoring them with parades and fanfare. However, many others come home individually, welcomed only by family and a few friends. Many veterans subsequently develop lives characterized by fear, distrust, and isolation. Accordingly, the third primary ST goal is to increase perceived social support, especially development of healthy family and community support systems. The ST facilitator's manual provides session-by-session clinical strategies and guidelines for implementation, using a predominantly present-centered motivation enhancement approach. The session-by-session themes include:

1. *Defining spirituality* broadly as "connecting to something outside the self."
2. *Building connections* by increasing the number and quality of social supports both within and beyond the group.
3. *Enhancing spiritual practices* by encouraging individual practices and "giving back" through community service.
4. *Addressing theodicy—the "why" question* to help members resolve possible conflicts in their images of their "higher power."
5. *Considering forgiveness of self and others* as important in reducing guilt and reestablishing positivity in life direction (two sessions).
6. *Redefining personal values* so that they are reflected in day-to-day behavior,
7. *Restoring or finding meaning in life* by "being meaningful" or finding ways to "matter" to other people.

Group Adaptation of Combat Operational Stress First Aid

Group adaptation of combat operational stress first aid (GCOSFA) is derived from combat and operational stress first aid (COSFA), a flexible early intervention for the care of psychological stress injuries in sailors and marines or their Navy and Marine Corps units (Nash, Westphal, Watson, & Litz, 2010). COSFA was derived from Psychological First Aid, which is a practical, modular approach to reducing acute stress reactions or problems in functioning and promoting adaptive coping and problem solving in post-disaster environments (Brymer et al., 2006). The development of COSFA was based on current best practices in early intervention research, expert consensus, and practical experience (Hobfoll et al., 2007); thus it is "evidence informed" in its current form. COSFA actions can serve as emergency interventions to preserve life and safety until more definitive specialized care can be provided. In milder cases of stress injury it may be the only care needed. Some components of COSFA can be delivered by almost anyone, whereas other components of COSFA require greater training and a higher initial level of skill in communication and leadership. COSFA consists of seven core actions grouped on three levels. Table 8.2 gives an overview of these elements and shows how they fit together (Nash et al., 2010).

COSFA is applied conservatively in a group format (GCOSFA), using one or more sessions as needed within the continuous and secondary aid levels depicted in Table 8.2. The core actions are applied, removing obstacles so that service members can connect with others and feel safer, calmer, more competent, and confident. The group should support unit cohesion and leadership functions and provide information on coping support. As is the case with individually applied COSFA, the focus is on providing opportunities to tailor coping information to members' needs without asking that participants share details of their losses or traumatic experiences. In each group situation, there may be a focus on one or more of the COSFA components depending on the current resources and challenges of the situation at hand.

Strengths of Group Approaches with Military Personnel

All types of group approaches have both general and specific strengths when used with military personnel.

General Strengths of All Types of Groups

1. *Familiarity:* They follow a team (small-group) training and operational model actually used by all military branches.
2. *Enhanced resources:* Participating as a group member provides social

TABLE 8.2. Overview of COSFA Levels and Core Actions

Level		Core Action	
Continuous aid	• *Ongoing* COSFA actions, performed throughout deployment cycles • Overlaps significantly with good small-unit leadership • Always individualized (one-on-one)	1.	Check	• Assess current level of distress and functioning (stress zone). • Assess immediate risks. • Assess need for additional COSFA interventions or higher levels of care. • Reassess progress.
		2.	Coordinate	• Call for help, if needed. • Decide who else should be informed of situation (e.g., commanding officer). • Refer for further evaluation or higher levels of care, if indicated. • Facilitate access to other needed care.
Primary aid	• *Acute* COSFA actions performed for a short time in response to intense distress or loss of function • Crisis management • Life-saving and health-saving • Often one-on-one	3.	Cover	• Ensure immediate physical safety of stress-injured person and others. • Foster a psychological sense of safety and comfort. • Protect from additional stress (ensure respite).
		4.	Calm	• Reduce physiological arousal (slow heart rate and breathing, relax). • Reduce intensity of negative emotions such as fear or anger. • Listen empathically if individual talks about experiences.
Secondary aid	• *Delayed* COSFA actions performed after the crisis has passed • Longer term procedures to promote healing, recovery, and return to full function • Often requires active participation by small-unit leaders	5.	Connect	• Facilitate access to primary support persons such as trusted unit or family members. • Help problem-solve to remove obstacles to social support. • Foster positive unit social activities.
		6.	Competence	• Mentor back to full functioning. • Collaborate with leaders to facilitate rewarding work roles and retraining, if necessary. • Encourage gradual reexposure to feared situations.
		7.	Confidence	• Mentor back to full confidence in self, leadership, mission, and core values. • Foster the trust of unit members and family members in the individual. • Instill hope.

support and team cohesion; groups conserve and enhance personal resources, thereby strengthening individuals' coping capacity and resilience.

3. *Efficiency and cost effectiveness:* They reduce costs when compared with individual services.
4. *Reduced stigma:* They normalize educational/preventive services being received with peers using a nonpathologizing model.

Specific Strengths of Different Types of Groups

The group formats with the strongest empirical support, TFGT and PCGT, are well suited for clinical use with veterans in treatment for chronic PTSD. For those veterans who have a preference for therapy involving direct exposure to their traumatic memories, TFGT or one of the other exposure-based approaches featured in Table 8.1 may be selected. PCGT is a better match for those preferring a "here and now" focus that does not include directly addressing traumatic memories. The ST group may be indicated as an adjunct when spiritual issues such as guilt, forgiveness, and meaning arise among veterans or active-duty members in PTSD treatment. GCOSFA, with its emphasis on early intervention or prevention, is advantageous because it may be adapted for use with active duty-members in predeployment, deployment, and postdeployment time frames. Using psychoeducation, normalization, and information to prepare for upcoming mission challenges, GCOSFA groups seem especially useful when major transitions in deployment status are imminent.

Limitations of Group Approaches with Military Personnel

A key potential risk in all the groups described is retraumatization, or unplanned activation of traumatic experiences through exposure to other members' recounting of their experiences. With the exception of TFGT, none of the group modalities includes systematic trauma narrative work by group members as a goal; however, members may inadvertently refer to their experiences in sufficient detail to elicit reactivation among other group members. Establishing firm group operating rules about remaining present-focused without recounting traumatic experiences in group discussions is essential for PCGT, ST, and GCOSFA formats.

When considering matching service members or veterans with an ST group, individual choice needs to be honored. Although most individuals recognize and value a spiritual dimension to their life experience, there may be some for whom this is not the case. For those, as well as others who do not wish to address broadly defined spiritual issues, the ST group is contraindicated.

For GCOSFA groups convened in the wake of a traumatic combat or deployment event involving deaths of comrades, timing and staging of the group are critical issues. In particular, GCOSFA planners need to consider that wide variation among individuals in grief reactions is normal and expected. Thus care should be taken so that natural, healthy denial among members is not challenged, nor is grief pathologized. Group leaders need to keep in mind that restabilization is the expected norm, and the risk for raising expectations of pathological outcomes should be minimized. Another risk to be managed involves the belief that therapy within the group is all that will be required to deal with members' experiences, so that individuals with greater needs will not seek further care. This particular risk applies to group leaders, as well as members. Finally, in keeping with the basic first-aid principle, GCOSFA should be timed to avoid inappropriate application in settings in which physical survival is a greater priority.

Therapeutic Considerations

There are key group therapist competencies that are critical to success in delivering the formats we have presented. Ideally, group facilitators will have extensive knowledge, experience, and skills in combat-related trauma issues, group therapy principles, and cognitive-behavioral techniques. For TFGT, group facilitators need specific skills in applying exposure and cognitive restructuring therapies. ST facilitators do not have to be members of the clergy, but they do need to value and respect diversity in personal experiences and expressions of spirituality. Ideally, an ST group might be co-led by a clergy member and a mental health professional. GCOSFA group facilitators need expertise in the application of the core skill areas of combat and operational stress first aid.

Treatment Fidelity and Supervision Issues

Three of the group formats we have presented offer manuals to guide facilitators—a major benefit with respect to fidelity and supervision considerations. Along with the manuals, adherence checklists are also available to ensure that key elements of each session are addressed. In field testing and more formal treatment outcome research, independent adherence ratings can be performed on session tapes to evaluate adherence more rigorously. The use of manuals and fidelity checks for routine session-by-session guidance allows supervision to focus more specifically on other group leadership issues that may arise.

Although it may not always be possible, our recommendation is that all of the group formats be co-led by two facilitators. The adage "two heads are better than one" applies here. We also recommend an immediate post-session debrief and critique between the facilitators. In addition to ongoing supervision for inexperienced group facilitators, ready consultative access to a more senior or "master" group therapist is also highly desirable.

Case Vignette

Sergeant James Jones (not his actual name) is a 25-year-old Marine who has recently completed a third tour of combat duty, this time in Afghanistan. James reports that he has been having problems, including severe anxiety, anger, and relationship problems with his parents and his girlfriend. Doctors are now telling him that he might have a mild traumatic brain injury (TBI) from a blast he survived during his last combat tour. A recent physical alter-cation with another Marine raised his command's attention to his adjust-ment problems, and Sergeant Jones was transferred to a warrior transition program for evaluation and treatment referral that could lead to a medical discharge.

In reflecting on his wartime experiences, James states that sometime during his second combat tour "something just died inside." He no longer felt fear or anxiety; he felt like a machine. He pushed his men and himself hard and was merciless in response to insurgent attacks and ambushes. He stopped calling home and withdrew from friends during downtime at the base in between missions. He reports that he spent much of his third tour in Afghanistan at a remote FOB (forward operating base) where conditions were harsh and Taliban attacks were frequent. His most difficult incident happened during a convoy returning from the FOB to Bagrahm air base just 2 weeks before they were scheduled to return to the states. He reports that his vehicle hit an improvised explosive device (IED) that blew off the front of the Humvee. The young lance corporal sitting in the front passenger seat was blown out of the vehicle. Sergeant Jones reports that he was dazed by the blast, and when he came to, it was to screams of "medic." He struggled out of the vehicle, hearing heavy machine gun fire being directed at them from a ridge above them. Two of his men had pulled Corporal Evans to safety and were frantically trying to bind his mangled leg and apply a tour-niquet to stop the spurting blood. Sergeant Jones reports that he screamed at the turret gunner to direct 50-caliber fire toward the insurgents and moved around to look at the other side of the vehicle. Corporal Smith was slumped at the back of the vehicle, almost like he was sleeping. He had somehow taken a round to the side of his head under his helmet and was dead. When they were able to direct sufficient fire to clear the insurgents and land a medevac (medical evaluation) helicopter, Corporal Evans was flown to the base hospital, where he was stabilized and later sent to the central medical facility in Landstuhl, Germany. Jones hasn't seen Evans since but heard that he lost his right leg.

During the memorial service for Corporal Smith, James found himself getting extremely angry at the presiding chaplain and walked away when the chaplain tried to approach him after the service. James states that he had lost much of his religious faith earlier in the war but that this event was like the straw that broke the camel's back—it has left him extremely angry at God for killing Corporal Smith. Now, the thought of going to church sends him into a rage, much to his family's dismay. James is tormented by the belief that he failed his men and should have been able to keep them safe, especially when they were so close to leaving the war zone. He believes that it is horribly unfair and a harsh trick by God that Smith died when he had a beautiful wife and baby boy that he never saw in person. James went to visit Smith's family to pay his respects, felt so guilty he could hardly look them in the face, then got very drunk afterward.

James's diagnosis is combat-related PTSD, and he is receiving cognitive processing therapy in an individual format. In addition, his psychologist suggested that James might benefit from participation in an eight-session ST group co-led by the transition program's social worker and chaplain. James was initially reluctant to accept referral to the ST group but decided that he would go for at least two sessions to "give it a try." After attending the first session, James checked in with his therapist on his experience.

THERAPIST: So what are your thoughts about the ST group so far?

JAMES: At first I didn't think it was for me, but the other group members were as skeptical as I was, and that helped me feel like maybe I belonged there after all. There are seven other group members and we come from different religious backgrounds—Catholic, Protestant, and Jewish. We agreed that the group ethic is to value each individual's personal faith tradition, so there's no "right" set of beliefs.

THERAPIST: We agreed that you were going to attend the first two sessions, but the group has seven more sessions. What have you decided about attending the rest of the sessions?

JAMES: Well, I think there may be something there for me to make it worthwhile to finish it. The next sessions deal with guilt and forgiveness, and I have to say that those are some of my issues.

THERAPIST: OK, then. We will keep checking in during our sessions to see how your experience in the ST group is going.

References

Adler, A. B., Bliese, P. D., McGurk, D., Hoge, C. W., & Castro, C. A. (2009). Battlemind debriefing and battlemind training as early interventions with soldiers returning from Iraq: Randomization by platoon. *Journal of Consulting and Clinical Psychology, 77*(5), 928–940.

Adler, A. B., Litz, B. T., Castro, C. A., Suvak, M., Thomas, J. L., Burrell, L., et al. (2008). A group randomized trial of critical incident stress debriefing provided to U. S. peacekeepers. *Journal of Traumatic Stress. 21*(3), 253–263.

Bolton, E. E., Lambert, J. F., Wolf, E. J., Raja, S., Varra, A. A., & Fisher, L. M. (2004). Evaluation of a cognitive-behavioral group treatment program for veterans with posttraumatic stress disorder. *Psychological Services, 1*(2), 140–146.

Brymer, M., Jacobs, A., Layne, C., Pynoos, R., Ruzek, J., Steinberg, A., et al. (2006). *Psychological first aid: Field operations guide* (2nd ed.). Retrieved from *www. nctsn.org* and *www.ncptsd.va.gov*.

Cook, J. M., Walser, R. D., Kane, V., Ruzek, J. I., & Woody, G. (2006). Dissemination and feasibility of a cognitive-behavioral treatment for substance use disorders and posttraumatic stress disorder in the veterans' administration. *Journal of Psychoactive Drugs, 38,* 89–92.

Creamer, M., Elliott, P., Forbes, D., Biddle, D., & Hawthorne, G. (2006). Treatment for combat-related posttraumatic stress disorder: Two-year follow-up. *Journal of Traumatic Stress, 19,* 675–685.

Donovan, B., Padin-Rivera, E., & Kowaliw, S. (2001). "Transcend": Initial outcomes from a posttraumatic stress disorder/substance abuse treatment program. *Journal of Traumatic Stress, 14,* 757–772.

Drescher, K. D., Ramirez, G., Leoni, J. J., Romesser, J. M., Sornborger, J., & Foy, D. W. (2004). Spirituality and trauma: Development of a group therapy module. *Group: The Journal of the Eastern Group Psychotherapy Society, 28(4),* 71–87.

Drescher, K. D., Smith, M. W., & Foy, D. W. (2007). Spirituality and readjustment following war-zone experiences. In C. R. Figley & W. P. Nash (Eds.), *Combat stress injury theory, research, and management* (pp. 486–511). New York: Routledge Press.

Dunn, N. J., Rehm, L. P., Schillaci, J., Souchek, J., Mehta, P. D., Ashton, C. M., et al. (2007). A randomized trial of self-management and psychoeducational group therapies for comorbid chronic posttraumatic stress disorder and depressive disorder. *Journal of Traumatic Stress, 20*(3), 221–237.

Dynes, J. B. (1945). Rehabilitation of war casualties. *War Medicine, 7,* 32–35.

Foy, D. W., Drescher, K. D., & Watson, P. J. (in press). Group interventions for trauma/disaster. In R. Conyne (Ed.), *Oxford handbook of group counseling.* New York: Oxford University Press.

Foy, D. W., Ruzek, J. I., Glynn, S. M., Riney, S. A., & Gusman, F. D. (2002). Trauma focus group therapy for combat-related PTSD: An update. *Journal of Clinical Psychology, 58*(8), 907–918.

Frueh, B. C., Turner, S. M., Beidel, D. C., Mirabella, R. F., & Jones, W. J. (1996). Trauma management therapy: A preliminary evaluation of a multicomponent behavioral treatment for chronic combat-related PTSD. *Behavior Therapy and Research, 34,* 533–543.

Gusman, F. D., Stewart, J., Hiley-Young, B., Riney, S. J., Abueg, F. R., & Blake, D. D. (1996). A multicultural developmental approach for treating trauma. In A. J. Marsella, M. J. Friedman, E. T. Gerrity, & R. M Scurfield (Eds.), *Ethnocultural aspects of postraumatic stress disorder: Issues, research, and clinical applications* (pp. 439–457). Washington, DC: American Psychological Association.

Hobfoll, S. E., Watson, P. J., Bell, C. C., Bryant, R. A., Brymer, M. J., Friedman, M. J., et al. (2007). Five essential elements of immediate and mid-term mass trauma intervention: Empirical evidence. *Psychiatry, 70*(4), 283–315.

Murphy, R. T., Thompson, K. E., Murray, M., Rainey, Q., & Uddo, M. M. (2009). Effect of a motivation enhancement intervention on veterans' engagement in PTSD treatment. *Psychological Services, 6*(4), 264–278.

Nash, W. P., Westphal, R. J., Watson, P. J., & Litz, B. T. (2010). *Combat and operational stress first aid: Caregiver training manual.* Washington, DC: U.S. Navy, Bureau of Medicine and Surgery.

Rademaker, A. R., Vermetten, E., & Kleber, R. J. (2009). Multimodal exposure-based treatment for peacekeepers with PTSD: A preliminary evaluation. *Military Psychology, 21,* 482–491.

Ready, D. J., Thomas, K. R., Worley, V., Backsheider, A. G., Harvey, L. A. C., Baltzell, D., et al. (2008). A field test of group based exposure therapy with 102 veterans with war-related posttraumatic stress disorder. *Journal of Traumatic Stress, 21*(2), 150–157.

Schnurr, P. P., Friedman, M. F., Foy, D. W., Shea, M. T., Hsieh, F. Y., Lavori, P. W., et al. (2003). Randomized trial of trauma-focused group therapy for posttraumatic stress disorder: Results from a Department of Veterans Affairs cooperative study. *Archives of General Psychiatry, 60,* 481–489.

Seidel, R. W., Gusman, F. D., & Abueg, F. R. (1994). Theoretical and practical foundations of an inpatient posttraumatic stress disorder and alcoholism treatment program. *Psychotherapy, 31*(1), 67–77.

Sipprelle, R. C. (1992). A vet center experience: Multievent trauma, delayed treatment type. In D. Foy (Ed.), *Treating PTSD: Cognitive-behavioral strategies* (pp. 13–38). New York: Guilford Press.

CHAPTER 9

Couple and Family Therapy

Danielle J. Maack
Judith A. Lyons
Kevin M. Connolly
Michael Ritter

Increasing numbers of service members and their loved ones are suffering the effects of military-related trauma experiences. When a veteran returns home following combat experience, he or she may be met with some uncertainty about changes or questions about how the partner and family will readjust to the new relationship. The veteran may feel particularly relieved and happy to be reunited with loved ones, but these feelings may also be coupled with feelings of guilt and shame from decisions or actions made while in combat and may cause confusion and insecurity about his or her identity (Erbes, Polusny, MacDermid, & Compton, 2008). Family or partner roles may have shifted while the veteran was separated from the family, and these relationships may need to be renegotiated. Under all these pressures, with high expectations following the veteran's return, potential for relationship difficulties is high. Effects of posttraumatic stress disorder (PTSD) can extend beyond the spouse to the family unit with difficulties seen in parenting, poor family functioning, and behavioral problems in children of parents with PTSD (Cloutier, Manion, & Walker, 2002).

Family systems theory states that families will respond to stress in one of four ways: the family may become distanced from one another, an individual may sacrifice his or her own level of functioning for the sake of the family, the family can become conflicted, or the family can bond in an adaptive way and move forward (Kerr & Bowen, 1988). Research on PTSD continually supports the idea that symptomatology affects functioning in a number of different functional domains. For example, relative to trauma without PTSD, veterans suffering from PTSD have increased likelihood of divorce, higher rates of verbal and physical aggression, greater variety of and more severe relationship problems, and more demonstrated difficulties with expressing emotions (Monson, Fredman, & Adair, 2008). The odds of veterans with PTSD being unemployed increase by 150%, those of marital instability by 60%, and their risk of suicide associated with PTSD is larger than with any other anxiety disorder (Kessler, 2000). PTSD has been associated with a myriad of difficulties in family and marital relationships, including aggression toward partners and children, emotional distancing, and sexual dysfunction. The corrosive effect of traumatization on intimate relationships emphasizes the need for conjoint and family therapies for PTSD (Monson et al., 2008; Riggs, 2000).

Including family in therapy has been shown to improve treatment outcomes of schizophrenia (Falloon, Roncone, Held, Coverdale, & Laidlaw, 2002), bipolar disorder (Miklowitz & Goldstein, 1990), and depression (Jacobson, Dobson, Fruzzetti, Schmaling, & Salusky, 1991). Similarly, evidence suggests that family and friends play a major role in recovery from PTSD (Brewin, Andrews, & Valentine, 2000). Family engagement in treatment has been shown to improve communication between family and the treatment team by helping to teach families ways to respond to the patient's illness (Liberman, 1988). A study by Sautter et al. (2006) sought to identify predictors of partner PTSD treatment engagement in a sample of Vietnam veterans and their partners. Results from this study demonstrated that income, partner/caregiver burden, and patient–partner involvement significantly relate to partner PTSD treatment engagement. Partners who reported being most engaged in the veteran's PTSD treatment also reported high involvement in other aspects of the veteran's daily life, such as providing transportation and doing chores together.

A study by Tarrier, Sommerfield, and Pilgrim (1999) found that the relationship between the client and his or her relative can have a significant impact on treatment, depending on the relative's expressed emotion. Exhibiting more hostility and criticism (high expressed emotion) was predictive of PTSD symptom levels in clients presenting for treatment. Negative family relationships accounted for about 20% of the variance in PTSD treatment outcome. Thus couples and family relationships can serve either as support or as a challenging obstacle to recovery from PTSD, and targeting the family context may enhance outcomes.

A study by Batten et al. (2009) assessed veteran interest in family treatment involvement. Veterans (N = 114) enrolled in a trauma recovery program at a VA medical center and completed a brief survey providing information about the extent to which they would like to see an emphasis on family-focused treatment for PTSD. Seventy-nine percent of the veterans surveyed expressed interest in greater family involvement in their treatment, and 72% thought a family member would be interested in attending a couples or family support group. This interest existed regardless of whether or not the veteran had a spouse or children. Taken as a whole, this line of research suggests the importance of the integration and/or focus of family relationships in the treatment of PTSD.

Overview of Couple Therapy

Couple/family therapy can help couples cope more effectively with PTSD symptoms, can assist partners in understanding and empathizing with confusing behavioral and emotional changes, and also can help to strengthen intimate relationships (Erbes et al., 2008; Johnson & Williams-Keeler, 1998). There are typically two different approaches to couple/family treatment for PTSD, as described by Riggs (2000): systemic treatment, using the traditional couples/marital therapy model to reduce relationship distress caused by the trauma and subsequent symptoms of PTSD, and (2) supportive therapies, or interventions with the aim of reducing PTSD symptoms of an individual by increasing his or her social support. Both approaches offer direction for the family to be a support system as opposed to an obstacle in the individual's treatment and recovery from PTSD. This is in line with family systems, as these approaches attempt to promote family or couple bonding and forward movement in the relationship(s). Systemic therapies include a focus on disruptions to the family system caused by the trauma and PTSD symptoms, with treatment focusing on repairing the family dynamic and decreasing stress to the family system. Systemic therapies draw from couples and family treatment, but a concern with these therapies is that the treatment focus marginalizes the treatment of PTSD itself. Supportive therapies, on the other hand, directly target PTSD symptoms and incorporate support of the partner or family in helping the individual to recover. Some support measures offer psychoeducation to the family members about the nature of PTSD, its symptoms, and treatment. Much research in the area of couple/family therapies and trauma has been conducted in the military sector, with civilian treatment based on evidence from therapy completed with veterans (Monson et al., 2008). Examples and descriptions of these types of family/couple therapies applied to individuals with PTSD follow.

Emotion-focused therapy (EFT) has been applied to couples in which one or both partners have experienced past sexual and/or physical abuse, violent crime, natural disasters, or chronic or terminal illness (Johnson & Williams-Keeler, 1998). Instead of focusing on communication and connecting with others, trauma survivors may focus on personal safety and protecting themselves. EFT is designed to help partners reprocess their emotional responses to one another and thus change their pattern of interaction, leading to a more secure attachment. EFT has demonstrated long-term benefit in couples, with continued improvements in marital functioning seen in couples with chronically ill children at 2-year follow-up (Cloutier et al., 2002), and, in couples with attachment injuries, benefits from EFT were maintained over a 3-year follow-up (Halchuk, Makinen, & Johnson, 2010).

The most recent version of cognitive-behavioral conjoint therapy for PTSD (CBCT; Monson et al., 2008) is based on the theory that the association between PTSD symptoms and distress in relationships is complex and dynamic. Symptoms of PTSD contribute to partner distress, which in turn maintains and exacerbates PTSD symptomatology. Underlying this association are communication skills deficits, as well as behavioral avoidance. Cognitively, the interaction between maladaptive thought processes and content related to the traumatic event(s) maintains this cycle of association. CBCT treats the couple as a unit. It is designed as a 15-session (75 minutes each) treatment consisting of three stages: (1) treatment orientation, psychoeducation about PTSD, and safety building; (2) behavioral interventions that increase approach behaviors, increase relationship satisfaction, and facilitate communication; and (3) cognitive interventions to address maladaptive cognitions that maintain PTSD symptoms, as well as relational difficulties. Although formal evaluation of the present model of CBCT has yet to be completed, in the previous iteration of CBCT (which was more present focused) veterans reported modest improvements in PTSD symptoms, with greater improvements seen in depression, anxiety, and social functioning. Veterans' spouses reported major improvements in relationship satisfaction, as well as improvements in social functioning (Monson, Schnurr, Stevens, & Guthrie, 2004).

Strategic approach therapy (SAT) is a 10-session, couple-based, manualized behavioral marital therapy designed to target avoidance symptoms of PTSD (Sautter, Glynn, Thompson, Franklin, & Han, 2009). This treatment uses partner-based interventions to reduce anxiety and effortful avoidance and behavioral exchange techniques to reduce emotional numbing. Sautter and colleagues recruited six Vietnam veterans diagnosed with PTSD and their partners to receive SAT. The treatment consisted of three phases: (1) psychoeducation about PTSD and motivational enhancement, (2) behavior activation to increase behaviors that promote positive emotions, and (3) partner-assisted anxiety reduction. Pre–post change in scores from self-report, partner-, and clinician-rated measures indicated significant decreases in emotional numbing, overall PTSD severity, and effortful avoidance. These findings lend additional support to the idea that the involvement of partners and family in mental health treatment can improve treatment outcome. Results indicate that SAT may prove helpful in reducing avoidance symptoms of PTSD, which generally function to maintain PTSD symptoms. This approach has been used with couples in which one partner is diagnosed with PTSD, but it has also been used with couples in which both partners have been diagnosed with PTSD. Sautter et al.'s (2009) study was the first to provide preliminary support for the use of SAT as treatment for PTSD avoidance symptoms; however, more research is needed. This pilot study included only six couples, using a pre–post design. Although preliminary findings suggest the usefulness and feasibility of SAT as a treatment for PTSD, larger, well-controlled studies with posttreatment follow-up are needed to evaluate efficacy.

Another treatment adapted for couples with a partner experiencing PTSD is integrative behavioral couple therapy (IBCT; Jacobson, Christensen, Prince, Cordova, & Eldridge, 2000; adaptation for PTSD, Erbes et al., 2008). The primary emphasis in IBCT is to help partners accept aspects of each other and their relationship that have come to be viewed as intolerable and obscure. IBCT emphasizes the balance between acceptance and change strategies to target relationship and individual problems faced by couples when a partner has PTSD. In addition, IBCT highlights the role of experiential avoidance as causing the individual to distance him- or herself from interpersonal relationships. This avoidance also prevents the individual from approaching opportunities to face any discomfort and thus hinders recovery. As described, IBCT for PTSD emphasizes four target areas for treatment. First, IBCT reduces conflict and increases partner intimacy, which may lead to reductions in stress for both partners and help promote social support and recovery. Second, IBCT promotes acceptance, tolerance, and expression of emotions that underlie anger, such as hurt, fear, and sadness—this aspect is seen as a functional opposite of experiential avoidance. Third, IBCT focuses on skills acquisition and generalizing strategies to improve communication and problem-solving skills. Finally, IBCT emphasizes intimacy and increased positive activities, fostering relational exposure to confront situations, feelings, and conversations that, when avoided, maintain PTSD symptomatology. In applying IBCT to PTSD, the goal is to enhance exposure to current life events and relationships that the individual(s) may be avoiding due to trauma, and not necessarily to work on exposure to past traumatic events.

For couples with marital problems, IBCT has demonstrated effectiveness as an acceptance-based treatment for marital discord (Jacobson et al., 2000). Christensen, Atkins, Baucom, and Yi (2010) reported follow-up results from a randomized control trial that assessed marital distress over 5 years following 8 months of either traditional behavioral couple therapy or IBCT. At 5-year follow-up, couples who stayed together demonstrated substantial improvement from their pretreatment satisfaction scores, suggesting that enduring changes were made during therapy and further offering support for IBCT for couple discord.

Strengths of Couple Therapy with Military Personnel

Family and/or couple treatment for trauma is a specific type of treatment that incorporates the family unit and encourages the family to come together with the service member in such a way that they do not feel alienated. It is common for families and friends to fail to understand the veteran's experience of war and how an individual's thoughts and feelings have changed. Greater social support has been identified as one of the strongest correlates of lower PTSD rates (Brewin et al., 2000). Incorporating the family into the treatment can, in a sense, bring the family unit closer as the veteran works through treatment. For many veterans, the stress and consequences of combat deployments do not resolve upon returning home; the application of therapy focused on couples has proved useful in treating combat-related stress (Erbes et al., 2008).

Limitations of Couple Therapy with Military Personnel

Although interventions and therapy incorporating couples and family in treatment appear promising to help alleviate the symptoms of PTSD, there are a number of limitations that may hinder treatment. First, a major barrier to couple and family treatment for PTSD is that participation rates for this type of treatment are low (Glynn et al., 1999; Sautter et al., 2006). This is not uncommon to family interventions across many different populations, and it certainly is not specifically related to military personal seeking treatment for PTSD.

This low family/partner engagement could arise from a myriad of issues. A study by Lyons and Root (2001) assessed members from family focus groups within VA PTSD clinics and reported that travel, distance, and scheduling conflicts were most frequently cited as reasons for not engaging in couple/family treatment. Scheduling conflicts were prominent, especially at sites that do not offer evening or weekend appointments. In another study, conflicting work schedules and lack of child care were reasons cited for nonattendance by family members (Glynn et al., 1999).

Research completed at the Oklahoma City VA (Sherman, Blevins, Kirchner, Ridener, & Jackson, 2008) assessed key factors involved in engaging significant others in the treatment of PTSD. This study focused on Vietnam veterans and their partners. Nine themes emerged demonstrating that family participation is a complex phenomenon that is not well understood.

Two areas of particular concern were participation and logistical barriers. Concerns about participation included the following: lack of awareness that such programs existed, unavailability of family members who lived close enough to participate, lack of family willingness to understand the Veteran, and fear of family member being exposed to upsetting information about the veteran's trauma. Logistical barriers included geographical distance from the hospital, parking difficulties, conflicts with work schedules, finances, and lack of child care.

To help break these treatment barriers, it is important to publicize the availability of services for the veterans and their families. In addition, emphasizing the potential benefits for both veteran and family members is crucial to eliciting treatment acceptance and to instilling hope. It is essential to be as flexible as possible in scheduling appointments to meet the family's needs. Offering evening clinic hours at least one day a week may increase the likelihood of partner availability to attend sessions. As research continues to demonstrate the benefits of couple/family-based therapies, working to overcome these obstacles to treatment becomes more vital.

Therapeutic Considerations

It is important to note that family involvement in treatment may not be appropriate in all cases. Thus there are a number of individual factors to consider before initiating couple-based therapy for PTSD. Acute behavioral problems, including the possibility of domestic violence, substance use, child abuse, and suicidal or homicidal tendencies often need to be addressed prior to beginning couple/family therapy for PTSD. Individual or group therapy focused on these issues may be needed prior to engaging in family/couple therapy.

Although the veteran's trauma may be addressed in the course of couple or family treatment, it may not be therapeutic to encourage specific disclosure of traumatic events within the context of the couple. This may be especially true regarding combat events in which the soldier was an active participant (Erbes et al., 2008). The therapist cannot control the partner's reaction to a service member's trauma disclosure and may not be able to provide a safe and corrective environment for such exposure.

Overall, the decision to provide treatment in a family or couple context needs to be made based on the individual's situation and available resources. If partner attendance is sporadic or if the partner is unable or unwilling to participate in therapy sessions, adaptation of these therapies may be warranted. In this way, a strategy is provided to address issues in the couple or family even while the family member is not present in session. In addition, many programs currently do not have the resources or personnel to offer couple/family therapy to veterans. An approach for working with the individual to incorporate a partner/family focus is presented in the following section of this chapter.

A Strategy for Addressing Family Functioning through Individual Therapy with the Veteran/Service Member

What options does a therapist have when family functioning is obviously impaired, yet the family cannot be engaged in treatment due to attendance barriers, concerns regarding secondary traumatization, or other factors? One option that has yielded encouraging clinical benefit (described later) incorporates training in goal setting with *in vivo* exposure exercises. This strategy focuses on the avoidance of crowded social and/or emotionally charged situations. Such avoidance frequently precludes participation in activities that involve more than immediate family (children's ball games, restaurant/movie/concert dates, family/class reunions, shopping, etc.). One of the most common complaints of spouses pertains to a sense of being "married but alone"—a social isolation that stems from their partners' unwillingness to participate in normative family and social activities (Lyons & Root, 2001). Increasing the trauma survivor's tolerance of challenging social environments and interactions aims to yield improved relationship functioning without requiring the direct engagement of the partner or children in therapy. Many PTSD programs are already incorporating Foa, Hembree, and Rothbaum's (2007) prolonged exposure protocol. That protocol trains clients to establish hierarchies of avoided activities and engage in imaginal and *in vivo* exposure. The prolonged exposure protocol emphasizes situations that are avoided because they trigger trauma memories. However, using Foa's framework or other behavioral goal-setting models, therapists can easily incorporate an emphasis on family-relevant goals and activities even if these are not already included in the person's trauma-trigger hierarchy. Thus incorporating specifically designed *in vivo* exposure exercises can improve not only PTSD symptoms but also the veteran's family situation. Following is a case vignette illustrating this method in practice.

Case Vignette

Eddie (not his actual name) had returned from combat in Iraq several years earlier. He was able to maintain employment but had withdrawn from nearly all social activities due to anxiety and overall fatigue stemming from frequent nightmares. He had divorced his wife several months earlier and was estranged from the two children from that marriage (ages 9 and 15), having had no contact in the previous 4 months. He had remarried a month earlier after a very brief courtship. Eddie had hoped his new marriage would end his loneliness, but the marriage was already showing strain, and he continued to feel alone and isolated.

Eddie enrolled in an 8-week Veterans Affairs residential program that emphasized imaginal and *in vivo* exposure. At admission, Eddie identified several activities that he was avoiding: hunting and fishing, "crowds" (i.e., son's ball games, wrestling matches), waiting in lines, driving, attending church, dining in restaurants, and visiting family members. Each of these activities is something he described as quite difficult and rarely (if ever) engaged in due to the associated anxiety. He reported that the ability to resume each of these activities would improve his quality of life and relationships.

Eddie lodged at the facility Sunday evening until midafternoon on Friday each week, and then spent weekends at home. While at the medical center during the week, he practiced sitting in public areas of the hospital and engaged in imaginal practice of his individual weekend goals. He learned to self-monitor his progress using the Subjective Units of Distress scale (SUDS). Each weekend, he tackled at least one previously avoided family activity. When he returned to the program Sunday evening, he reported on his accomplishment of these goals and on the challenges he encountered. During the subsequent week, additional group sessions helped him identify ways to address similar challenges in the future and extend his goals for the next weekend. As treatment progressed, group and individual sessions and interdisciplinary treatment team rounds each reinforced his progress and helped him refine his understanding of the principles underlying hierarchical goal setting and imaginal plus *in vivo* exposure.

During the first week of his admission, Eddie contacted his estranged son and quickly received a positive response. For his first weekend home, he planned to watch his son play football on Saturday and to take his wife to a restaurant on Sunday. When he returned to the facility, he reported that he had met both goals. He reported a distress rating of 6–7 on a 0–10 scale while at his son's football game. Reminding himself of why he was there helped him to tolerate the anxiety. Dinner with his wife was difficult as well. He asked to sit in the back of the restaurant and needed a few moments to himself, but he was able to stay at the restaurant in spite of a distress rating of 8.

On subsequent weekends, Eddie continued to attend portions of his son's high school football games, beginning by staying on the fringe of the crowd for very short periods. As his son's team kept advancing in the playoffs, the crowds at games got larger. By the end of the 8-week admission, Eddie was able to be present during a portion of his son's championship game. Activities with his wife followed a similar progression.

The final session of his goal-setting group discussed how to continue self-directed progress on his goals and how to avoid relapse. He left with a plan to visit his parents regularly on his way home from work, to call his children and continue to schedule activities with them, and to reserve time each evening to spend with his wife. He identified fishing, movies, going to the park, and shopping as activities he planned to share with his wife and children after discharge.

Eddie continued to increase his outings with family during his first week at home; however, by the third week after discharge, he had reverted to his old habits. Peers in his long-term outpatient group encouraged him to resume family activities and gave examples of the personal costs of their own struggles with anxiety and isolation. He was reminded to maintain contact with peers from his residential cohort for mutual encouragement. He acknowledged that he had not been able to maintain the same level of effort once he returned to the daily demands of job, chores, and so forth. He was also discouraged that family expectations were increasing at a trajectory that was steeper than his incremental progress. Gradually, he began to regain, on an outpatient basis, the momentum he had begun while in the residential program.

Strengths of Goal Setting
and *In Vivo* Practice in Improving Family Functioning

This treatment strategy offers a mechanism for influencing family functioning even when family members are unable to participate in the therapy. When families are separated because of deployment, this option remains available by setting goals for shared communication. Similarly, it provides an alternative when scheduling, travel burden, or other barriers interfere with family treatment engagement. The emphasis on behavior change may be particularly helpful if resentment on the part of a family member is the primary factor impeding his or her treatment engagement; witnessing objective changes in behavior can facilitate resolution of anger and trust issues.

Limitations of Goal Setting
and *In Vivo* Practice in Improving Family Functioning

As seen in Eddie's case, behavior change can be difficult to sustain even after excellent initial progress. Unrealistic family expectations may undermine maintenance of treatment gains—a risk that is likely to be greater when family members are not involved in treatment discussions.

In a classic study that helped launch the field of behavioral marital therapy, Wills, Weiss, and Patterson (1974) demonstrated systematic inaccuracies in each spouse's ability to identify what behavior changes would please his or her mate. The goals set by the patient may not match family priorities for behavior change. One way that family input can be obtained, even in the context of individual therapy, is to have the client generate the list of behavior change goals and then ask the family to identify (within that list) the behaviors that are highest priority, as well as any planned behaviors that would be *un*welcome rather than desired.

Therapeutic Considerations of Goal Setting and *In Vivo* Practice in Improving Family Functioning

Most therapists are already familiar with goal-setting models for behavior change (setting objectively measurable, incremental goals). Many therapists working in PTSD programs are also familiar with the basics of imaginal and *in vivo* exposure therapy. Both models require clinical judgment to determine the pacing of increasingly challenging tasks. Ability to help the patient anticipate likely obstacles and brainstorm effective coping strategies is important.

When combined with trauma-focused prolonged exposure, the therapist must have a clear understanding of where family-related behavior change goals converge or diverge from *in vivo* tasks within the prolonged exposure protocol. In exposure therapy, the emphasis is on maintaining awareness of anxiety and tolerating that anxiety until it dissipates; deliberate distractions from the anxiety are discouraged. However, during homework assignments in which the goal is to improve social functioning, distraction or other anxiety-mitigating coping strategies can sometimes be appropriate. For example, if the veteran is attending a child's graduation ceremony, the emphasis may be on staying at least until the child crosses the stage, even if relaxation or distraction tactics must be utilized to empower the veteran to stay. Helping the veteran differentiate times at which exposure is the priority (long-term goal of overcoming anxiety) from those at which social functioning is the priority (short-term goal of performing a social task successfully) can clarify the occasions when these two contradictory tactics are each appropriate.

Conclusion

As illustrated, PTSD symptoms do not affect only the individual but can also have dramatic consequences on relationships and families. An increasing number of service members are facing the difficulty of reintegrating into their homes and communities while dealing with these symptoms.

Research is beginning to assess the difficulties of living with and treating PTSD within the context of family systems. Preliminary findings regarding family- and couple-oriented interventions support the efficacy of tailoring these approaches to the treatment of PTSD. However, concerns about incorporating family or partners into treatment are evident. Lack of awareness of existing programs, unavailability of family members who live close enough to participate, and unwillingness of family to try to understand the veteran are common barriers to this type of treatment. A case example was provided offering options for a treatment approach that can influence family functioning even when family members are unable to participate in the therapy. Taken as a whole, the literature provides support for using couple/family interventions in the treatment of PTSD. In this way, not only is the individual receiving help with his or her PTSD symptoms, but this dynamic intervention also provides help with navigating the difficult transition of integrating back into the family and community.

Acknowledgments

This chapter is the result of work supported with resources and the use of facilities at the G. V. (Sonny) Montgomery VA Medical Center, Jackson, Mississippi, with additional support from VA South Central Mental Illness Research, Education and Clinical Center. The views expressed here represent those of the authors and do not necessarily represent the views of the Department of Veterans Affairs or the University of Mississippi Medical Center.

References

Batten, S. V., Drapalski, A. L., Decker, M. L., DeViva, J. C., Morris, L. J., Mann, M. A., et al. (2009). Veteran interest in family involvement in PTSD treatment. *Psychological Services, 6*(3), 184–189.

Brewin, C. R., Andrews, B., & Valentine, J. D. (2000). Meta-analysis of risk factors for posttraumatic stress disorder in trauma-exposed adults. *Journal of Consulting and Clinical Psychology, 68*(5), 748–766.

Christensen, A., Atkins, D. C., Baucom, B., & Yi, J. (2010). Marital status and satisfaction five years following a randomized clinical trial comparing traditional versus integrative behavioral couple therapy. *Journal of Consulting and Clinical Psychology, 78*(2), 225–235.

Cloutier, P. F., Manion, I. G., & Walker, J. G. (2002). Emotionally focused interventions for couples with chronically ill children: A 2-year follow up. *Journal of Marital and Family Therapy, 28*(4), 391–398.

Erbes, C. R., Polusny, M. A., MacDermid, S., & Compton, J. S. (2008). Couple therapy with combat veterans and their partners. *Journal of Clinical Psychology: In Session, 64*(8), 972–983.

Falloon, I. R. H., Roncone, R., Held, T., Coverdale, J. H., & Laidlaw, T. M. (2002). An international overview of family interventions: Developing effective treatment strategies and measuring their benefits for patients, carers, and communities. In H. P. Lefley & D. L. Johnson (Eds.), *Family interventions in mental illness: International perspectives* (pp. 3–23). Westport, CT: Praeger.

Foa, E. B., Hembree, E. A., & Rothbaum, B. O. (2007). *Prolonged exposure therapy for PTSD: Emotional processing of traumatic experiences: Therapist guide.* New York: Oxford University Press.

Glynn, S. M., Eth, S., Randolph, E. T., Foy, D. W., Urbaitis, M., Boxer, L., et al. (1999). A test of behavioral family therapy to augment exposure for combat-related posttraumatic stress disorder. *Journal of Consulting and Clinical Psychology, 67*(2), 243–251.

Halchuk, R., Makinen, J., & Johnson, S. (2010). Resolving attachment injuries in couples using emotionally focused therapy: A three-year follow-up. *Journal of Couple and Relationship Therapy, 9,* 31–47.

Jacobson, N. S., Christensen, A., Prince, S. E., Cordova, J., & Eldridge, K. (2000). Integrative behavioral couple therapy: An acceptance-based, promising new treatment for couple discord. *Journal of Clinical and Consulting Psychology, 68*(2), 351–335.

Jacobson, N. S., Dobson, K., Fruzzetti, A. E., Schmaling, K. B., & Salusky, S. (1991). Marital therapy as a treatment for depression. *Journal of Consulting and Clinical Psychology, 59*(4), 547–557.

Johnson, S. M., & Williams-Keeler, L. (1998). Creating healing relationships for couples dealing with trauma: The use of emotionally focused marital therapy. *Journal of Marital and Family Therapy, 24,* 25–40.

Kerr, M. E., & Bowen, M. (1988). *Family evaluations.* New York: Norton.

Kessler, R. C. (2000). Posttraumatic stress disorder: The burden to the individual and to society. *Journal of Clinical Psychiatry, 61*(Suppl. 5), 4–12.

Liberman, R. P. (1988). *Psychiatric rehabilitation for chronic mental patients.* New York: American Psychiatric Press.

Lyons, J. A., & Root, L. P. (2001). Family members of the PTSD veteran: Treatment needs and barriers. *National Center for Posttraumatic Stress Disorder Clinical Quarterly, 10*(3), 48–52.

Miklowitz, D. J., & Goldstein, M. J. (1990). Behavioral family treatment for patients with bipolar affective disorder. *Behavior Modification, 14*(4), 457–490.

Monson, C. M., Fredman, S. J., & Adair, K. C. (2008). Cognitive-behavioral conjoint therapy for posttraumatic stress disorder: Application to Operation Enduring and Iraqi Freedom veterans. *Journal of Clinical Psychology, 64*(8), 958–971.

Monson, C. M., Schnurr, P. P., Stevens, S. P., & Guthrie, K. A. (2004). Cognitive-behavioral couples treatment for posttraumatic stress disorder: Initial findings. *Journal of Traumatic Stress, 17*(4), 341–344.

Riggs, D. S. (2000). Marital and family therapy. In E. Foa, T. Keane, & M. Friedman (Eds.), *Effective treatments for PTSD: Practice guidelines from the International Society for Traumatic Stress Studies* (pp. 280–301). New York: Guilford Press.

Sautter, F., Lyons, J., Manguno-Mire, G., Perry, D., Han, X., Sherman, M., et al.

(2006). Predictors of partner engagement in PTSD treatment. *Journal of Psychopathology and Behavioral Assessment, 28*(2), 123–130.

Sautter, F. J., Glynn, S. M., Thompson, K. E., Franklin, L., & Han, X. (2009). A couple-based approach to the reduction of PTSD avoidance symptoms: Preliminary findings. *Journal of Marital and Family Therapy, 35*(3), 343–349.

Sherman, M. D., Blevins, D., Kirchner, J., Ridener, L., & Jackson, T. (2008). Key factors involved in engaging significant others in the treatment of Vietnam Veterans with PTSD. *Professional Psychology: Research and Practice, 39*(4), 443–450.

Tarrier, N., Sommerfield, C., & Pilgrim, H. (1999). Relatives' expressed emotion (EE) and PTSD treatment outcome. *Psychological Medicine, 29*, 801–811.

Wills, T. A., Weiss, R. L., & Patterson, G. R. (1974). A behavioral analysis of the determinants of marital satisfaction. *Journal of Consulting and Clinical Psychology, 42*, 802–811.

CHAPTER 10

Psychopharmacological Treatment

William M. Sauvé
Stephen M. Stahl

When it comes to the psychopharmacological treatment and management of posttraumatic stress disorder (PTSD), there are a limited number of agents that are formally approved for its treatment, namely, sertraline and paroxetine. Although generally other serotonin-specific reuptake inhibitors, as well as other classes of antidepressants, can be included, a look to the literature is required to expand one's armamentarium of rational choices in the management of this exceptionally challenging disorder. Additionally, careful attention must always be paid to some unique requirements of the active-duty patient. Some agents, although potentially efficacious, can have a negative impact on the members' fitness for duty; hence this consideration must be included in any risk–benefit discussion.

PTSD manifests in multiple ways and includes many divergent symptoms, mandating that the clinician be able to use multiple pharmacological agents simultaneously, with the goal of managing multiple types of symptomatology as they arise. The first type is "reexperiencing," which can include intrusive recollections, nightmares, and flashbacks, as well as significant distress at exposure to internal or external cues reminiscent of the traumatic event. Next is "avoidance," which can include actively avoiding thoughts, activities, or any other stimuli reminiscent of the event, as well as significant numbing of affect. Finally, there is "hyperarousal," which can include insomnia, irritability, poor concentration, hypervigilance, and exaggerated startle (American Psychiatric Association, 2000).

Based on this breakdown of symptomatology, some types can certainly be addressed psychopharmacologically, beginning with significant anxiety and affective components, for which the main indicated agents tend to be first-line treatments. The first symptom cluster that one might approach with psychopharmacological management for PTSD could logically be anxiety.

Psychopharmacological Treatment of Anxiety Symptoms in PTSD

Anxiety symptoms of PTSD include hyperarousal, hypervigilance, exaggerated startle, insomnia, and symptoms of avoidance. These are addressed on a first-line basis with the indicated agents sertraline (Stahl, 2009, p. 497) or paroxetine (Stahl, 2009, p. 409). Paroxetine is often favored because of its mild hypnotic properties, which tend to make it more acutely anxiolytic. As a selective serotonin reuptake inhibitor (SSRI), however, its efficacy over the long term is likely to be equivalent to that of all the other drugs in this class. Another consideration when starting SSRI medications in any patient with anxiety is to remember that several of these drugs have the property of being acutely activating, which can appear to exacerbate anxiety in the very near term. Titrating these medications up very slowly can often mitigate this side effect. Withdrawal effects, particularly notorious with paroxetine, can be similarly mitigated by very slow down titration when discontinuing SSRIs.

Second-line considerations include the serotonin–norepinephrine reuptake inhibitors (SNRIs), such as venlafaxine, desvenlafaxine, and duloxetine (Stahl, 2009, pp. 579, 133, 165), the tricyclic antidepressants, and consideration of both gabapentin and pregabalin (Stahl, 2009, pp. 221, 445), which have had some evidence of efficacy for anxiety in recent studies, especially for pregabalin (Montgomery, Herman, Schweizer, & Mandel, 2009; Pae, Marks, Han, Masand, & Patkar, 2009; Pande et al., 2003; Pohl, Feltner, Fieve, & Pande, 2005; Rickels, et al., 2005). Although the possible mechanism of action for these drugs is not particularly well understood, it may be that gabapentin and pregabalin, which are alpha 2 delta ligands, may modulate activity in neurons with excessive activity by binding selectively to open voltage sensitive calcium channels (Stahl & Grady, 2010, p. 100). Note that pain is very often a comorbid condition with PTSD, and it may be particularly elegant to consider these agents when treating this comorbidity in that they all have demonstrated efficacy in pain syndromes (Stahl & Grady, 2010, p. 153). Additionally, SNRIs are often found to be somewhat activating in the near term, so once again a slow titration may be in order. As with SSRIs, slow down titration can mitigate withdrawal effects, often observed after discontinuing SNRIs, especially venlafaxine.

Third-line treatment of the anxiety symptoms may involve the use of benzodiazepines, but this class of medications should be used with caution due to abuse and dependency issues. No studies to date have demonstrated efficacy of these medications in PTSD, and co-occurring substance abuse and dependence considerations with PTSD are known to be a major issue.

Psychopharmacological Treatment of Affective Symptoms in PTSD

Affective symptoms in PTSD are the next consideration. Most remarkably, these symptoms include irritability, detachment/numbing of affect, a sense of foreshortened future, and an overall depressed mood. These can be addressed on a first-line basis once again by the indicated agents, the most studied having been sertraline and paroxetine, but once again serotonin specific reuptake inhibitors as a class are likely to be similarly efficacious. Second-line considerations include the SNRIs, as well as the tricyclic antidepressants. Additionally, for affective symptoms, particularly those that overlap with depression, the clinician may choose to augment the use of an antidepressant with the dopamine partial agonist aripiprazole or with low doses of quetiapine, both now approved for this use for the treatment of major depression that fails to respond to an SSRI or an SNRI (Stahl, 2009, pp. 45, 459). Aripiprazole has recently been indicated for augmentation of antidepressants in the treatment of depression at low doses, generally in the 5- to 10-mg range. In the treatment of PTSD, aripiprazole has been started on open-label basis as monotherapy (average dosing in the 10-mg range), with some encouraging results (Mello, Costa, Schoedl, & Fiks, 2008), and some case reports exist noting aripiprazole being used to augment antidepressant medications and the treatment of PTSD. Quetiapine has also been recently approved for this same use in bipolar depression, possibly because of the norepinephrine reuptake inhibitor properties of quetiapine/norquetiapine (Stahl & Grady, 2010, p. 114). Third-line consideration for the treatment of affective symptoms would be the monoamine oxidase inhibitors (MAOIs), known for efficacy in depressed mood, though some of the dietary restrictions warranted with the use of these medications are not particularly practical for the active-duty service member (see Table 10.1).

Psychopharmacological Treatment of Reexperiencing Symptoms in PTSD

The third major consideration in the treatment of PTSD symptoms is reexperiencing symptoms, particularly nightmares. Nightmares can be extremely distressing, leading to a literal fear of sleep. When nightmares

TABLE 10.1. Suggested Tyramine Dietary Modifications for Monoamine Oxidase Inhibitors

Food to avoid	Food allowed
• Dried, aged, smoked, fermented, spoiled, or improperly stored meat, poultry, and fish • Broad bean pods • Aged cheeses • Tap and nonpasteurized beers • Marmite, sauerkraut • Soy products/tofu	• Fresh or processed meat, poultry, nd fish • All other vegetables • Processed and cottage cheese, ricotta cheese, yogurt • Canned or bottled beers and alcohol (have little tyramine) • Brewer's and baker's yeast

Note. No dietary modifications needed for low doses of transdermal selegiline or for low oral doses of selective MAO-B inhibitors. From Stahl (2008, p. 1117). Copyright 2008 by the Neuroscience Education Institute. Reprinted by permission.

are particularly vivid, they can be potentiating of the initial trauma. It has been suggested, in fact, that biochemically there is no difference between dreaming and real experience, suggesting that severe nightmares about a prior traumatizing event are in fact as retraumatizing to the patient as if the initial event were happening over and over. Additionally, severely disrupted sleep, often brought about and/or exacerbated by nightmares, significantly impedes any recovery efforts in the mental health arena. No formal indications exist, but some of the most promising data to date suggest the first-line use of prazosin. Prazosin is a centrally acting alpha-adrenergic antagonist (more centrally acting secondary to its lipophilicity) appearing to have a significant positive effect not only in the reduction of nightmare frequency and intensity but also in the overall quality of sleep and, in some studies, even in the improvement in the overall symptomatology of PTSD (Raskind et al., 2003, 2007; Taylor et al., 2008; Thompson, Taylor, McFall, Barnes, & Raskind, 2008). Although no specific indication has been generated for this agent and, therefore, no published dosing recommendations exist, available studies indicate that the effective dose lies somewhere between 5 and 15 mg per day. Dosing of this medication is, of course, a challenge—the prominent negative effect is hypotension and dizziness, which can have significant consequences for the service member in the deployed setting. Based on that, the recommendation is to start at a minimum dose and titrate the patient up to a minimum of 5 mg as quickly as possible, as tolerated.

Second-line treatment options for nightmares and the above-noted sleep difficulties are trazodone (Stahl, 2009, p. 547), typically used in low doses for its hypnotic properties, and hydroxyzine (Stahl, 2009, p. 243), which is indicated both for sleep and anxiety, making it useful in PTSD not only in larger doses (50–150 mg) for the initiation of sleep but also in smaller doses (25 mg) on an as-needed basis throughout the day for anxiety. Additionally, the nonbenzodiazepine sedative hypnotics, sometimes called "Z" drugs, including zolpidem, zaleplon, and eszopiclone (Stahl, 2009, pp. 595,

585, 181), may be considered but must be used with caution. Sleep difficulties and PTSD are typically long-term issues, and at least one study indicates that over the long term these drugs as a class are not particularly helpful in improving sleep quality (Alderman & Gilbert, 2009). Also, keeping in mind once again that PTSD is often comorbid with substance abuse and dependence, the usual precautions should be applied. Finally, the sedative hypnotic drugs are often associated with risk for amnesia, which can be severely upsetting to the sufferer of PTSD. Although the desire for sleep is often very high in the sufferer of PTSD (indeed, it is often the chief complaint), if the methods of inducing sleep leave the patient feeling out of control, amnestic, or somehow cognitively impaired, the symptoms of hyperarousal and anxiety will be severely exacerbated. Eszopiclone may have a slightly smaller risk for this, secondary to its higher selectivity on the gamma-aminobutyric acid receptor, possibly secondary to its being the more selective enantiomer of zopiclone (Stahl, 2008, p. 842).

Third-line consideration for the treatment of nightmares and sleep disturbance can involve the use of quetiapine, which is primarily a hypnotic drug in low doses (25–300 mg range) and may also have some positive effect on the reduction of nightmare frequency and severity, secondary to alpha-adrenergic antagonist properties. It is important to keep in mind, however, that this agent comes with some significant metabolic risks that are not dose dependent, and therefore the patient should be monitored for weight gain, lipids, and glucose metabolism, just as when treating with high doses for bipolar disorder and schizophrenia. It is interesting to note, however, that recent trends in the military medical community indicate a greater acceptance of using the second-generation antipsychotics in small doses for off-label use, when previously the use of these drugs at any dose for any reason often resulted in significant problems with fitness-for-duty considerations. Finally, benzodiazepines may be a third-line consideration for the initiation of sleep, but all the same precautions exist as noted previously, and these medications should also be used with caution.

Also of note, the beta blockers have shown some potential in the secondary prevention of PTSD (some studies indicate that beta blockers used within 6 hours following a traumatic event have resulted in some reduced symptomatology at the 3-month follow-up,); however, the usefulness of this particular strategy in the combat theater may be somewhat limited.

Summary of Psychopharmacological Treatment of Symptom Domains in PTSD

In summary, the psychopharmacological treatment of PTSD involves an approach from at least three different areas, encompassing anxiety, affective symptoms, and reexperiencing symptoms. Achieving any success with monotherapy is unlikely, but outcomes may improve with a rational approach that addresses each of the aforementioned areas with the symptom-based psychopharmacological agent—for example, using a serotonin-specific reuptake inhibitor as first line to address anxiety and affective symptoms, in conjunction with a rapid titration of prazosin to address sleep and nightmares.

Research on Psychopharmacological Treatment with Civilian Populations

Antidepressants

In 2005, Davidson and colleagues showed, in PTSD sufferers who had responded to fluoxetine and were randomized to placebo, that relapse rates on fluoxetine were 22% compared with 50% per placebo. It was also noted that time to relapse was improved. Two studies by Stein and colleagues, both in 2006, indicated that serotonin-specific reuptake inhibitors were superior to placebo. The first of these was a meta-analysis in which 35 short-term trials were reviewed, whereas the second is a reanalysis of two previously published trials (Stein, Ipser, & Seedat, 2006; Stein, van der Kolk, Austin, Fayyad, & Clary, 2006). In 2007, Marshall and colleagues showed, in a controlled trial of paroxetine versus placebo, that paroxetine was superior on the Clinician-Administered PTSD Scale (CAPS), showing improvement over the course of 10 weeks. In 2006, Davidson and colleagues also showed that venlafaxine separated from both sertraline and placebo. In 2007, Becker and colleagues found no difference from placebo in a study involving 30 patients, in which augmentation of an antidepressant with bupropion was compared with placebo. In 2003, Davidson and colleagues showed mirtazapine to be more effective than placebo on the Global Improvement item of the Short PTSD Rating Interview (SPRINT) but noted no improvement on SPRINT in its entirety.

Prazosin

In 2008, Taylor and colleagues, in a double-blind placebo-controlled crossover study involving 13 civilian participants, showed that prazosin was superior to placebo for sleep, nightmares, and overall scores using the PTSD Checklist (PCL).

Beta-Blockers

In 2002, Pitman and colleagues, using 41 subjects, studied the administration of propanolol versus placebo given within 6 hours of a traumatic event in the emergency room. No significant change was shown in the CAPS at 1 month, but there was a decrease in response in 3 months. In 2007, Stein, Kerridge, Dimsdale, and Hoyt, studying 48 patients in a surgical trauma center, administered propanolol versus gabapentin versus placebo in the context of trauma but demonstrated no significant difference on follow-up.

Second-Generation Antipsychotics

In 2004, Reich, Winternitz, Hennen, Watts, and Stanculescu studied 19 women suffering from PTSD related to childhood abuse, showing that risperidone, administered with flexible dosing, led to improvement on CAPS-2. In 2006, Padala and colleagues studied risperidone versus placebo in women with sexual or domestic abuse-related PTSD. The Treatment Outcome PTSD Scale (TOP-8) total score was improved over the course of 12 weeks, as well as ratings on CAPS, the Hamilton Depression Scale (HAM-D), and the Hamilton Anxiety Scale (HAM-A). In 2008, Rothbaum and colleagues demonstrated that 25 patients with PTSD who had not remitted after treatment with sertraline showed an equivocal response when treatment was augmented with risperidone.

Research on Psychopharmacological Treatment with Military Populations

Antidepressants

In 2002, Zohar and colleagues demonstrated that Israeli combat veterans showed no significant improvement on sertraline versus placebo. Similarly, a multicenter trial using sertraline showed no significant superiority to placebo in combat-related PTSD (Friedman, Marmar, Baker, Sikes, & Farfel, 2007). In 2004, however, Davis and colleagues demonstrated nefazodone to be superior to placebo in male combat veterans, as measured by CAPS. In 2006, Martenyi and Soldatenkova, in a trial involving Balkan war veterans, demonstrated fluoxetine to be superior to placebo on the TOP-8, as well as being superior on relapse prevention (it has been suggested that the subjects in the study were much younger and that older combat veterans tended to be more treatment resistant on previous studies). A recent study investigated duloxetine in a naturalistic study involving 21 treatment-refractory patients with combat-related PTSD and comorbid depression, finding that there was a significant improvement in both PTSD and depressive symptoms; it also noted nightmare improvement (Walderhaug et al., 2010).

Prazosin

Raskind et al. (2003), in a double-blind crossover trial using prazosin versus placebo in Vietnam veterans, demonstrated prazosin to be significantly superior for nightmares and in general improvement on CAPS. In 2007 Raskin and colleagues, in a parallel group trial with 40 veterans using prazosin versus placebo, demonstrated again that prazosin was superior for nightmares and sleep. In this study improvement was also noted on the overall CAPS, but the separation was not found to be statistically significant (Raskind et al., 2007). In 2008, a study involving 22 veterans showed that prazosin, in an average dose of 9.6 mg per day, reduced nightmare frequency and intensity, as well as the frequency of non-nightmare distressed awakenings, suggesting that increased brain adrenergic activity contributes to both nightmares and non-nightmare distressed awakenings in PTSD (Thompson et al., 2008). A study involving 23 refugees treated with prazosin for 8 weeks resulted in improvement in nightmares, as well as in Global Impression, with 6 patients reporting "marked improvement," 11 patients reporting "moderate improvement," and 6 patients reporting "minimal improvement" (Boynton, Bentley, Strachan, Barbato, & Raskind, 2009).

Second-Generation Antipsychotics

In 2005, a study by Bartzokis, Lu, Turner, Mintz, and Saunders involving 73 combat veterans demonstrated that using risperidone to augment sertraline resulted in improvement versus placebo, which was consistent with previous findings with olanzapine on a smaller scale (Stein, Kline, & Matloff, 2002). However, in a recent 6-month, randomized, double-blind, placebo-controlled multicenter trial of veterans diagnosed with military-related PTSD, Risperidone performed no better than placebo on measures of PTSD, depression, and anxiety in SRI resistant cases (Krystal et al., 2011).

Nonbenzodiazepine Sedative–Hypnotic "Z-Drugs"

In 2009, Alderman and Gilbert investigated the long-term use of zopiclone in Vietnam veterans with PTSD in a 6-month follow-up cohort study. Although the risk for dependence was not found to be significantly increased, efficacy for sleep quality over the long term was low.

Battlefield Morphine

Analogous to civilian studies of beta blockers administered shortly after the onset of a traumatic event, a study of soldiers who did or did not receive morphine demonstrated that use of morphine during trauma care may result in reduced risk for PTSD (Holbrook, Galarneau, Dye, Quinn, & Dougherty, 2010).

Summary of PTSD Psychopharmacology Research

In summary, research involving the psychopharmacological treatment of PTSD, both combat and noncombat related, supports the use of antidepressant agents, specifically serotonin-specific reuptake inhibitors, as well as SNRIs as first-line treatment for PTSD, with very encouraging data pointing to the use of prazosin for the treatment of nightmares and sleep and possible improvement across all the symptoms of PTSD. Additionally there are some encouraging, yet mixed, results involving augmentation with the second-generation antipsychotics. More study is clearly warranted.

Strengths and Limitations of Psychopharmacological Treatment with Military Personnel

When treating the active-duty service member, one of the clinician's primary considerations must be symptom chronicity and severity when thinking about future potential for active-duty status. However, it remains a fact that in the military system, the simple fact of being on certain psychiatric medications can also have a negative impact on the member's active-duty status, which the clinician must also consider. Keeping these things in mind, specific advantages and disadvantages of the various psychopharmacological agents listed previously follow. Should the clinical situation indicate that continued active duty will not be possible, some considerations can be ignored (such as the need to obtain a waiver when using psychotropics), and a more aggressive approach may be warranted.

First-Line Approach

Selective Serotonin Reuptake Inhibitors

This class of medication is generally well accepted in the military setting, in the combat theater, and between deployments. These medications are a low risk to cloud the sensorium or cause excessive sedation, which can be very problematic in the military setting where members are expected to be able to use weapons, to be awake for extended periods of duty, to be able to function and wake up in emergency situations, to utilize heavy equipment, or simply to be able to wake up on time very early in the morning. They require minimal monitoring, and sudden discontinuation of the medication is generally not thought to be dangerous—an important consideration for deploying military members, who sometimes suffer significant logistical challenges. Most of these agents tend to be ubiquitous in most settings, making them easy to obtain and use in the combat theater, as well as between deployments. As one limitation, however, the use of any psychotropic medications requires obtaining a waiver for the use of small arms in the military setting, and the SSRIs are no exception. Although it is not commonly difficult to obtain a waiver, it is important that this matter be attended to while treatment plans are being made. Also consider that some of the more exclusive military communities (e.g., aviation, undersea) consider the use of any psychotropic medications to be disqualifying by definition. Waivers can be obtained only in certain situations. Additionally, once a medication such as this is started, simply stopping it will not solve the administrative problem (such communities may require that a member be free of all psychotropic medications for a year, even after only a few days or weeks of use). Thus serious attention must be paid to the actual nature of the service member's job before making treatment plans that involve psychotropic medications.

Prazosin

A major advantage of this medication is that it is not classified as psychotropic; hence the stigma attached to its use is limited, and administrative concerns are less significant. This medication has the potential to reduce nightmare intensity and frequency, in addition to improving total sleep quality, without causing excessive sedation, which as noted previously is particularly important in the active-duty military population, even more so when deployed to potentially hazardous areas. As long as the medication is well tolerated, minimal monitoring is required, and it tends to be available, making it easy to obtain and use in and out of the combat theater. The only significant disadvantage to the use of this medication in the military population is the discomfort that may surface from sudden discontinuation, although risk of serious rebound hypertension is low. Some attention must be paid by the clinician as to possible future deployments and whether or not this agent is going to be available in certain situations. Plans should be made for its gradual tapering and discontinuation if need be.

Second-Line Approach

Serotonin–Norepinephrine Reuptake Inhibitors

Advantages of using this class of medications are similar to those of SSRIs in that once again they are generally well accepted in the military setting and in the combat theater, as well as between deployments. They do not usually present a risk of clouding the sensorium or causing excessive sedation, and they require minimal monitoring in terms of safety. Again, sudden discontinuation is not particularly dangerous, though significantly more uncomfortable than with other medications. These drugs may not be quite as ubiquitous as SSRIs, but they remain largely easy to obtain. Disadvantages of this class of medications include the waiver process, noted earlier, and the fact that certain exclusive military communities do not accept the use of these medications; once again, close attention must be paid to these issues by the clinician.

Pregabalin

The advantage of using this medication in the military population is that, like prazosin, it is not generally seen as a psychotropic medication, thus reducing stigma and administrative burden. It can potentially reduce anxiety and improve sleep without being excessively sedating, which is advantageous for all the aforementioned reasons. Disadvantages of the use of pregabalin include that it is relatively new, and therefore expensive, and not easily obtainable on most formularies; nonformulary consultations are sometimes difficult to justify for a strict off-label use of this medication. Additionally, an agent such as this one is likely to be very hard to come by in the combat theater, possibly creating an obstacle to its consistent use with active-duty members.

Aripiprazole

Therapeutically, this medication is advantageous because of its rapid onset of action should it prove efficacious. This can be an advantage in the treatment of the military patient, in that presentations are often acute and results may need to be obtained within a short period of time. It is well tolerated and not excessively sedating, and, of all the second-generation antipsychotics, it has one of the better metabolic profiles. Therefore it does not create as much of a risk for weight gain, which can be extremely problematic in the active-duty military member. This medication, however, is still classified as an antipsychotic medication. Although the use of antipsychotic medications for other than the treatment of psychosis is becoming more accepted in the military population, a waiver for small-arms use is still required and could certainly engender more resistance from an administrative standpoint. If the treatment plan involves returning the member to duty, the clinician would be well advised in this case to seek such a waiver prior to actually starting this medication.

Trazodone

This medication can be helpful for sleep in small doses, and, although it is significantly more sedating than other medications listed, it is still unlikely to cause amnesia or to significantly impair the military member's ability to function. Additionally, this medication is inexpensive and largely ubiquitous, again making it easy to obtain and use in and out of the combat theater. The disadvantage to the use of this medication is the potential side effect of priapism, which, although very rare, is still a possibility and which, in the case of the deployed active-duty male service member who may have limited access to surgical care, could prove devastating.

Hydroxyzine

Another ubiquitous agent, this medication is advantageous for the active-duty military member, is easy to obtain and use, and is not a controlled substance. It has the additional advantage of being formally indicated for use in anxiety and sleep and carries with it very few risks. Once again, although it is more sedating, it remains very unlikely to cause amnesia or to render the individual unable to function while taking it. No significant disadvantage specific to the use of this medication in the military member is noted, and although its therapeutic actions are not normally seen as being particularly dramatic, it can be a very useful agent, particularly in addition to other treatments.

Third-Line Approach

Benzodiazepines

These medications can be somewhat advantageous in that their effect is unmistakable and often dramatic, giving them some utility in severe, acute situations. However, these medications are controlled substances and have the potential to cause significant impairment in cognitive functioning, making them extremely problematic in active-duty military members who need to be able to handle weapons, be awake for extended periods of time in dangerous situations, and possibly handle heavy equipment. Also, noting the significant comorbidity of substance abuse in the patient suffering from PTSD, these medications should be considered only with significant caution.

Monoamine Oxidase Inhibitors

Although these medications are advantageous because of an excellent record of efficacy, their use in the active-duty military member is somewhat problematic secondary to dietary constraints, as well as some risk when using it with other medications or switching to other antidepressants. Particularly in the combat theater, having any dietary restrictions may be a significant problem. It is also noted, once again, that a waiver would have to be obtained to use the psychotropic medication, which is a constant consideration.

Nonbenzodiazepine Hypnotic "Z Drugs"

These medications can be useful in the military population, particularly for brief sleep problems often brought about by travel or acute stress. However, they have significant capacity to cause amnesia, to make it difficult for the member to wake up quickly from sleep, and possibly even to result in complex sleep behaviors. Complex sleep behaviors (such as sleepwalking), may be annoying or even upsetting to the civilian patient suffering from them in his or her home, but imagine the consequences associated with sleepwalking in the service member who sleeps in an area surrounded by concertina wire and fighting holes! Additionally, as noted in regard to the benzodiazepines, substance abuse or dependency comorbidity is a common concern and should be considered when these medications are to be used.

Quetiapine

It has recently been expressed in military administrative circles that the use of antipsychotic medications in small doses for nonpsychotic symptoms can be acceptable, and waivers for their use can be obtained. The off label use of this medication for sleep and possible reduction of nightmares can be somewhat helpful for the military member, and, although sedating, it is not known for causing amnesia or significant impairment. However, it still carries with it significant risks of weight gain and other metabolic problems, which are not known to be dose dependent. This can be a significant problem for active-duty military members, and they should be monitored very closely, which may not always be particularly practical in the combat theater.

Case Vignette

History

A 50-year-old active-duty member with 30 years of reserve service as a physician who had obtained the rank of colonel, with one deployment to OIF, presented with a previously determined diagnosis of PTSD after experiencing significant suicidal ideation. This occurred in the context of increasing occupational and marital stressors over the previous 10 days and a threat of divorce. The man left work to attempt to reconcile but ended up threatening to shoot himself; he then spent several hours in the woods feeling suicidal before he called some friends for help.

Reported symptoms at the time of presentation were depressed mood, anhedonia, insomnia, nightmares (related to prior combat experience), anergia, poor concentration, and feelings of worthlessness, worsening for several months. Additionally, he had suffered from hypervigilance, exaggerated startle, avoidance of stimuli reminiscent of his combat experience, and intrusive thoughts ever since returning from combat. As a physician riding with convoys during his combat tour, he had experienced multiple firefights and explosions from improvised explosive devices (IEDs).

Past Psychiatric History

The patient did seek the help of a psychiatrist after returning from combat, was diagnosed with PTSD, and treated with venlafaxine and alprazolam, which he was still using at presentation. He terminated with the psychiatrist (who was no longer seeing patients) 4 years later, but he continued on the medications through his primary care physician. He reports that the medications have been largely helpful, but he has never been symptom free, and recently symptoms have been severely exacerbated in light of new occupational and social stressors.

Past Medical History

Hyperlipidemia (with history of significantly elevated hepatic enzymes, on statin medications).

Spondylolysis left L5 with full workup and residual weak anterior compartment muscles, paresthesia over L5 dermatome.

Right rotator cuff tear treated with two surgeries, all resulting in chronic pain.

Current Medications

Alprazolam 0.5 mg at 11:00 A.M. and 5:00 P.M., and 1 mg in the evening.

Venlafaxine extended release 300 mg in the morning.

Pregabalin 150 mg twice daily (for ongoing pain).

Topiramate 50 mg each evening (for migraines).

Omeprazole 20 mg each morning.

Herbal over-the-counter medications: saw palmetto daily, glucosamine–chrondroitin daily, fish oil tablets daily.

Family Psychiatric History

The patient reports multiple family members suffering from attention-deficit/hyperactivity disorder, bipolar disorder, major depressive disorder, and alcohol dependence.

Psychosocial History

The patient was born to an intact family; he states that, although his family members have psychiatric issues throughout, they are all very close, and he had a great childhood. He denies any history of childhood abuse or neglect. He did well in school, but was "too fast" to have many friends; he usually had one or two friends in high school but has been a loner ever since. He completed college, medical school, and residency training without problems. His first marriage lasted 25 years; his current marriage is his second. His current occupational problems are somewhat related to his concerns about practicing as a physician while regularly using alprazolam.

Substance History

Tobacco: Denies use.
Caffeine: approximately 200 mg a day.
Supplements: Denies use.
Alcohol: Last drink 6 months ago (two drinks on that occasion).
Illicit drugs: Denies use.
Other/over-the-counter: Denies use.

Treatment Course

Augmentation of venlafaxine with aripiprazole, 5 mg daily was recommended. He tapered and discontinued alprazolam over 4 weeks after adding aripiprazole. The patient reported significantly reduced anxiety, as well as improvement in anergia/anhedonia. He had no suicidal ideation after admission to the hospital. Combat-related nightmares continued; low-dose quetiapine was initiated, and the patient reported improvement in sleep, as well as reduced intensity of nightmares. Prior to discharge, the patient was offered psychotherapy (prolonged exposure) for chronic PTSD in addition to his pharmacological management, which no longer included any benzodiazepine (benzodiazepines are contraindicated in prolonged exposure therapy). At monthly follow-ups for medications, the patient reported continued improved sleep, minimal nightmares, reduced anxiety, and great improvement in affective symptoms. He remains engaged in psychotherapy and finds it helpful. His scores on PTSD Checklist—Military Version (PCL-M) and Clinician Administered PTSD Scale (CAPS) improved significantly. Upon follow-up, he reported no benzodiazepine use for over 3 months.

References

Alderman, C. P., & Gilbert, A. L. (2009). A qualitative investigation of long-term zopiclone use and sleep quality among Vietnam war veterans with PTSD. *Annals of Pharmacotherapy, 43*(10), 1576–1582.

American Psychiatric Association. (2000). *Diagnostic and statistical manual of mental disorders* (4th ed., text rev.). Washington, DC: Author.

Bartzokis, G., Lu, P. H., Turner, J., Mintz, J., & Saunders, C. S. (2005). Adjunctive risperidone in the treatment of chronic combat-related posttraumatic stress disorder. *Biological Psychiatry, 57*(5), 474–479.

Becker, M. E., Hertzberg, M. A., Moore, S. D., Dennis, M. F., Bukenya, D. S., & Beckham, J. C. (2007). A placebo-controlled trial of bupropion SR in the treatment of chronic posttraumatic stress disorder. *Journal of Clinical Psychopharmacology, 27*(2), 193–197.

Boynton, L., Bentley, J., Strachan, E., Barbato, A., & Raskind, M. (2009). Preliminary findings concerning the use of prazosin for the treatment of posttraumatic nightmares in a refugee population. *Journal of Psychiatric Practice, 15*(6), 454–459.

Davidson, J., Rothbaum, B. O., Tucker, P., Asnis, G., Benattia, I., & Musgnung, J. J. (2006). Venlafaxine extended release in posttraumatic stress disorder: A sertraline- and placebo-controlled study. *Journal of Clinical Psychopharmacology, 26*(3), 259–267.

Davidson, J. R., Connor, K. M., Hertzberg, M. A., Weisler, R. H., Wilson, W. H., & Payne, V. M. (2005). Maintenance therapy with fluoxetine in posttraumatic stress disorder: A placebo-controlled discontinuation study. *Journal of Clinical Psychopharmacology, 25*(2), 166–169.

Davidson, J. R., Weisler, R. H., Butterfield, M. I., Casat, C. D., Connor, K. M., Barnett, S., et al. (2003). Mirtazapine vs. placebo in posttraumatic stress disorder: A pilot trial. *Biological Psychiatry, 53*(2), 188–191.

Davis, L. L., Jewell, M. E., Ambrose, S., Farley, J., English, B., Bartolucci, A., et al. (2004). A placebo-controlled study of nefazodone for the treatment of chronic posttraumatic stress disorder: A preliminary study. *Journal of Clinical Psychopharmacology, 24*(3), 291–297.

Friedman, M. J., Marmar, C. R., Baker, D. G., Sikes, C. R., & Farfel, G. M. (2007). Randomized, double-blind comparison of sertraline and placebo for posttraumatic stress disorder in a Department of Veterans Affairs setting. *Journal of Clinical Psychiatry, 68*(5), 711–720.

Holbrook, T. L., Galarneau, M. R., Dye, J. L., Quinn, K., & Dougherty, A. L. (2010). Morphine use after combat injury in Iraq and posttraumatic stress disorder. *New England Journal of Medicine, 362*(2), 110–117.

Krystal, J.H., et al. (2011). Adjunctive risperidone treatment for antidepressant-resistant symptoms of chronic military service-related PTSD: A randomized trial. *Journal of the American Medical Association, 306* (5), 493–502.

Marshall, R. D., Lewis-Fernandez, R., Blanco, C., Simpson, H. B., Lin, S. H., Vermes, D., et al. (2007). A controlled trial of paroxetine for chronic PTSD, dissociation, and interpersonal problems in mostly minority adults. *Depression and Anxiety, 24*(2), 77–84.

Martenyi, F., & Soldatenkova, V. (2006). Fluoxetine in the acute treatment and relapse prevention of combat-related posttraumatic stress disorder: Analysis of the veteran group of a placebo-controlled, randomized clinical trial. *European Neuropsychopharmacology, 16*(5), 340–349.

Mello, M. F., Costa, M. C., Schoedl, A. F., & Fiks, J. P. (2008). Aripiprazole in the treatment of posttraumatic stress disorder: An open-label trial. *Revista Brasileira de Psiquiatria, 30*(4), 358–361.

Montgomery, S. A., Herman, B. K., Schweizer, E., & Mandel, F. S. (2009). The efficacy of pregabalin and benzodiazepines in generalized anxiety disorder presenting with high levels of insomnia. *International Clinical Psychopharmacology, 24*(4), 214–222.

Padala, P. R., Madison, J., Monnahan, M., Marcil, W., Price, P., Ramaswamy, S., et al. (2006). Risperidone monotherapy for posttraumatic stress disorder related to sexual assault and domestic abuse in women. *International Clinical Psychopharmacology, 21*(5), 275–280.

Pae, C. U., Marks, D. M., Han, C., Masand, P. S., & Patkar, A. A. (2009). Pregabalin augmentation of antidepressants in patients with accident-related posttraumatic stress disorder: An open label pilot study. *International Clinical Psychopharmacology, 24*(1), 29–33.

Pande, A. C., Crockatt, J. G., Feltner, D. E., Janney, C. A., Smith, W. T., Weisler, R., et al. (2003). Pregabalin in generalized anxiety disorder: A placebo-controlled trial. *American Journal of Psychiatry, 160*(3), 533–540.

Pitman, R. K., Sanders, K. M., Zusman, R. M., Healy, A. R., Cheema, F., Lasko, N. B., et al. (2002). Pilot study of secondary prevention of posttraumatic stress disorder with propranolol. *Biological Psychiatry, 51*(2), 189–192.

Pohl, R. B., Feltner, D. E., Fieve, R. R., & Pande, A. C. (2005). Efficacy of pregabalin in the treatment of generalized anxiety disorder: Double-blind, placebo-controlled comparison of BID versus TID dosing. *Journal of Clinical Psychopharmacology, 25*(2), 151–158.

Raskind, M. A., Peskind, E. R., Hoff, D. J., Hart, K. L., Holmes, H. A., Warren, D., et al. (2007). A parallel group placebo-controlled study of prazosin for trauma nightmares and sleep disturbance in combat veterans with posttraumatic stress disorder. *Biological Psychiatry, 61*(8), 928–934.

Raskind, M. A., Peskind, E. R., Kanter, E. D., Petrie, E. C., Radant, A., Thompson, C. E., et al. (2003). Reduction of nightmares and other PTSD symptoms in combat veterans by prazosin: A placebo-controlled study. *American Journal of Psychiatry, 160*(2), 371–373.

Reich, D. B., Winternitz, S., Hennen, J., Watts, T., & Stanculescu, C. (2004). A preliminary study of risperidone in the treatment of posttraumatic stress disorder related to childhood abuse in women. *Journal of Clinical Psychiatry, 65*(12), 1601–1606.

Rickels, K., Pollack, M. H., Feltner, D. E., Lydiard, R. B., Zimbroff, D. L., Bielski, R. J., et al. (2005). Pregabalin for treatment of generalized anxiety disorder: a 4-week, multicenter, double-blind, placebo-controlled trial of pregabalin and alprazolam. *Archives of General Psychiatry, 62*(9), 1022–1030.

Rothbaum, B. O., Killeen, T. K., Davidson, J. R., Brady, K. T., Connor, K. M., & Heekin, M. H. (2008). Placebo-controlled trial of risperidone augmentation for selective serotonin reuptake inhibitor-resistant civilian posttraumatic stress disorder. *Journal of Clinical Psychiatry, 69*(4), 520–525.

Stahl, S. M. (2008). *Stahl's essential psychopharmacology: Neuroscientific basis and practical applications* (3rd ed.). Cambridge, UK: Cambridge University Press.

Stahl, S. M. (2009). *Stahl's essential psychopharmacology: The prescriber's guide* (3rd ed.). Cambridge, UK & New York: Cambridge University Press.

Stahl, S. M., & Grady, M. M. (2010). *Stahl's illustrated anxiety, stress, and PTSD*: Cambridge, UK: Cambridge University Press.

Stein, D. J., Ipser, J. C., & Seedat, S. (2006). Pharmacotherapy for post trau-matic stress disorder (PTSD). *Cochrane Database of Systematic Reviews*(1), CD002795.

Stein, D. J., van der Kolk, B. A., Austin, C., Fayyad, R., & Clary, C. (2006). Efficacy of sertraline in posttraumatic stress disorder secondary to interpersonal trauma or childhood abuse. *Annals of Clinical Psychiatry, 18*(4), 243–249.

Stein, M. B., Kerridge, C., Dimsdale, J. E., & Hoyt, D. B. (2007). Pharmacotherapy to prevent PTSD: Results from a randomized controlled proof-of-concept trial in physically injured patients. *Journal of Traumatic Stress, 20*(6), 923–932.

Stein, M. B., Kline, N. A., & Matloff, J. L. (2002). Adjunctive olanzapine for SSRI-resistant combat-related PTSD: A double-blind, placebo-controlled study. *American Journal of Psychiatry, 159*(10), 1777–1779.

Taylor, F. B., Martin, P., Thompson, C., Williams, J., Mellman, T. A., Gross, C., et al. (2008). Prazosin effects on objective sleep measures and clinical symptoms in civilian trauma posttraumatic stress disorder: A placebo-controlled study. *Biological Psychiatry, 63*(6), 629–632.

Thompson, C. E., Taylor, F. B., McFall, M. E., Barnes, R. F., & Raskind, M. A. (2008). Non-nightmare distressed awakenings in veterans with posttraumatic stress disorder: Response to prazosin. *Journal of Traumatic Stress, 21*(4), 417–420.

Walderhaug, E., Kasserman, S., Aikins, D., Vojvoda, D., Nishimura, C., & Neumeis-ter, A. (2010). Effects of duloxetine in treatment-refractory men with posttrau-matic stress disorder. *Pharmacopsychiatry, 43*(2), 45–49.

Zohar, J., Amital, D., Miodownik, C., Kotler, M., Bleich, A., Lane, R. M., et al. (2002). Double-blind placebo-controlled pilot study of sertraline in military veterans with posttraumatic stress disorder. *Journal of Clinical Psychopharma-cology, 22*(2), 190–195.

CHAPTER 11

Psychosocial Rehabilitation

Walter E. Penk
Dolores Little
Nathan Ainspan

In the past, combat veterans leaving Vietnam, those who had been drafted and had served 13 months in battle, ended their war by catching a plane in Vietnam and then, a day or so later, arriving home in the United States without much fanfare and sometimes without enough regard. Many Vietnam-era veterans felt that they had never received the support they needed to learn how to transition home from war.

Today, homecoming warriors from Iraq and Afghanistan go through a standardized reacclimation program. Returning home from war now means that soldiers prepare for peace just as they readied to fight in war (Dao, 2010).

Nowadays, transitioning home from war means that the families of soldiers are attending seminars about problems with acute posttraumatic stress disorder (PTSD), anxiety, suicidal thoughts, and sleep. During the first days after arriving home, soldiers themselves receive legal counseling, along with medical and psychological screenings. Then, after a month of leave, soldiers reconvene in units to enter what is called a "restoration" phase—sitting through workshops about such topics as marital relationships and chronic PTSD, refurbishing their equipment, and exercising in high-adrenaline activities such as rock climbing and skydiving.

One must prepare for peace as one does for war (Technical Cooperation Program, 2008). Such reacclimation and restoration training—which may later might be expanded to include psychosocial rehabilitation, as explained later—is accomplished in many different ways. One way is *reset training*, the term used to designate a process in which military forces, after battle, reassess gains and losses and begin planning for the next battle. Similarly, after leaving the military, veterans undergo a type of reset training, either as part of a personal plan for resuming life as a civilian or by talking with peers and friends about coming home (e.g., Kudler, Straits-Troster, & Jones, 2006). As a sign that times have changed, now even those practitioners in private practice can be trained in new approaches to provide services for military personnel returning home (see Moore & Jongsma, 2009, and Berghuis & Jongsma, 2010).

One of the images that signifies the return home from war can be seen near the U.S.S. Midway, berthed in San Diego Harbor, where there stands a towering 50-foot statue illustrating the photo cover page of the August 1945 issue of *Life* magazine that was published to mark the end of World War II. It is a tall statue of a Navy corpsman in dark blue kissing a military nurse in white. The statue reminds us all that it is time for new relationships to start. In the present time combat operations in Iraq have ended. It is time to stop fighting and to start living. Times keep changing, but the challenges are the same. Returning home is a time to find peace.

Coming Home

What do warriors need to do to transition home? We learn from the Technical Cooperative Program that soldiers need to engage in building resilience (Bowles & Bates, 2010) to help themselves and their families to recover from traumas and stresses of war. In this chapter we review studies that guide recovery and resilience. We focus on resources that lead to deeper understandings of how psychosocial rehabilitation produces benefits for those recovering from experiences and wounds of war. We examine naturalistic and clinical observations and randomized controlled trials invesstigating how health services produce favorable adjustments in everyday living. Psychosocial rehabilitation is about learning skills for adjustment. And learning to function at home is what peace is about, as Criterion F for PTSD focuses our attention on overcoming interferences in social and occupational functioning.

Psychosocial Rehabilitation and Criterion F for PTSD

Psychosocial rehabilitation works to restore functioning. Psychosocial rehabilitation is well designed and frequently practiced, but unfortunately it is insufficiently tested in comparative effectiveness research. We know there are many kinds of psychosocial rehabilitation that appear beneficial; but we have not as yet integrated treating trauma into psychosocial rehabilitation. During World War II and the Vietnam War, the draft conscripted citizens for military service. Treatments for PTSD were kept separate from psychosocial rehabilitation. Now, those who fought in Iraq and Afghanistan must learn how to integrate treatments for stress and trauma into interventions for psychosocial rehabilitation.

Today is a new age of sweeping changes in occupational needs, of a professional military, of more families and more women in the military, and of new technologies that guide new demands in home and family life, communities, and work.

And new forces are gathering around health care delivery—accountability, clinical practice guidelines, transparency, and cost–benefits analyses. The federal government is taking on a newe role to monitor and ensure healthcare. Developments of such forces in healthcare are changing the delivery of care, demanding that practitioners design and deliver services tailored specifically for individuals as individuals. Healthcare systems, including the Department of Defense (DoD) and the Veterans Health Administration (VHA), are now championing best practices as the standards to guide planning and operationalizing decisions in treatment and rehabilitation. Best practices require evidence-based results, preferably results based on randomized clinical trials (RCTs). And best practices must now integrate treatments for combat-related disorders into psychosocial rehabilitation (Penk & Flannery, 2000; Penk, Drebing, & Schutt, 2002; Sayer, Carlson, & Schnurr, 2010; Glynn, Drebing, & Penk, 2009).

Emphasis on best practices, clinical practice guidelines, and empirically based evidence in both the Department of Veterans Affairs (DVA) and the DoD started in the 1990s. Algorithms were written for persons with serious mental disorders and were summarized in modules L–Z of the VA/DoD *Clinical Practice Guidelines for Management of Psychoses* (Office of Quality and Performance and Patient Care Services, 2004). Later, best practices for psychosocial rehabilitation were expanded to include major depressive disorder, PTSD, and substance use disorders. Decisions about the benefits of psychosocial rehabilitation techniques formerly were founded on clinical observation and naturalistic evaluations, using findings from many VA sites to assess treatment outcomes (e.g., North East Program Evaluation Center [NEPEC] at the VA Connecticut Health Care System in West Haven; the Program Evaluation Research Center [PERC], in Palo Alto; VA Health Services Research and Development [HSR&D], Center for Health Quality, Outcomes, and Economic Research [CHQOER], Mental Illness Research, Education and Clinical Center [MIRECC], etc.). And now randomized controlled trials on psychosocial rehabilitation are being funded by the Defense

Centers of Excellence for Psychological Health and Traumatic Brain Injury (*www.dcoe.health.military*) and the VA's Rehabilitation Research and Development section (*www.rehab.va.gov*, *www.ncptsd.va.gov*).

DoD and VA outcome evaluation centers have amassed findings from treatment and rehabilitation. Moreover, DoD and VA Rehabilitation Research and Development are funding RCTs of the efficacy of psychosocial rehabilitation. We summarize such results in this chapter. DoD and VHA are amassing a national treasury of results based on standardized, objective measurement that continues to grow as DoD and the VA continue to build their computer-based clinical records system.

Clinical Practice Guidelines for Psychosocial Rehabilitation

Best practices for psychosocial rehabilitation are set out in the clinical practice guidelines adopted as policy by both the DoD and the VHA Office of Mental Health Services:

> Each rehabilitation goal and treatment approach must be established with the veteran's active involvement.

> > The safety of the veteran must be paramount.
> > A proper discharge plan includes an arrangement for safe, stable housing.
> > Each and every veteran should have the option of work or productivity of some kind.
> > Each and every veteran and family should be educated about his/her disorder(s), resources for both the veteran and the family, and support groups.
> > Each veteran should be assigned a case manager, if needed.
> > Each veteran should obtain access to job skills training, if so chosen.
> > Each veteran should be assigned to a primary care team, either in a medical or mental health setting, to monitor medical conditions which may be masked by mental disorders.
> > Each veteran should have access to psychiatrists, psychologists, social workers, and nurses, as indicated, for medical management and to provide other needed services. (Office of Quality and Performance and Patient Care Services and the Department of Defense, March 2004, *www.oqp.med.va.gov/cpg/cpg.htm*.)

Each of these objectives applies to soldiers in the military, as well as to veterans. Embedded in these key elements of the VA/DoD clinical practice guidelines are the services that are advocated in the VA's Mental Health Strategic Plan, highlighted by the President's New Freedom Initiatives, and that guide the VA's Office of Mental Health Services Veterans Health Administration Handbook 1160 (2009).

These key elements include such psychosocial rehabilitation services as patient education services; training in self-care and independent living skills; social skills training; supported housing, education, and employment; family psychoeducation; peer counseling; vet-to-vet services; and intensive case management. Each of these key elements constitutes its own unique form of clinical service, on a par with other elements in the system of healthcare that are more familiar, such as inpatient hospitalization or community-based outpatient clinics. We summarize empirically based findings on each of these interventions designed to support and to foster recovery and resilience among combat veterans returning home from war.

The DoD/VA's policy on key elements in psychosocial rehabilitation begins with the phrase "with the veteran's active involvement," a mandate that providers must form active partnerships with veterans receiving services. The center of treatment and rehabilitation is always the person for whom and with whom services are tailored and provided.

Theories Guiding Types of Psychosocial Rehabilitation

Why, nowadays, are active-duty military personnel and veterans seeking treatment and rehabilitation? To cite one among many theorists who provide a theoretical framework to guide development and evaluation of rehabilitation services, Albert Bandura (2006), in his seminal article, "Toward a Psychology of Human Agency," describes the theoretical foundation for "the veteran's active involvement." Bandura describes principles of human nature that facilitate partnerships between providers and those receiving services as they form alliances to address their problems and learn behaviors to overcome difficulties that impair and/or reduce recovery following illnesses and disease. Bandura identifies services such as psychosocial rehabilitation techniques as the kinds of experiences necessary to unleash what he calls the "agency of humans" so that they may be not just onlookers of events that shape their lives or products of life circumstances. Rather, Bandura proposes that those receiving treatment and rehabilitation services, including those returning home from war, must be seen by their providers as at the center of events that influence their functioning. Psychosocial rehabilitation must be person centered, recognizing that changes in behaviors to become prohealth and risk averse are carried out only by human agents who have become "self-organizing, proactive, self-regulating, and self-reflecting" (p. 172). Psychosocial rehabilitation techniques must center on and engage the human agent to bring about changes that improve functioning.

What Bandura describes as the "psychology of human agency" is similar to the values and character strengths that are at the center of being in the military, summarized so well in the seven U.S. Army values: loyalty, duty, respect, selfless service, honor, integrity, and personal courage (U.S. Army, 1999). These are the values in military doctrine that must be transferred from one's career in the military to one's life as a civilian. They guide adaptation and performance as a civilian within oneself, in relationship with one's family, in actualization of worth in work, and in contributing to the community.

Such values and character strengths are embedded principles for psychosocial rehabilitation. Another theorist, William Anthony, developed themes for practicing psychosocial rehabilitation—each person sets his or her own goals, changes his or her behaviors to actualize his or her preferences, and partners with providers through processes of psychosocial rehabilitation featuring self-determination. These themes are based on theories and training first developed by William Anthony and colleagues at Boston University's Center for Psychiatric Rehabilitation (Anthony, 1993; Anthony & Blanch, 1987; Anthony, Cohen, & Farkas, 1990). William Anthony's approach to psychosocial rehabilitation evolved while he served as a military officer at Walter Reed Army Medical Center during the Vietnam War, pioneering psychosocial rehabilitation techniques for combat veterans returning home from wars in Vietnam. Anthony later generalized his notions about psychosocial rehabilitation to civilians recovering from mental disorders.

Military values are embedded in character strengths and moral values prized in what now is called "positive psychology" (Peterson & Seligman, 2004; Duckworth, Peterson, Matthews, & Kelly, 2007; Matthews, 2007; see also Penk & Robinowitz, 2008). Positive psychology is an approach to living expressed through techniques of psychosocial rehabilitation in three areas of adjustment: developing positive emotions, developing personal individual traits, and designing positive institutions. (For more details, see Matthews, 2009, on the soldier's mind, motivation, mindset, and attitudes; see also Peterson, 2006. For one approach to assessment that each reader can self-administer, see tests available from the University of Pennsylvania Positive Psychology Center at *www.ppc.sas.upenn.edu* and the Authentic Happiness website for training at *www.authentichappiness.com*.)

Designing and implementing positive psychology processes in psychosocial rehabilitation assumes that military personnel and veterans face a unique set of challenges. Psychosocial rehabilitation must not only address symptoms associated with response to trauma but likewise multiple diagnoses. Comorbidities—serious mental illness, addictions, suicidal and homicidal inclinations, PTSD and complications of traumatic brain injury (TBI)—need to be addressed in planning rehabilitation.

Finally, psychosocial rehabilitation needs to add prevention techniques to approaches that incorporate therapy into interventions (Harpine, Nitza, & Conyne, 2010). DoD and the VA must promote a generalized approach to recovery from traumatic experiences based on procedures for preventing disease and illness. DoD and VA psychosocial rehabilitation must be centered on techniques training stressed and traumatized soldiers in how to prevent combinations of disorders as they struggle to cope with "learned helplessness."

Past History of Recovering from Traumas of War

Literature over the centuries is replete with the collective wisdom of human experience that promotes psychosocial rehabilitation: Education and work still pave the royal road that leads to coping with illness and disease and assuaging symptoms of trauma experienced in war. Although times may change, the nature of rehabilitation remains the same. To cite but a few among thousands of examples, St. Benedict, in coping with the ravages of war in the sixth century, founded his monastic order on Monte Cassino with the premise "Ora et Labora" ("pray and labor"). The benefits of work and having a sense of mission have long been acknowledged as essential for effectively coping with illness and trauma.

And "moral therapies" practiced in 19th-century New England certainly have prepared the way for the development of psychosocial rehabilitation techniques in the 20th and 21st centuries. The current interventions used by the DoD and VHA are indebted to "moral therapies." Prototypes of current psychosocial rehabilitation techniques, such as intensive case management, supported education, supported employment, peer counseling, supported housing, and social skills training can be found in practices of the 19th century (Military and Community and Family Policy at *www.prhome. defense.gov/MCFP*; the Yellow Ribbon Program at *www.yellowribbon.mil*; and the Center for the Study of Traumatic Stress at *www.usuhs.mil/csts* and *www.cstsonline.org*; Veterans Health Administration, 2009).

Examples of techniques developed by past generations of practitioners can be found in many archives. For example, techniques promoting sublimation in response to illness and to trauma were designed and developed after the Great Fire of 1871 in the Boston area by disaster response programs for citizens and new immigrants devastated by the disaster. Ideas from New England transcendentalism and the St. Louis movement in 19th-century American education were operationalized for thousands placed in harm's way when large sections of Boston were burned to the ground. Concurrently, psychosocial interventions were also extended to other vulnerable populations in Massachusetts—the seriously mentally ill, the incarcerated, the unemployed mill workers displaced by advances in 19th-century technology (see Prochnik, 2006, on "moral therapies").

DoD and the VA are directly indebted to moral therapies. Such traditions in rehabilitation are apparent in the Veterans Affairs committee room of the U.S. House of Representatives that is dominated by the portrait of Edith Nourse Rogers. For it was Edith Nourse Rogers who served as the primary author of the Servicemen's Readjustment Act of 1944 and shepherded it through the House to be signed by Franklin Delano Roosevelt on June 22, 1944. Rogers was the daughter of mill-owning families in Saco, Maine, married into mill-owning families in Lowell, Massachusetts, and represented citizens from the Fifth District in Massachusetts in the U.S. House of Representatives from 1927 until 1960. She became the first chair of the Veterans Affairs committee when the House was reorganized in 1947, and she led the writing of every major bill legislating the VA until her death in 1960. Her family was a victim of trauma: Her great-great-great-grandmother, Goody Nourse, was pressed to death in the Salem witch trials.

The Servicemen's Readjustment Act of 1944, better known as the GI Bill, empowered the VA to provide medical, education, and employment training for veterans of World War II and subsequent eras. Such legislation funded education and employment as psychosocial rehabilitation to heal medical and mental disorders as residuals of trauma (e.g., Bruun & Crosby, 1999).

Histories of the VA and of how psychosocial rehabilitation were developed along with histories of medical treatments for serious mental disorders are now being published (e.g., Baker & Pickren, 2007; Baker, 2007). Archives and oral histories are being collected about the stewardship of General Omar Bradley, George Kelly, James Grier Miller, Harold Hildreth, Lee Gurel, and Cecil Peck (see Waldrop, 2007, on the history of counseling services in the VA and accounts of early outcome evaluations of VA psychosocial programs in the 1960s).

But times change. Now it is highly likely that those who wish to learn techniques for recovering from traumas and rebuilding resiliencies within themselves will do so by connecting with expert advice and peer interactions on the Internet (cf. Penk & Ainspan, 2009). Now so many evidence-based practices comparing the effects of devices and chemicals, cognitive-behavioral techniques and psychoeducational interventions are explained in complete detail in a variety of places on the Web or through Facebook, Twitter, Cisco, and other Internet-based social networks.

Psychosocial rehabilitation techniques were designed not just to serve combat veterans classified as meeting criteria for DSM-IV-TR mental disorders. Rather, such approaches have been shown to benefit the adjustment of those who have not experienced any form of mental disorders. The U.S. military has established a number of agencies to keep the American military fit and able for many deployments and redeployments (see, e.g., Military One Source, *www.MilitaryOneSource.com*, for resiliency training, and the Center for Deployment Psychology, *www.deploymentpsych.org*). Psychosocial rehabilitations are not just techniques for reset training; they are rather techniques that each and every one of us may use to continue our education as we lead our everyday lives. Defense Centers of Excellence for Psychological Health and Traumatic Brain Injury (DCoE) is an excellent resource for information about agencies and their collaborations to promote resilience among soldiers and veterans (*www.dcoe.health.mil*). It disseminates tools for best practices among medical and educational agencies that can provide services to military and to veterans (see also Moore & Jongsma, 2009; Berghuis & Jongsma, 2010).

Psychosocial rehabilitation techniques are now being written into manuals to guide collaborations between clinicians and soldiers, along with families, who are rebuilding resiliencies to adapt to the stress and trauma of war resulting from multiple deployments. Such manualized approaches may be used by clinicians varying in professional training from physicians and psychologists to clergy, social workers, intensive case managers, and peer volunteers seeking to facilitate recovery among military personnel and veterans (Harris & Fallot, 2001). Next we summarize frequently used forms of psychosocial rehabilitation that have been found to be beneficial for military personnel and for veterans. More detailed analyses of outcomes are given in Glynn et al. (2009) and Sayer et al. (2010), along with assessment of standardized effect sizes of results obtained under conditions of randomized clinical trials (Insitute of Medicine, 2007). A list of organizations and programs for resilience building are summarized in Bowles and Bates (2010).

Self-Education and Self-Management

For soldiers who are not fully informed about aspects of health needs and who engage in high-risk behaviors (e.g., heavy use of alcohol, high drug use, overuse of prescription drugs, suicide attempts), clinicians should recommend patient education techniques. Review of empirical literature by Glynn et al. (2009, pp. 396–399) showed in 30 studies that were mainly naturalistic but included three randomized clinical trials that patient education techniques concerning recovery from trauma indeed are beneficial. Between-groups standardized effect sizes (based on gains in reducing symptoms of PTSD using interactions delivered through the Internet) were recorded as high as 1.48 (Lange et al., 2003).

Results from such comparative effectiveness research (Turpin, Downs, & Mason, 2005; Glodich, 2001) should encourage clinicians to learn about existing and newly published self-help techniques. Clinicians should continually review agencies and websites that produce self-management resources for clients, such as the National Center for PTSD (*www.ncptsd.va.gov*) and the VA's My HealtheVet program (*www.myhealth.va.gov/mhvportal*). Raymond B. Flannery's (1992) *Posttraumatic stress disorder: The victim's guide to healing and recovery* (New York: Crossroad) is an excellent guide for self-help and self-management.

Supported Education

As mentioned earlier, the GI Bill remains one of the most important forms of psychosocial rehabilitation available for combat veterans. Many soldiers invest portions of their military wages to be used for education once they retire. But a new GI Bill that expands supported education services was written and funded by the U.S. Congress in 2009. The new GI Bill provides opportunities for new training and new careers once military careers have ended. And it might be noted that state governments likewise provide educational benefits for veterans (e.g., the Hazelwood Act in Texas.).

Several models of supported education have been developed and tested for outcomes among psychiatric patients who are returning to college after treatment for mental disorders (e.g., Collins, Mowbray, & Bybee, 2000; Mowbray, Gutierrez, Bellamy, & Szilvagyi, 2003). Supported education approaches are not standardized with regard to services provided but generally include educational training in reading and mathematics, teaching how to cope with emotions and cognitive conflicts, stress management, training in social interactions, and support and therapy from clinicians who are available for students attending college.

Adaptations of supported education for PTSD are available from the VHA and the Veterans Benefits Administration (VBA) as the new GI Bill of 2009 goes into effect (see *www.gibill.va.gov*). Program descriptions are available (Sabatier, 2008; Glynn et al., 2009). Several investigators are carrying out RCTs among Iraq and Afghanistan combat veterans who have returned to college while simultaneously receiving treatment in VA settings and/or from private practitioners. Leaders in supported education health services research include Alexa Smith-Osborne at the University of Texas in Arlington, Lisa Mueller, and Marsha Ellison at the Edith Nourse Rogers Memorial Veterans Hospital in Bedford, Massachusetts, and Audrey Sorrells, Associate Dean of Students for Research at the University of Texas at Austin.

Supported Employment

Return to work remains one of the most effective forms of psychosocial rehabilitation (Penk, 2000; Penk et al., 2002). Manuals for vocational rehabilitation have been developed (e.g., Becker & Drake, 2003; VHA Uniform Mental Health Services, 2009; see also SAMHSA evidence-based toolkits at *www.mental-health.samhsa.gov/cmhs/communitysupport/toolkits/employment*). Studies are under way to demonstrate effective outcomes among persons meeting criteria for mental disorders, including PTSD (e.g., Glynn et al., 2009, pp. 409–413). Resources are available for interventions that integrate PTSD treatments into VA's Compensated Work Therapy (CWT) programs (see findings from RCTs in Davis, Drebing, Parker, & Leon, 2010). DoD likewise supports training to improve careers in the military. DCoEs for psychological health and traumatic brain injury are among many centralized resources (*www.dcoe.health.mil*).

Self-help approaches in supported employment for military personnel returning to duty are presented in Bates, Bowles, Kilgore, & Solursh (2008). Models are presented by types of injuries, by lists of stressors in recovering from wounds, by recovery processes, and by services available to achieve fitness to return to duty in the military. For veterans wishing to return to work, Ainspan and Penk (2008) have summarized resources on supported employment, as well as on workplace accommodations for military personnel with disabilities.

Family Psychoeducation

Though the numbers of RCTs testing efficacy of family therapy for PTSD and other trauma-related conditions are few, nevertheless favorable findings from case studies and naturalistic studies are overwhelmingly positive about the importance of such interventions for Iraq and Afghanistan combat veterans and their families (Glynn et al., 2009). Effect sizes are favorable, averaging around 0.30, empirically validating use of family therapy and family psychoeducation among combat veterans. Additional evidence, with effect sizes averaging 0.50, can be found in results from RCTs for couple therapy among combat veterans (Monson, Schnurr, Stevens, & Guthrie, 2004).

Changes in time underscore the importance of developing new forms of psychosocial rehabilitation for a military has been transformed over the years. Whereas the demographics of the Vietnam era included many military and veterans who were less than 21 years of age and unmarried, now far more veterans are in their 20s and 30s, married and with families. As a consequence, new forms of family therapy, couple therapy, and family psychoeducation are required. DoD sponsors the Military Community and Family Policy (MC&FP) section that is directly responsible for programs and policies to support life programs for military personnel and their families (see the DoD website Military OneSource [MOS] *www.militaryonesource*; also *www.defenselink.mil/prhome/mcfp.html*). The Yellow Ribbon Program (YRP) centers its family interventions for National Guard and Reserve military personnel and families (see *www.yellowribbon.mil*; also, Glynn [2008] and Darwin [2008]).

Several centers are active within the VA in developing interventions for families. In 2010, the VA expanded eligibility for VA mental health and psychosocial rehabilitation services to include families in keeping with scope of services already provided by DoD through TRICARE, the health program for active and retired service members and their families. The VISN 16 MIRECC follow-up program is but one example of multisite collaborations among VA clinicians and health services investigators who are writing manuals for family psychoeducational and family/couple therapies and who are testing the efficacy of such techniques in RCTs (e.g., Sherman, 2008; Sherman, Sautter, Jackson, Lyons, & Han, 2006; Sherman, Fisher, Bowling, et al., 2009; Sherman, Fisher, Sorvico, & McFarlane, 2009; Bowling & Sherman, 2008). Manuals have been written for clinicians and clients on such topics as family psychoeducation about PTSD, techniques for avoiding domestic violence, and family therapy to increase safety and security (see, for example, www.uohsc.edu/VetParenting)

Supported Housing

Varying forms of supported housing among active-duty military personnel and veterans are needed, even more so in the 21st century, as the U.S. housing market has faltered and home foreclosures are increasing for hundreds of thousands of Americans, including military personnel and veterans. Secretary of Veterans Affairs Eric Shinseki has announced a 5-year program for DVA to eliminate homelessness for 130,000 homeless veterans.

Among the military who fought in Iraq and Afghanistan, specialized housing is needed by thousands of seriously wounded active-duty military members who are not able to navigate the average U.S. home with narrow entrances, hallways, doors, and barriers in kitchens and bathrooms. Nonprofit, nonpartisan national 501(c)(3) organizations build homes designed to accommodate the needs of those whose wounds require specialized constructions (*www.HomesForOurTroops.org*). Monies are available for donations to pay for the $63,780 funded by the VA's Specially Adapted Housing grants for wounded veterans.

Programs to train military and veterans in housing are available from SAMHSA (see Homelessness Resources Center at *www.SAMHSA.gov*). Supported housing rehabilitation has been developed for some who are homeless and for those veterans and active-duty military personnel who are not living in safe, stable, affordable housing (see Rog, 2006, for a description of supported housing techniques, including descriptions of different types of housing for different veterans with specialized needs; see also Mares,

Kasprow, & Rosenheck, 2004). VA has devised a system of supported housing interventions that has included, over the years, long-term-care inpatient hospitalization and domiciliaries. But times are changing in the VA as well, as new forms of housing services have been designed and are proving to be effective, such as CWT/TR Compensated Work Therapy/Transitional Residence (CWT/TR). CWT/TR is a form of supported housing in which, in order to live for a limited period of time, a homeless unemployed veteran must accept a job from which he or she pays in part for housing (Schutt, Rosenheck, Penk, Drebing, & Seibyl, 2005). VA's North East Program Evaluation Center (NEPEC) at the West Haven, Connecticut, VA has found excellent outcomes for CWT/TR (i.e., continuing in work and in treatment and successfully relocating to independently paid housing in the community).

Health services research has demonstrated that supported housing interventions reduce homelessness. Effect sizes exceed 1.00 for not returning to shelters over a 2-year period for such models as the "evolving consumer household" supported housing (Goldfinger et al., 1999; Schutt, 2010).

Intensive Case Management

Intensive case management has proven to be an extremely effective form of psychosocial rehabilitation (see review in Glynn et al., 2009, pp. 413–415). Efficacy is more pronounced under conditions in which interventions go beyond brokering and linking to services (i.e., simple case management) to those in which case managers have been trained to deliver specialized skills when relating to clients (i.e., intensive case management). Examples of intensive case management are provided in Karls and Wandrei (2000) and include assigning case managers to provide services to reduce addictions; facilitating access to primary care services among wounded veterans who need medical services; and training clients to access services for which veterans are eligible within the VHA and the VBA (see, e.g., VAH, 2009).

Case managers (e.g., registered nurse [RN]) case managers in the U.S. Army, clinical primary care managers or RN clinical case managers in the U.S. Navy, and primary care managers in the U.S. Air Force) provide valued leadership to ensure that military combatants get adequate medical care (Bates, Bowles, Kilgore, & Solursch, 2008). Such specialized support from case managers is vital in recovery and in returning to duty. Similarly, DVA has developed and provides a variety of intensive case management, the most recent type of case manager being specialists for Iran and Afghanistan combat veterans, who guide such veterans through an array of resources for themselves and their families available both in DVA (i.e., VHA and VBA) and in other federal and state agencies (such as the Departments of Labor,

Education, etc.). Recent improvements in the form of case management include adding peers as counselors from among those who have recovered from stress and trauma (e.g., Gregory, 2008)

Physical Health, Exercise, and Nutrition

Physical fitness remains central in psychosocial rehabilitation, just as it is vital in "boot camp" when entering the military and for remaining fit during a military career. DVA provides resources and ways of recording progress for improving health (see VA's MyHealth*e*Vet web site at *www.va.gov* or *www. myhealth.va.gov*). The mission of the DVA includes supporting physical health, exercise, and nutrition among veterans through participation in VA medical center programs. Physical and mental fitness is essential in the military, as evidenced by the many requirements to meet standards and the need for continuing training to stay fit. Active-duty military members undergo periodic Medical Evaluation Board (MEB) assessments (Bates, Bowles, Kilgore, & Solursch, 2008) as well as, in selected instances, examination by the Physical Evaluation Board to determine physical fitness to return to duty or to be retrained for another job in the military (Dole & Shalala, 2007)

Guidelines to Assess Functioning for Psychosocial Rehabilitation among Military Personnel and Veterans

Techniques to assess the impact of PTSD and other combat-related disorders continue to be developed (e.g., Weathers, Keane, & Foa, 2009). One major change in diagnostic criteria—adding functioning to classification—required redesign and revalidation of many earlier measures, such as the Clinician-Administered PTSD Scale (CAPS), the Structured Clinical Interview for DSM-IV (SCID-IV), and PTSD checklists. Criterion F (functioning) was added to DSM-IV-TR (2000) criteria: Clinicians now must plan treatment to reduce symptoms but likewise evaluate interferences in social and occupational functioning resulting from trauma. Longitudinal studies of combat veterans have shown that whereas PTSD symptoms may reduce over time, such symptoms persist in negatively affecting functioning. Ro and Clark (2009) document at least four factors for assessment that characterize functioning: well-being, basic functioning, self-mastery, and interpersonal and social adjustment. Marx is developing new measures for interferences in functioning among combat veterans (Marx et al., 2009; see also McQuaid et al., in press; Holowka & Marx, 2011, in press; and Sayer et al., 2010 for reviews of assessment literature on functioning and PTSD). Such shifts in PTSD criteria mean that clinicians must assess functioning and must provide services—psychosocial rehabilitation—that reduce symptoms and improve functioning (see the Deployment Resources and Resiliency Inventory [DRRI], King, King, Vogt, Knight, & Sawyer, 2006).

Case Vignette

Charles Lenfant (not his actual name) grew up in Houston, Texas. After graduating from high school, the only decent job he could find was with Parks and Recreation for the City of Houston. He learned landscaping and was frequently called on to design and cultivate green spaces, much needed after periodic flooding, as well as new construction in Houston's new neighborhoods. Work was steady, but, with just a high school education, Lenfant never rose in the ranks of city employment.

To increase his income and get more independence, and honoring advice from his grandfather, he joined the National Guard. And Lenfant also enrolled part-time in community college taking business and computer courses. By adding education and the Guard, he was hoping to be promoted.

But, unexpectedly, Lenfant's Texas National Guard unit was mobilized and deployed to Iraq. In Iraqi warzones, Lenfant quickly rose in rank and in responsibilities in the military, soon becoming a sergeant working in supply. Although not exposed directly to combat, Lenfant was consistently under fire and was jolted by roadside bomb blasts while overseeing equipment, monitoring transfers of supplies, and directing supply clerks. He rose in rank as he replaced soldiers in his unit who were wounded or killed. His military job not only increased in complexity, but he performed well, with distinction, while constantly exposed to trauma, suffering minor wounds and seeing comrades killed.

Lenfant safely returned home. He discovered that unemployment was high. The best he could do was to return to the same job he had had before in Houston's parks and recreation department, again at low pay, without much responsibility. In Iraq Lenfant had had a highly demanding job with many responsibilities under dreadful conditions. Returning home, he found the same job he had before at low pay, but he also found peace.

Though Lenfant's life was much the same at home and at work, his emotional life was not the same. Lenfant found himself not talking much about his war experiences, even though his parents, brothers and sisters, and friends often asked about what happened. He found that he was increasingly irritated at work when his coworkers would not carry out orders as fast as he was responding to tasks. He discovered that he was beginning to dislike being around crowds, wanting to work alone more and more often, unhappy when he was asked to work among crowds on holidays when many families had gathered and filled up the parks. He disliked going to the home store to buy replacements for equipment, not being able to stand and wait in long lines to complete purchases. More and more, he found himself starting to hate driving in long traffic lines going to and from work in the mornings and evenings. And he found himself becoming angrier and angrier about things he did not understand, a slow fury growing within himself that he had been cheated by life because he was not paid enough and not promoted to better positions with more responsibilities.

At the same time, he became increasingly fearful, and he began to sleep less as nightmares about acquaintances wounded in war increased. Periodically during the day, he would experience ordinary events that brought back the intense feelings of fear he felt in Iraq, reminding him of times when friends were hurt by explosions.

Eventually, he decided that he would follow advice from friends and his parents to talk things over with clinicians in a PTSD clinic in a local VA medical center. He met with a psychiatrist who offered medication to settle him down and with a psychologist who wanted to enroll him in a course of 20 sessions of prolonged exposure. But these interviews had brought back so many intense reminders of events in combat that he was trying to forget that he never went back for treatment. He did request an appointment about eligibility for service-connected status, an application that is still pending.

But, luckily, Lenfant had a very spry and perky 90-year-old grandfather who had served in World War II who had good memories of using the GI Bill and had had some favorable outcomes in his later investments. This was the same grandfather who had encouraged him to join the National Guard and had encouraged him to reduce his military pay for future education while serving in Iraq. And this was the same grandfather who offered to help by paying some expenses in case Lenfant decided to return to college and access GI Bill assistance allowances, as well as attend a university in Texas where tuition and other assistance was paid for under the Hazelwood Act.

And, with no guarantee that he would ever work in anything other than in landscaping, Charles Lenfant took the chance: He reduced his work to part-time with the city and returned to college, full time, with expenses paid in part under the GI Bill and the Texas Hazelwood Act, as well as by his grandfather.

Lenfant specialized in urban planning/city design and civil engineering. He loved college, but he was quickly overwhelmed by many stresses from studying, which further intensified feelings of anger and depression and anxieties he had been trying to control. But on this occasion he discovered that there was a group of Iraq and Afghanistan combat veterans who likewise had enrolled in college, were stressed by school, remembered traumas, and concluded that they needed to talk with a professional. The clinician they found was, in a sense, a peer, but a peer who happened to be a neuropsychologist in the military and was retired, having himself returned to college to add clinical expertise to his qualifications as a clinical psychologist. He was now seeing veterans at the counseling center in the university. And this time, attending group therapy, Lenfant felt relief. Part of his good feelings came from feeling the return of another sense of belonging. He suddenly realized that he had missed the sense of belonging to a community, to a unit, as in the military, and a sense of belonging with others that he did not feel earlier at his work. And so, returning to college and being in group therapy with veterans brought back a sense of belonging to a unit. Besides, at college and in his group, there were women who had served in Iraq and Afghanistan.

Although he never benefited much from practicing relaxation techniques or expressing his distress, nonetheless he had to admit that some of his fears were subsiding, his anger was lessening, and certainly his nightmares were decreasing. He still avoided medications, but that was not surprising: He never liked smoking, did not experiment much with drugs, and just never liked the disorientation of drinking. His relief came from actions, and he readily fell into swimming at the university. And he thoroughly enjoyed the "co-op" phase of his college education in civil engineering, when he began to add work to his classes. He was learning what he needed to solve his personal problems through his actions, and not talking about his feelings.

For Lenfant, changes for the positive were very slow, in part because he actually found that he had increased the work that he was doing. Surprisingly, he had not reduced the time he was working, once he added up the time it took for classes, as well as working part time for the city. So, by the end of the second year at college, he took another profound step, although it was costly given the limitations in his budget to support himself: He quit his part-time job with the city, but not without obtaining a promise that he might return once he graduated. And, of course, there was always the fear that his National Guard unit would be redeployed to Iraq or to Afghanistan.

Earning less, now living on the GI Bill, the college co-op plan, and gifts from his grandfather, Lenfant initiated a comparatively well-balanced schedule, taking time for exercise, watching his diet, sitting in on group therapy, taking courses, working at practicum assignments, and even adventuring on outings with a female combat veteran whom he had met in one of his classes.

Slowly but consistently, he regained social contacts that he had lost. He found himself meeting new people. He certainly was growing in new skills; one of his co-op jobs was an assignment to work in engineering and maintenance at the university, a huge campus in Houston, which required much maintenance in air-conditioning most of the year.

And he graduated. Again, Lenfant found that few jobs were available. He consulted with the university's career center to see what sorts of jobs he now might qualify for. He even contacted his former supervisor at parks and recreation in Houston to see what was available. What was available, as it turned out, was, surprisingly, an offer from the university's engineering and maintenance department, a job he immediately took. The pay was much better than with the city. He could also continue to attend his group therapy, and the university was offering graduate school.

Lenfant felt more content, more at ease, and was sleeping better. It was now time to talk with his grandfather about World War II. His grandfather had never talked about the war; Lenfant had never talked about Iraq. It was time to get together and talk about their wars. And Lenfant would bring his girlfriend; she, too, had served in Iraq.

References

Ainspan, N. B., & Penk, W. E. (Eds.). (2008). *Returning wars' wounded, injured, and ill.* Westport, CT: Greenwood.

American Psychiatric Association. (2000). *Diagnostic and statistical manual of mental disorders* (4th ed., text rev.). Washington, DC: Author.

Anthony, W. A. (1993). Recovery from mental illness: The guiding vision of the mental health service system in the 1990s. *Psychosocial Rehbilitation Journal, 16,* 11–23.

Anthony, W. A., & Blanch, A. (1987). Supported employment for persons who are psychiatrically disabled: An historical and conceptual perspective. *Psychosocial Rehabilitation Journal, 2,* 4–23.

Anthony, W. A., Cohen, M., & Farkas, M. (1990). *Psychiatric rehabilitation.* Boston: Center for Psychiatric Rehabilitation.

Baker, R. R. (Ed.). (2007). *Stories from VA psychology.* Bloomington, IN: Author House. Available from *www.authorhouse.com.*

Bandura, A. (2006). Toward a psychology of human agency. *Perspectives on Psychological Science, 1,* 164–180.

Bates, M. J., Bowles, S. V., Kilgore, J. A., & Solursh, L. P. (2008). Fitness for duty, recovery, and return to service. In N. D. Ainspan & W. E. Penk (Eds.), *Returning wars' wounded, injured, and ill.* Westport, CT: Greenwood/Praeger Security International.

Becker, D. R., & Drake, R. E. (2003). *A working life for people with severe mental illness.* New York: Oxford University Press.

Berghuis, D. J., & Jongsma, A. E. (2010). *The veterans and active duty military psychotherapy progress notes planner.* New York: Wiley.

Bowles, S. V., & Bates, M. J. (2010). Military organizations and programs contributing to resilience building. *Military Medicine, 175,* 382–384.

Bowling, U. B., & Sherman, M. D. (2008). Welcoming them home: Supporting soldiers and their families in navigating the tasks of re-integration. *Professional Psychology: Research and Practice, 39,* 450–458.

Bruun, E., & Crosby, J. (1999). *Our nation's archives: The history of the United States in documents.* New York: Black Dog & Leventhal.

Collins, M. E., Mowbray, C. T., & Bybee, D. (2000). Characteristics predicting successful outcomes of participants with severe mental illness in supported education. *Psychiatric Services, 51,* 774–780.

Dao, J. (2010, August 21). Returning to civilian life. *New York Times,* p. A10.

Darwin, J. (2008). Disabilities and injuries among the members of the National Guard and Reserve Units. In N. D. Ainspan & W. E. Penk (Eds.), *Returning wars' wounded, injured, and ill.* Westport, CT: Greenwood/Praeger Security International.

Davis, L. L., Drebing, C., Parker, P. E., & Leon, A. L. (2010, November). *Occupations in persons with PTSD.* Paper presented at ISTSS Conference, Montreal, Quebec, Canada.

Dole, B., & Shalala, D. (2007). Serve, support, simplify: Report of the President's Commission on Care for America's Returning Wounded Warriors. Available at *www.pccuw.gov.*

Duckworth, A. K., Peterson, C., Matthews, M. D., & Kelly, D. R. (2007). Grit: Perseverance and passion for long-term goals. *Journal of Personality and Social Psychology, 92,* 1087–1101.

Glodich, A. (2001). Protocol for a trauma-based psychoeducational group intervention to decrease risk-taking, reenactment, and further violence exposure. *Journal of Child and Adolescent Group Therapy, 11*(2–3), 87–107.

Glynn, S. M., Eth, S., Randolph, E. T., Foy, D. W., Urbaitis, M., & Boxer, L. (1999). A test of behavioral family therapy to augment exposure for combat-related PTSD. *Journal of Consulting and Clinical Psychology, 67,* 243–251.

Glynn. S. (2008). Impact on families and friends. In N. D. Ainspan & W. E. Penk (Eds.), *Returning wars' wounded, injured, and ill.* Westport, CT: Greenwood/Praeger Security International.

Glynn, S., Drebing, C., & Penk, W. E. (2009). Psychosocial rehabilitation. In E. B. Foa, T. M. Keane, M. J. Friedman, & J. A. Cohen (Eds.), *Effective treatments for PTSD: Practice guidelines from the International Society for Traumatic Stress Studies* (2nd ed.). New York: Guilford Press.

Goldfinger, S. M., Schutt, R. K., Tolomiczenko, G. S., Seidman, L., Penk, W. E., Turner, W., et al. (1999). Housing placement and subsequent days homeless among formerly homeless adults with mental illness. *Psychiatric Services, 50,* 674–679.

Gregory, W. (2008). Peer support services. In N. D. Ainspan & W. E. Penk (Eds.), *Returning wars' wounded, injured, and ill.* Westport, CT: Greenwood/Praeger Security International.

Harpine, E. C., Nitza, A., & Conyne, R. (2010). Prevention groups: Today and tomorrow. *Group Dynamics: Theory, Research, and Practice, 14,* 268–280.

Harris, M., & Fallot, R. D. (Eds.). (2001). *Using trauma theory to design service systems.* San Francisco: Jossey-Bass.

Holowka, D. W., & Marx, B. P. (2011, in press). *Assessing PTSD-related functional impairment and quality of life.* In G. Beck & D. M. Sloan (Eds.). Oxford handbook of traumatic stress studies. New York: Oxford University Press.

Institute of Medicine. (2007). *Treatment of posttraumatic stress disorder: An assessment of evidence*. Washington, DC: National Academies Press.

Karls, J. N., & Wandrei, K. E. (2000). P-I-E as a new tool for more effective case management. In J. Williams (Ed.). *Person-in-environment*. Washington, DC: National Association of Social Work.

King, L. A., King, D. W., Vogt, D. S., Knight, J. A., & Sawyer, A. (2006). Deployment Resources and Resiliency Inventory: A collection of measures for study of deployment-related experiences of military personnel and veterans. *Military Psychology, 18*, 89–120.

Kudler, H., Straits-Troster, K., & Jones, E. (2006, April). *Strategies in the service of new combat veterans*. Paper presented at the VISN 17 PTSD Conference, San Antonio, Texas. (Available from howard.kudler@va.gov)

Lange, A., Rietkijk, D., Hudcovicova, M., van den Ven, J. P., Schrieken, B., & Emmelkamp, P. M. G. (2003). Interapy: A controlled randomized trial of the standardized treatment of posttraumatic stress through the Internet. *Journal of Consulting and Clinical Psychology, 71*, 901–909.

Mares, A. S., Kasprow, W. J., & Rosenheck, R. (2004). Outcomes of supported housing for homeless veterans with psychiatric and substance abuse problems. *Mental Health Services Research, 6*, 199–211.

Marx, B. P., Schnurr, P. P., Rodriguez, P., Holowka, P., Lunney, C., Weathers, F., etc. (2009, November). Development of a functional impairment scale for active-duty service members and veterans. In K. N. Lester (Chair), *Beyond PTSD symptom reduction: Social and health-related benefits of trauma-focused treatments*. Symposium conducted at the meeting of the International Society of Traumatic Stress Studies, Atlanta, Georgia.

Matthews, M. D. (2007). [Using character strengths to adapt to combat deployments]. Unpublished raw data.

Matthews, M. D. (2009). The soldier's mind: Motivation, mindset, and attitude. In S. Freeman, B. Moore, & A. Freeman (Eds.), *Living and surviving in harm's way: A psychological treatment handbook for pre- and postdeployment of military personnel* (pp. 9–26). New York: Routledge.

McQuaid, J. R., Marx, B. P., Rosen, M.J., Bufka, L. F., Tenhula, W., Cook, W., & Keane, T. M. (in press). Mental health assessment in rehabilitation research. *Journal of Rehabilitation Research and Development*.

Monson, C. M., Schnurr, P. P. Stevens, S. P., & Guthrie, K. A. (2004). Cognitive-behavioral couple's treatment for PTSD: Initial findings. *Journal of Traumatic Stress, 17*, 341–344.

Moore, B. A., & Jongsma, A. E. (2009). *The veterans and active duty military psychotherapy: Treatment planner*. New York: Wiley.

Mowbray, C. T., Gutierrez, L. M., Bellamy, C. D., & Szilvagyi, S. (2003). Replication of psychosocial rehabilitation program: A case study analysis of supported education. *Journal of Community Psychology, 31*, 437–445.

Office of Quality and Performance and Patient Care Services and the Department of Defense. (2004). *www.oqp.med.va.gov/cpg/cpg.htm*.

Penk, W. E. (2000). Designing work experiences for persons with serious mental disorders. In F. J. Frese (Ed.), *The role of organized psychology in treatment of the seriously mentally ill* (pp. 17–26). San Francisco: Jossey-Bass.

Penk, W. E., & Ainspan, N. D. (2009). Community response to returning military. In S. Freeman, B. Moore, & A. Freeman (Eds.), *Living and surviving in harm's way: A psychological treatment handbook for pre- and postdeployment of military personnel.* New York: Routledge.

Penk, W. E., Drebing, C., & Schutt. R. (2002). PTSD in the workplace. In J. C. Thomas & M. Hersen (Eds.), *Handbook of mental health in the workplace* (pp. 215–248). Thousand Oaks, CA: Sage.

Penk, W. E., & Flannery, R. B. (2000). Psychosocial rehabilitation. In E. B. Foa, T. M. Keane, & M. J. Friedman (Eds.), *Effective treatments for PTSD: Practice guidelines from the International Society for Traumatic Stress Studies* (pp. 388–426). New York: Guilford Press.

Penk, W. E., & Robinowitz, R. (2008). The psychological impact of disabilities. In N. D. Ainspan & W. E. Penk (Eds.), *Returning wars' wounded, injured, and ill* (pp. 205–222). Westport, CT: Greenwood/Praeger Security International.

Peterson, C. (2006). *A primer in positive psychology.* New York: Oxford University Press.

Peterson, C., & Seligman, M. E. P. (2004). *Character strengths and virtues: A handbook and classification.* New York: Oxford University Press.

Prochnik, G. (2006). *Putnam Camp: Sigmund Freud, James Jackson Putnam, and the purpose of American psychology.* New York: Other Press.

Ro, E., & Clark, C. (2009). Psychosocial functioning in the context of diagnosis. *Personality Assessment, 21,* 313–324.

Rog, D. J. (2006). The evidence on supported housing. *Psychiatric Rehabilitation Journal, 29,* 334–344.

Sabatier, C. J. (2008). Education options. In N. D. Ainspan & W. E. Penk (Eds.), *Returning wars' wounded, injured, and ill.* Westport, CT: Greenwood/Praeger Security International.

Sayer, N. A., Carlson, K. F., & Schnurr, P. P. (2010). Assessment of functioning and disability in assessment of PTSD. In D. M. Benedek & G. H. Wynn (Eds.), *Clinical manual for management of PTSD.* Washington, DC: American Psychiatric Association.

Schutt, R. (2010). Evolving consumer households. Cambridge, MA: Harvard University Press.

Schutt, R. K. (2010). *Homelessness, housing, and mental illness.* Cambridge, MA: Harvard University Press.

Schutt, R. K., Rosenheck. R., Penk, W. E., Drebing, C., & Seibyl, C. L. (2005). The social environment of work residence programs. *Psychiatric Rehabilitation Journal, 26,* 291–300.

Sherman, M. D., Sautter, F., Jackson, H., Lyons, J., & Han, X. (2006). Domestic violence in veterans with posttraumatic stress disorder who seek couples therapy. *Journal of Marital and Family Therapy, 32,* 429–434.

Sherman, M. D., Fisher, L. P., Bowling, U. D., Dixon, L. B, Ridener, L., & Harrison, D. (2009). A new engagement strategy in a new VA-based family psychoeducation program. *Psychiatric Services, 60,* 254–257.

Sherman, M. D., Fisher, L. D., Sorvico, K., & McFarlane, W. (2009). Adapting the multi-family group model for the VA system: The REACH program. *Professional Psychology: Research and Practice, 40,* 593–600.

Technical Cooperation Program. (2008). *Defining resilience: An international perspective.* Paper presented at the International Military Testing Association annual meeting, Amsterdam, The Netherlands.

Turpin, G., Downs, M., & Mason, S. (2005). Effectiveness of providing self-help information following acute traumatic injury: Randomized clinical trial. *British Journal of Psychiatry, 187*(1), 76–82.

U.S. Army. (1999). *US Army Field Manual 22-100.* Washington, DC: Department of the Army.

Veterans Health Administration. (2009). *Veterans Health Administration Handbook 1160.* Washington, DC: Department of Veterans Affairs.

Waldrop, R. S. (2007). The beginning of counseling psychology in VA hospitals. In R. R. Baker (Ed.), *Stories from VA psychology* (pp. 127–134). Bloomington, IN: Author House.

Weathers, F. W., Keane, T. M. & Foa, E. B. (2009). Assessment and diagnosis of adults. In E. B. Foa, T. M. Keane, M. J. Friedman, & J. A. Cohen (Eds.), *Effective treatments for PTSD* (2nd ed., pp. 23–61). New York: Guilford Press.

PART II

SPECIFIC CLINICAL ISSUES ASSOCIATED WITH PTSD

CHAPTER 12

Co-Occurring Affective and Anxiety Disorders

Eric C. Meyer
Nathan A. Kimbrel
Matthew T. Tull
Sandra B. Morissette

Overview of Research

Prior research suggests a high rate of co-occurrence between posttraumatic stress disorder (PTSD) and other anxiety and affective disorders in both civilian (Brown, Campbell, Lehman, Grisham, & Mancill, 2001; Kessler, Chiu, Demler, & Walters, 2005; Kessler, Sonnega, Bromet, Hughes, & Nelson, 1995) and military/veteran populations (Hoge et al., 2004; Kulka et al., 1990; Orsillo et al., 1996). For example, among a large sample of community outpatients diagnosed with mood and anxiety disorders, Brown and colleagues (2001) found that, among individuals diagnosed with PTSD, 62% met criteria for another anxiety disorder and 77% met criteria for an affective disorder. Among individuals diagnosed with PTSD, the most common co-occurring anxiety disorders were generalized anxiety disorder (GAD [DSM-IV hierarchical rules not applied]; 38%), panic disorder (PD; 23%), and obsessive–compulsive disorder (OCD; 23%). The most common co-occurring affective disorders were major depressive disorder (MDD; 69%) and dysthymia (23%). Hierarchy-free, co-occurring DSM-IV diagnoses in the past 12 months were examined in the National Comorbidity Survey Replication (Kessler et al., 2005). Moderate to high tetrachoric correlations were found between PTSD and other anxiety diagnoses (0.43–0.57) and between PTSD and affective diagnoses (0.44–0.50).

High rates of co-occurrence between PTSD and other anxiety and affective disorders have also been found among military and veteran populations (Hoge et al., 2004; Kulka et al., 1990; Orsillo et al., 1996). For example, Orsillo et al. (1996) found that veterans with PTSD were significantly more likely to be diagnosed with additional affective and anxiety disorders than veterans without a diagnosis of PTSD. PD (25%) was the most common co-occurring anxiety disorder. Interestingly, the rates of co-occurring GAD (7%) and OCD (5%) among veterans diagnosed with PTSD were much lower than the rates reported for a large civilian sample (Brown et al., 2001), likely indicating some combination of population-based and methodological differences. In contrast, MDD (55% among veterans) was clearly the most common co-occurring disorder among individuals diagnosed with PTSD in both civilian and military samples. PTSD is also quite common among veterans diagnosed with depression, as 36% of a large sample of randomly selected veterans diagnosed with depression also had a probable PTSD diagnosis (Campbell et al., 2007). Moreover, in this study, veterans diagnosed with co-occurring MDD and PTSD reported more severe depressive symptoms and were significantly more likely to report suicidal ideation than MDD-only veterans, highlighting the importance of assessing co-occurring conditions.

A wide array of biological, psychological, and environmental risk factors likely contribute to the co-occurrence of PTSD and other anxiety and affective disorders. We highlight three factors—genetic factors, personality factors, and traumatic brain injury (TBI)—that are believed to play significant roles in the co-occurrence of PTSD and other anxiety/affective disorders among military personnel.

Genetic Contributions

There is growing evidence that much of the overlap between PTSD and depression may be accounted for by genetic factors. For example, Koenen et al. (2008) reported that a common genetic liability accounted for 62.5% of the variance in MDD–PTSD comorbidity among a large sample of male Vietnam-era veterans. Kilpatrick et al. (2007) identified a gene x environment interaction suggesting a similar genetic profile for PTSD and depression. Specifically, Kilpatrick and colleagues noted that a polymorphism in the serotonin transporter gene (SLC6A4) interacted with trauma exposure and social support to predict both PTSD and MDD. Carriers of the low-expression variant of the serotonin-transporter polymorphism were 4.5 times more likely to develop both PTSD and depression if exposed to high levels of trauma (hurricane exposure) and low levels of social support. This finding suggests that genetic vulnerability confers increased risk for the development of PTSD and depression following traumatic exposures and that this risk may be further increased by low levels of social support.

There has been considerably less research addressing possible genetic overlap between PTSD and affective and anxiety disorders other than MDD. However, these limited data do suggest that genes that influence risk for other affective and anxiety disorders may also influence risk for PTSD (Koenen, 2007). Additional support for common genetic vulnerability between PTSD and other affective and anxiety disorders comes from a study by Hettema, Neale, Myers, Prescott, and Kendler (2006) who found "substantial, but not complete, overlap between the genetic factors that influence individual variation in neuroticism and those that increase liability across the internalizing disorders" (p. 857). Thus it may be the case that genetic factors influence the development of personality traits such as neuroticism and negative emotionality that, in turn, interact with environmental factors (e.g., trauma, social support) to influence risk for PTSD and co-occurring affective and anxiety disorders.

Personality Factors

Miller and colleagues have investigated the role of personality factors in the co-occurrence of PTSD and other anxiety and affective disorders (e.g., Miller, Greif, & Smith, 2003). Miller et al. (2003) identified three personality-based subtypes of responses among combat veterans, termed "resilient," "externalizing," and "internalizing." The internalizing subtype was characterized by co-occurring PTSD and depression and is therefore of particular relevance to the current chapter. The externalizing subtype was characterized by high levels of PTSD and co-occurring substance use problems. By contrast, the resilient subtype was characterized by lower levels of psychopathology. Relative to the resilient subtype, the internalizing subtype was characterized by lower Positive Emotionality (PEM), higher Negative Emotionality (NEM), and lower Constraint (CON), as measured by the Multidimensional Personality Questionnaire (MPQ; Patrick, Curtin, & Tellegen, 2002). The internalizing subtype also differed from the externalizing subtype in reporting lower PEM and NEM and higher CON than the externalizing subtype, with the biggest difference occurring in PEM. Taken together, these findings suggest that personality factors likely influence the type of co-occurring disorders that military personnel develop following traumatic exposure and that lower levels of PEM may be a key factor distinguishing veterans with PTSD and co-occurring anxiety and affective disorders from veterans exhibiting more externalizing psychopathology following trauma exposure.

Traumatic Brain Injury

TBI is considered a "signature" injury of the Operation Enduring Freedom and Operation Iraqi Freedom (OEF/OIF) conflicts and has been found to increase risk for both PTSD and depression (Hoge et al., 2008). For example, a large RAND survey (Tanelian & Jaycox, 2008) reported that 37% of returning OEF/OIF soldiers with probable TBIs also reported probable PTSD, probable MDD, or both. In addition, of individuals reporting probable TBIs and co-occurring PTSD or MDD, the majority (78%) reported all three conditions. Similarly, Hoge and colleagues (2008) found that TBI with loss of consciousness was associated with significantly increased risk for both PTSD (odds ratio = 2.98) and depression (odds ratio = 3.67). In addition, studies with civilian populations suggest that TBI may be associated with increased risk for PTSD, PD, social phobia, and agoraphobia (Bryant et al., 2010), as well as MDD (Jorge et al., 2004; Seel et al., 2003). Although additional research is needed in this important area, evidence suggests that TBI may play a key role in the co-occurrence of PTSD and other anxiety and affective disorders among military personnel.

Summary and Future Directions for Etiological Research

Prior research suggests that PTSD frequently co-occurs with other anxiety and affective disorders, particularly MDD. It is likely that genetic factors, personality factors, and TBI all contribute to the co-occurrence of these disorders; however, it is likely that other factors not discussed here also contribute to this co-occurrence (e.g., Green, Grace, Lindy, Gleser, & Leonard, 1990). For example, a study of Vietnam veterans conducted by O'Toole, Marshall, Schureck, and Dobson (1998) suggests that some anxiety and affective disorders (e.g., MDD, dysthymia, specific phobia) may reflect vulnerability for the development of PTSD, whereas other anxiety and affective disorders (e.g., PD, GAD) may develop secondary to PTSD. Additional prospective research is needed to untangle the complex etiological relationships among PTSD and other anxiety and affective disorders.

Assessment

Accurate assessment and diagnosis of PTSD is complicated by high rates of co-occurrence between PTSD and other affective and anxiety disorders, as well as symptom overlap. For example, the DSM-IV-TR (American Psychiatric Association, 2000) Criterion C symptom for PTSD of diminished interest or participation in significant activities overlaps with depression. Consequently, it is important that the assessment approach facilitates differential diagnosis. Here we present an overview of commonly used semistructured clinical interviews for the assessment of PTSD and other affective and anxiety disorders, focusing on the different methods and extents to which these measures facilitate differential diagnosis. We then briefly review relevant self-report assessments.

Structured Clinical Interview for DSM-IV

The Structured Clinical Interview for DSM-IV (SCID-IV; First, Spitzer, Gibbon, & Williams, 1996) is likely the most commonly used clinical interview for the assessment of anxiety and affective disorders, as well as for other DSM-IV diagnoses. Each module includes detailed prompts and inquiries to establish a diagnosis of a specific DSM-IV disorder. To aid in making differential diagnoses, at the end of each module, interviewers are instructed to consider whether symptoms may be better accounted for by another disorder, and a list of other potential diagnoses is provided. For example, at the conclusion of the PD module, interviewers rate their levels of confidence regarding whether anxiety and phobic avoidance more accurately reflects avoidance of stimuli associated with a traumatic event (i.e., PTSD) or avoidance of social situations due to fear of embarrassment (i.e., social phobia). In the SCID-IV PTSD module, respondents are asked to describe their symptoms as they relate to their worst traumatic experience, which reduces the chances that they may report symptoms of another anxiety or affective disorder on the PTSD module. In addition, the modular structure of the SCID-IV allows clinicians and researchers to target assessment of disorders that may aid in making an accurate differential diagnosis with regard to PTSD (Friedman, Keane, & Resick, 2007). A limitation of the SCID-IV is that it assesses only the presence or absence of symptoms, as opposed to symptom frequency and intensity. Therefore, the SCID-IV does not provide a continuous assessment of the severity of PTSD symptoms (or other disorders).

Anxiety Disorders Interview Schedule for DSM-IV

The Anxiety Disorders Interview Schedule for DSM-IV (ADIS-IV; Brown, Di Nardo, & Barlow, 1994) is a semistructured clinical interview designed to assess DSM-IV anxiety disorders, including PTSD. The ADIS-IV was specifically developed to facilitate differential diagnoses across the anxiety disorders, as well as to provide relevant, clinically useful information over and above that required to make a diagnosis. For example, the ADIS-IV assesses the history of the respondent's symptoms, situational and cognitive factors associated with symptoms, and detailed symptom ratings. The ADIS-IV also assesses for the presence of other psychiatric conditions, including substance use disorders and major depression, and it instructs the interviewer to make a distinction between a principal diagnosis and additional diagnoses, based on symptom severity and the degree of life interference associated with each diagnosis. These represent definite advantages of the ADIS-IV, aiding in case conceptualization and treatment planning, especially when working with patients with complex symptom presentations. For instance, a patient with PTSD can also be rated on his or her level of avoidance of social situations even if he or she does not meet criteria for social anxiety disorder, providing clinicians with information that may be useful in gaining additional understanding of a patient's primary diagnosis and current symptom presentation, as well as in developing a comprehensive treatment plan.

Clinician–Administered PTSD Scale–IV

As noted by Castro, Hayes, and Keane (Chapter 2, this volume), the Clinician-Administered PTSD Scale-IV (CAPS; Blake, Weathers, Nagy, & Kaloupec et al., 1995) is a 30-item clinical interview designed to provide both a categorical and a dimensional assessment of PTSD. Multiple psychometric studies have supported the robust psychometric properties of the CAPS with a variety of samples (see review by Weathers, Keane, & Davidson, 2001), making it the gold standard in PTSD assessment. However, an important limitation of using the CAPS is that it assesses only PTSD and associated features. Consequently, the CAPS must be used in conjunction with other clinical interviews to assess for the presence of co-occurring affective and anxiety disorders.

Self-Report Measures

A number of self-report measures provide dimensional assessments of PTSD severity. In addition, many have established cutoffs that indicate whether an individual is experiencing PTSD symptoms at a level indicative of a PTSD diagnosis. Some of the most common and well-established self-report measures include the PTSD Checklist (PCL; Weathers, Litz, Herman, Huska, & Keane, 1993), the Mississippi Scale for Combat-Related Posttraumatic Stress Disorder (Mississippi Scale; Keane, Caddell, & Taylor, 1988), the Posttraumatic Diagnostic Scale (PDS; Foa, Cashman, Jaycox, & Perry, 1997), and the Revised Impact of Event Scale (IES-R; Weiss & Marmar, 1997). Because self-report measures are necessarily limited in their ability to aid in making differential diagnoses, it is important to assess for the presence of symptoms of other affective and anxiety disorders. Self-report measures with strong psychometric properties include the Beck Depression Inventory–II (BDI-II; Beck, Steer, & Brown, 1996), the Center for Epidemiologic Studies Depression Scale (CES-D; Radloff, 1977), the Generalized Anxiety Disorder Questionnaire–IV (GADQ-IV; Newman et al., 2002), the Panic Disorder

Self-Report (PDSR; Newman, Holmes, Zuellig, Kachin, & Behar, 2006), the Social Phobia Scale (SPS) and the Social Interaction Anxiety Scale (SIAS; Mattick & Clark, 1998), and the Obsessive–Compulsive Inventory (OCI; Foa, Kozak, Salkovskis, Coles, & Amir, 1998).

Treatment Approaches

Understanding the impact of co-occurring disorders on treatment for PTSD is crucial, given that the modal PTSD case involves one or more co-occurring diagnoses (Kessler et al., 1995). In addition, the effectiveness of cognitive-behavioral therapy (CBT) and prolonged exposure (PE; Foa, Hembree, & Rothbaum, 2007) for PTSD is limited by the presence of co-occurring disorders, including depression (Taylor et al., 2001), GAD (Tarrier, Sommerfield, Pilgrim, & Faragher, 2000), and panic attacks (Falsetti & Resnick, 1997). Another important consideration is that use of benzodiazepines during treatment for PTSD has been associated with poorer treatment outcome for PTSD (van Minnen & Hagenaars, 2002). In their review of psychosocial and pharmacological treatments for PTSD and a broad range of co-occurring disorders, Najavits and colleagues (2009) concluded that the preferred treatment approach involves integrated treatment in which co-occurring disorders are treated at the same time, preferably by the same provider, thus allowing for flexible attention to all disorders and the links among them. Alternate approaches include the targeted treatment of one disorder with the expectation that the other condition will also improve, sequential treatment of disorders, and parallel treatment in which disorders are treated concurrently by separate providers or clinics. There are few data to inform the question of which approach is the most effective, as this relatively recent literature largely reflects early stages of treatment development. The current section focuses on studies examining military and veteran samples and studies published since the review by Najavits et al. (2009).

Integrated Treatment

PTSD and PD

Multiple-channel exposure therapy (M-CET; Falsetti, Resnick, & Davis, 2005, 2008) is based on cognitive processing therapy (CPT; Resick & Schnicke, 1992), an existing empirically supported treatment for PTSD, and panic control treatment (PCT; Craske, Barlow, & Meadows, 2000), an empirically supported treatment for PD. M-CET is composed of psychoeducation, breathing retraining, cognitive restructuring, and interoceptive and *in vivo* exposure conducted in twelve 90-minute group sessions. The developers of M-CET randomized a sample of women diagnosed with PTSD and panic attacks following a variety of potentially traumatic events to either M-CET or to a minimal-attention control condition of bimonthly telephone consultation (Falsetti et al., 2005, 2008). At posttreatment, among treatment completers ($n = 48$), a significantly higher proportion in the M-CET group no longer met criteria for PTSD (75%) compared with controls (17%). In addition, a significantly higher proportion of the M-CET group no longer met criteria for PD (75%) compared with controls (39%), and a significantly higher proportion of the M-CET group reported experiencing no panic attacks within the past month (50% vs. 13%). The M-CET group also reported significantly greater reductions in PTSD symptoms, number of panic attacks, fear of panic attacks, distress and interference associated with panic attacks, and depressive symptoms. M-CET was also associated with improved marital, occupational, economic, and overall adjustment. Each of these findings favoring M-CET was also found in more conservative intent-to-treat analyses, with the exception of depression. Individuals who completed M-CET maintained improvements in all areas at 3 and 6 months posttreatment.

These results provide strong preliminary support for M-CET as a treatment for PTSD and co-occurring PD. Changes in diagnostic status for PTSD compare favorably with studies that examined treatment for PTSD alone (e.g., Foa et al., 1999; Resick, Nishith, Weaver, Astin, & Feuer, 2002; Resick et al., 2008). Methodology by Falsetti and colleagues (2005, 2008) was strong, including a sample with exposure to multiple and diverse traumatic events, clinical assessors blind to treatment condition, and good fidelity and competence in providing the treatments. Further research on M-CET with larger and more diverse samples, including military and veteran samples, is warranted. One potential area of concern was that the drop-out rate for M-CET (36.4%) was somewhat higher than previously reported for CPT (26.8%) or PE (27.3%) for PTSD (Resick et al., 2002), although the overall drop-out rate did not differ between groups. It is certainly possible that the co-occurring panic disorder led to the increased dropout rate.

Sensation reprocessing therapy (SRT) is a cultural adaptation of individual CBT for PTSD and PD for Southeast Asian individuals developed by Hinton, Hofmann, Pitman, Pollack, and Barlow (2008). SRT is delivered in 12 individual sessions and comprises culturally appropriate education, visualization, cognitive restructuring, and mindfulness techniques, combined with existing methods of treating each disorder (e.g., Falsetti & Resnick, 2000; Foa & Rothbaum, 1998). Two samples of individuals diagnosed with PTSD and panic attacks were randomly assigned to SRT or to a waitlist control group, first a pilot sample of Vietnamese refugees, followed by survivors of the Cambodian genocide of 1970. These samples, which were characterized as treatment resistant, were subsequently combined, and large effects were observed for the SRT group (n = 28) compared to the wait-list control (n = 28) in terms of reductions in PTSD symptoms and panic severity (Hinton et al., 2008). Changes in panic severity partially mediated the effect of treatment on PTSD severity. Overall, SRT appears to be a promising integrative treatment for PTSD and PD, and its cultural awareness and sensitivity is noteworthy. Limitations of this research are that participants continued to receive supportive psychotherapy in parallel with SRT or wait-list, medication use was not controlled, a single clinician administered all treatment, and treatment adherence was not assessed. Additional research is needed in light of these methodological limitations.

PTSD and OCD

Integrative treatment for OEF/OIF combat veterans with PTSD and obsessive checking behavior related to traumatic experiences encountered in theater was examined in a recent case series with two male veterans diagnosed with PTSD who did not meet criteria for co-occurring OCD due to the diagnostic exclusion that compulsions may not be restricted to the context of another Axis I disorder (Tuerk, Grunbaugh, Hamner, & Foa, 2009). The authors present data suggesting that these cases represent a common symptom presentation among OEF/OIF veterans diagnosed with PTSD. Treatment involved a combination of PE and *in vivo* exposure with response prevention (Foa, Steketee, Grayson, Turner, & Latimer, 1984) to address compulsive checking. In both cases, PE was moderately effective in reducing the frequency and intensity of intrusive memories. However, the checking behaviors persisted in both cases, and the authors posited that negative reinforcement associated with checking was interfering with *in vivo* exposure, thereby constraining the effectiveness of PE. Exposure with response prevention, including a single in-home session, was conducted in both cases to address the overlearned checking behaviors. This additional component led to reductions in checking and urges to check, and neither veteran met criteria for PTSD by the end of treatment (12–15 sessions). This approach appears to be indicated for veterans whose multiple, repetitive checking behaviors have been repeatedly reinforced by superiors and peers during their war zone service.

Treatments for PTSD That Impact Co-Occurring Conditions

Depression/MDD

As noted by Najavits et al. (2009), given the high rate with which depression co-occurs with PTSD, virtually all PTSD treatment studies include individuals with co-occurring depression. However, studies often do not indicate the proportion of individuals who meet criteria for MDD or whether the treatment has differential effectiveness for individuals with MDD. In fact, we found no published studies in which differential treatment response for PTSD was reported for the subgroup who met criteria for a co-occurring mood disorder or that reported on the interaction between treatment condition and presence of co-occurring disorders. However, because of the importance and high rate of co-occurrence of PTSD and depression, we review select studies in veteran and military samples that examined the effect of treatment for PTSD on depression.

Monson et al. (2006) conducted a randomized clinical trial (RCT) examining the efficacy of CPT compared with wait-list control for 60 veterans diagnosed with military-related PTSD. The index trauma for the majority of participants was combat, whereas minority reported sexual and nonsexual assault. The rate of co-occurring mood disorders was 88%. Treatment was delivered in 12 individual sessions. There was a trend toward a decrease in level of depressive symptoms for CPT compared with wait-list control ($p < .08$), which represented a large effect at posttreatment and a medium effect at 1-month follow-up. The CPT group reported a significantly greater reduction in PTSD symptoms than the wait-list group, which corresponded to large effects at posttreatment and medium-to-large effects at 1-month follow-up for clinician- and self-reported symptoms. Distress associated with trauma-related guilt decreased in the CPT group compared with wait-list control at posttreatment, corresponding to a large effect. Strengths of this study include relatively liberal inclusion and exclusion criteria, in which veterans with current substance abuse and a moderate level of suicidal ideation were enrolled, and high treatment fidelity.

PE for veterans with chronic PTSD following service in Vietnam, OEF/OIF and sexual trauma during military service was examined in a recent case series (Rauch et al., 2009). Of these 10 veterans (8 men, 2 women), 50% met criteria for current MDD. Participants received between 7 and 21 individual sessions, with treatment ending based on mutually agreed-upon symptom remission ($n = 8$) and logistical problems ($n = 2$). In terms of PTSD symptoms, significant reductions (large effect) were observed. Reliable change in PTSD symptoms was observed for 90% of the veterans, and clinically significant change was observed for 80%. Similarly, in terms of depressive symptoms, significant reductions were observed (large effect), with reliable reductions in 40% of cases, and clinically significant reductions in 40% of cases. An interesting aspect of this research with respect to dissemination of evidence-based treatments was that half of the cases served as the first training cases for therapists who had no previous experience with PE and minimal CBT training. However, no treatment adherence data were collected.

GAD and MDD

Only one study has addressed treatment of co-occurring PTSD and GAD, with no studies of military or veteran samples. In a RCT examining individual CBT for 78 motor vehicle accident survivors with full or subsyndromal PTSD, Blanchard et al. (2003) reported on subsets of participants who also met criteria for GAD (35%) and MDD (49%). This form of CBT included psychoeducation, relaxation training, *in vivo* exposure, exposure-based homework, behavioral activation, and cognitive restructuring. Treatment did not address symptoms of GAD or MDD directly. CBT was compared with supportive psychotherapy and a wait-list control. In terms of reducing PTSD symptoms, CBT was superior to supportive psychotherapy, which was superior to wait list. These results were maintained at 3-month follow-up. In terms of addressing symptoms of GAD and MDD, CBT was superior to the two comparison conditions, which did not differ. Of the participants who met criteria for GAD at pretreatment, only 25% (2 of 8) in the CBT group met criteria at posttreatment compared to 79% for the comparison conditions combined. Similarly, for MDD, 18% (2 of 11) in the CBT group met criteria at posttreatment, compared with 63% in the comparison conditions. This treatment appears to be effective for PTSD following motor vehicle accidents and possibly for co-occurring GAD and MDD.

Treatments for Co–Occurring Conditions That Affect PTSD

Panic Disorder

A recent study examined CBT for PD among veterans with a primary diagnosis of chronic PTSD (Teng et al., 2008). A sample of 35 veterans meeting diagnostic interview criteria for PTSD and PD with or without agoraphobia were randomly assigned to 10 individual sessions of PCT, which consists of education, cognitive restructuring, and behavioral exercises, or to an active control treatment, psychoeducational and supportive treatment (PE-SUP). The proportion of panic-free participants did not differ between groups at posttreatment but did differ at 3-month follow-up, with 63% panic-free in the PCT group compared with 19% in PE-SUP. The PCT group reported significantly greater reductions in panic attack severity and panic disorder severity at posttreatment (moderate to large effects). However, these statistically significant differences were not maintained at 3-month follow-up, although effect sizes remained small to moderate. The PCT group reported significantly less fear of panic at follow-up (moderate effect) and less anxiety sensitivity at posttreatment and follow-up (moderate effects). However, there were no significant group differences in terms of symptoms of PTSD, anxiety, or depression at posttreatment or follow-up. In addition, PCT had a higher dropout rate (33%) than PE-SUP (12%), although the small number of dropouts overall limits interpretation of this finding.

Depression

It is frequently assumed that co-occurring depression is secondary to PTSD and that treating PTSD will lead to concomitant reductions in depression. One study examined whether treatment for co-occurring depression may lead to reductions in PTSD (Dunn et al., 2007). This study examined self-management therapy (SMT), an evidence-based group treatment for depression, compared with a psychoeducational group therapy (PGT) among 101 male veterans diagnosed with chronic, combat-related PTSD and MDD or dysthymia. In addition, approximately half of participants across treatment groups met criteria for personality disorders. Participants were randomized to 14 weekly sessions of SMT ($n = 51$) or PGT ($n = 50$). Drop-out rates were significantly higher for SMT than for PGT, although participants rated the helpfulness of both interventions equally. No group differences were observed in terms of changes in depression or PTSD symptom severity by 12-month follow-up.

Obsessive–Compulsive Disorder

This area remains largely unexplored, although Najavits et al. (2009) reported on two studies of inpatient treatment for OCD among individuals with co-occurring PTSD (Gershuny, Baer, Jenike, Minichiello, & Wilhelm, 2002; Gershuny, Baer, Radomesky, Wilson, & Jenike, 2003), concluding that primary behavioral treatment for OCD (i.e., exposure with response prevention) appears to be contraindicated for individuals with co-occurring PTSD. These findings highlight the importance of explicitly addressing co-occurring conditions (i.e., integrative treatment).

Limitations of and Future Directions for Treatment Approaches

We concur with the findings of Najavits et al. (2009) that integrated treatment of PTSD and co-occurring affective and anxiety disorders appears to be the most effective treatment approach. Currently, however, there are few studies that have examined integrated treatment for PTSD and co-occurring disorders. Preliminary results are promising for M-CET for PTSD and PD and for PE combined with exposure with response prevention for PTSD and co-occurring compulsions related to traumatic events encountered in the war theater. Findings to date suggest that single-diagnosis treatments for PTSD, which make up the majority of widely disseminated treatments for PTSD within VA and DoD (e.g., PE, CPT), have positive results for co-occurring depression, with one study also finding positive results for co-occurring GAD. Treatments that target co-occurring diagnoses do not appear to be effective in reducing PTSD symptoms. Another finding is that manualized interventions appear to be an effective treatment modality for treating individuals with PTSD and co-occurring affective and anxiety disorders.

Evidence suggests that the development and further refinement of integrated treatment approaches that directly address PTSD and co-occurring conditions would add significant clinical utility in terms of increasing the proportion of individuals with PTSD who benefit from psychosocial interventions. Currently, only one integrated treatment approach for PTSD and a co-occurring affective or anxiety disorder, M-CET for PTSD and PD, has undergone a single rigorous clinical trial with a moderate sample size (Falsetti et al., 2008). A small case series with OEF/OIF veterans examining the integration of PE and exposure with response prevention for PTSD and trauma-congruent checking behaviors found that integrating these two empirically supported approaches yielded encouraging results (Tuerk et al., 2009). This integrated approach may yield positive results with other clinical presentations in which obsessions or compulsions are thematically related to, or serve to relieve anxiety stemming from, trauma exposure. In addition, empirically supported treatments for PTSD have demonstrated positive results in reducing symptoms of depression with veterans (e.g., Monson et al., 2006; Rauch et al., 2009) and civilians (Blanchard et al., 2003). Integrating treatment components that target depressive symptoms more specifically (e.g., behavioral activation) may enhance the ability of these treatment approaches to reduce co-occurring depression. Finally, there is no published research on integrated treatment for PTSD and GAD or PTSD and social phobia.

Implications for Military Service and Integration into the Civilian Community

Co-occurring PTSD and anxiety or affective disorders can significantly influence whether military personnel continue their military careers and their reintegration into civilian life. Although mental health disorders do not necessarily lead to discharge, Hoge and colleagues found that they are the most common reason for early military attrition and also contribute to high rates of health care utilization (Hoge et al., 2002; Hoge et al., 2005). PTSD and co-occurring anxiety or affective disorders may also contribute to worse functional outcomes and poorer quality of life. This is particularly concerning in light of findings by Ginzburg, Ein-Dor, and Solomon (2010), who conducted a longitudinal study of 664 veterans of the 1982 Lebanon war and found that rates of co-occurring PTSD, anxiety, and depressive symptoms (26.7–30.1%) were higher than rates of PTSD only (9.3–11.1%), PTSD plus depression (1.2–4.5%) or PTSD plus anxiety (2.9–4.5%). This trifecta of illnesses was associated with worse functioning compared with PTSD alone or the presence of two co-occurring disorders. These findings are consistent with those of Mittal, Fortney, Pyne, Edlund, and Netherell (2006), who found that, compared with VA primary care patients diagnosed with MDD alone, patients with co-occurring GAD, PTSD, and MDD had worse health-related quality of life. In a study conducted nationwide, following hospitalization for traumatic injuries, patients with co-occurring PTSD and depression had a five- to sixfold increased risk of not returning to employment compared with a threefold increased risk of not returning to work when only one disorder was present (Zatzick et al., 2008). Thus, in addition to challenges associated solely with mental health problems, veterans with co-occurring PTSD and affective disorders may face even greater obstacles to reintegrating and returning to the workforce. This difficulty with returning to work among those with co-occurring disorders presents significant hardship for the families to whom veterans return.

The impact of war zone deployments, mental health disorders, and associated functional impairment clearly extends beyond military personnel and veterans to their families. Caregiver burden related to caring for veterans with physical or "invisible" wounds can be tremendous. Moreover, when the veteran returns home, symptoms of PTSD and co-occurring disorders can be quite confusing for families, particularly when they represent clear changes from predeployment. Data on the impact of co-occurring PTSD and affective and anxiety disorders on family functioning are lacking. However, parental mental health issues clearly have the potential to negatively affect child and family functioning (e.g., Stallard, Norman, Huline-Dickens, Salter, & Cribb, 2004). Conversely, children's mental health issues can negatively affect parental and family functioning (Kim, Viner-Brown, & Garcia, 2007). This is notable given that deployments alone have been demonstrated to have detrimental effects on children, including elevated rates of impairment in school, peer relationships, and family relationships (Chandra et al., 2009). After veterans are redeployed home, problems with children can affect how they reintegrate into the family, which may have learned new ways of functioning in the veteran's absence. High rates of divorce are observed among veterans with PTSD (Cook, Riggs, Thompson, Coyne, & Sheikh, 2004; Jordan et al., 1992), and a vicious cycle may ensue in which family structure transitions (e.g., divorce, remarriage, etc.) can further negatively affect functioning among children (Fomby & Cherlin, 2007).

Conclusion

In summary, after serving our country, both military personnel and the families to whom they return face diverse challenges, including coping with physical injuries and emotional wounds, finding employment in a struggling economy, and reintegrating into the family system. PTSD, affective disorders, and anxiety disorders can each independently influence ongoing military service and reintegration into the civilian community; synergistic effects associated with co-occurring disorders appear to intensify these problems. Thus it is imperative for health care providers to assess postdeployment functioning over time among both military personnel and their family members. In addition, treatment programs that target co-occurring mental health disorders and associated functional impairment are needed for military personnel and their families. Finally, empirically informed interventions that consider the dynamic influence of family members and military personnel on readjustment following return from the war zone would be particularly welcome. Development of such family-based interventions would augment the development of additional integrative treatment approaches for individuals diagnosed with PTSD and co-occurring disorders.

References

American Psychiatric Association. (2000). *Diagnostic and statistical manual of mental disorders* (4th ed., text rev.). Washington, DC:Author.

Beck, A. T., Steer, R. A., & Brown, G. K. (1996). *Manual for the Beck Depression Inventory* (2nd ed.). San Antonio, TX: Psychological Corporation.

Blanchard, E. B., Hickling, E. J., Malta, L. S., Jaccard, J., Devineni, T., Veazey, C. H., et al. (2003). Prediction of response to psychological treatment among motor vehicle accident survivors with PTSD. *Behavior Therapy, 34*, 351–363.

Blake, D., Weathers, F., Nagy, L., & Kaloupek, D. (1995). The development of a Clinician-Administered PTSD Scale. *Journal of Traumatic Stress, 8*, 75–90.

Brown, T. A., Campbell, L. A., Lehman, C. L., Grisham, J. R., & Mancill, R. B. (2001). Current and lifetime comorbidity of the DSM-IV anxiety and mood disorders in a large clinical sample. *Journal of Abnormal Psychology, 110*, 585–599.

Brown, T. A., Di Nardo, P. A., & Barlow, D. H. (1994). *Anxiety Disorders Interview Schedule for DSM-IV (ADIS-IV)*. San Antonio, TX: Psychological Corporation.

Bryant, R. A., O'Donnell, M. L., Creamer, M., McFarlane, A. C., Clark, R. C., & Silove, D. (2010). The psychiatric sequelae of traumatic injury. *American Journal of Psychiatry, 167*, 312–320.

Campbell, D. G., Felker, B. L., Liu, C.-F., Yano, E. M., Kirchner, J. E., et al. (2007). Prevalence of depression-PTSD comorbidity: Implications for clinical practice guidelines and primary care-based interventions. *Journal of General Internal Medicine, 22,* 711–718.

Chandra, A., Lara-Cinisomo, S., Jaycox, L. H., Tanielian, T., Burns, R. M., Ruder, T., et al. (2009). Children on the homefront: The experience of children from military families. *Pediatrics, 125,* 13–22.

Cook, J. M., Riggs, D. S., Thompson, R., Coyne, J. C., & Sheikh, J. I. (2004). Posttraumatic stress disorder and current relationship functioning among World War II ex-prisoners of war. *Journal of Family Psychology, 18,* 36–45.

Craske, M. G., Barlow, D. H., & Meadows, E. (2000). *Mastery of your anxiety and panic: Therapist guide for anxiety, panic, and agoraphobia* (2nd ed.). San Antonio, TX: Psychological Corporation.

Dunn, N. J., Rehm, L. P., Schillaci, J., Souchek, J., Mehta, P., Ashton, C. M., et al. (2007). A randomized trial of self-management and psychoeducational group therapies for comorbid chronic posttraumatic stress disorder and depressive disorder. *Journal of Traumatic Stress, 20,* 221–237.

Falsetti, S. A., & Resnick, H. S. (1997). Frequency and severity of panic attack symptoms in a treatment-seeking sample of trauma victims. *Journal of Traumatic Stress, 10,* 683–689.

Falsetti, S. A., & Resnick, H. S. (2000). Cognitive behavioral treatment for PTSD with comorbid panic attacks. *Journal of Contemporary Psychotherapy, 30,* 163–179.

Falsetti, S. A., Resnick, H. S., & Davis, J. (2005). Multiple channel exposure therapy: Combining cognitive-behavioral therapies for the treatment of posttraumatic stress disorder with panic attacks. *Behavior Modification, 29,* 70–94.

Falsetti, S. A., Resnick, H. S., & Davis, J. (2008). Multiple channel exposure therapy for women with PTSD and comorbid panic attacks. *Cognitive Behaviour Therapy, 37,* 117–130.

First, M., Spitzer, R., Gibbon, M., & Williams, J. (1996). *Structured Clinical Interview for DSM-IV.* Washington, DC: American Psychiatric Press.

Foa, E. B., Cashman, L., Jaycox, L., & Perry, K. (1997). The validation of a self-report measure of posttraumatic stress disorder: The Posttraumatic Diagnostic Scale. *Psychological Assessment, 9,* 445–451.

Foa, E. B., Dancu, C. V., Hembree, E. A., Jaycox, L. H., Meadows, E. A., & Street, G. P. (1999). A comparison of exposure therapy, stress inoculation training, and their combination for reducing posttraumatic stress disorder in female assault victims. *Journal of Consulting and Clinical Psychology, 67,* 194–200.

Foa, E. B., Hembree, E. A., & Rothbaum, B. O. (2007). *Prolonged exposure therapy for PTSD: Emotional processing of traumatic experiences: Therapist guide.* New York: Oxford University Press.

Foa, E. B., Kozak, M. J., Salkovskis, P. M., Coles, M. E., & Amir, N. (1998). The validation of a new obsessive–compulsive disorder scale: The Obsessive–Compulsive Inventory. *Psychological Assessment, 10,* 206–214.

Foa, E. B., & Rothbaum, B. O. (1998). *Treating the trauma of rape: Cognitive-behavioral therapy for PTSD.* New York: Guilford Press.

Foa, E. B., Steketee, G., Grayson, J. B., Turner, R. M., & Latimer, P. (1984). Deliberate exposure and blocking of obsessive-compulsive rituals: Immediate and long-term effects. *Behavior Therapy, 15,* 450–472.

Fomby, P., & Cherlin, A. J. (2007). Family instability and child well-being. *American Sociological Review, 72,* 181–204.

Friedman, M. J., Keane, T. M., & Resick, P. A. (2007). *Handbook of PTSD: Science and practice.* New York: Guilford Press.

Gershuny, B. S., Baer, L., Jenike, M. A., Minichiello, W. E., & Wilhelm, S. (2002). PeriodicalComorbid posttraumatic stress disorder: Impact on treatment outcome for obsessive–compulsive disorder. *American Journal of Psychiatry, 159,* 852–854.

Gershuny, B. S., Baer, L., Radomesky, A. S., Wilson, K. A., & Jenike, M. A. (2003). Connections among symptoms of obsessive–compulsive disorder and posttraumatic stress disorder: A case series. *Behaviour Research and Therapy, 41,* 1029–1041.

Ginzburg, K., Ein-Dor, T., & Solomon, Z. (2010). Comorbidity of posttraumatic stress disorder, anxiety, and depression: A 20–year longitudinal study of war veterans. *Journal of Affective Disorders, 123,* 249–257. ˙

Green, B. L., Grace, M. C., Lindy, J. D., Gleser, G. C., & Leonard, B. A. (1990). Risk factors for PTSD and other diagnoses in a general sample of Vietnam veterans. *American Journal of Psychiatry, 147,* 729–733.

Hettema, J. M., Neale, M. C., Myers, J. M., Prescott, C. A., & Kendler, K. S. (2006). A population-based twin study of the relationship between neuroticism and internalizing disorders. *American Journal of Psychiatry, 163,* 857–864.

Hinton, D. E., Hofmann, S. G., Pitman, R. K., Pollack, M. H., & Barlow, D. H. (2008). The panic attack–posttraumatic stress disorder model: Applicability to orthostatic panic among Cambodian refugees. *Cognitive Behaviour Therapy, 37,* 101–116.

Hoge, C. W., Castro, C. A., Messer, S. C., McGurk, D., Cotting, D. I., & Koffman, R. L. (2004). Combat duty in Iraq and Afghanistan, mental health problems, and barriers to care. *New England Journal of Medicine, 351,* 13–22.

Hoge, C. W., Lesikar, S. E., Guevara, R., Lange, J., Brundage, J. F., Engel, C. C., Messer, S. C., et al. (2002). Mental disorders among U. S. military personnel in the 1990s: Association with high levels of health care utilization and early military attrition. *American Journal of Psychiatry, 159,* 1576–1583.

Hoge, C. W., McGurk, D., Thomas, J. L., Cox, A. L., Engel, C. C., & Castro, C. A. (2008). Mild traumatic brain injury in U. S. soldiers returning from Iraq. *New England Journal of Medicine, 358,* 453–463.

Hoge, C. W., Tobani, H. E., Messer, S. C., Bell, N., Amoroso, P., & Orman, D. T. (2005). The occupational burden of mental disorders in the U. S. military: Psychiatric hospitalizations, involuntary separations, and disability. *American Journal of Psychiatry, 162,* 585–591.

Jordan, B. K., Marmar, C. R., Fairbank, J. A., Schlenger, W. E., Kulka, R. A., Hough, R. L., et al. (1992). Problems in families of male Vietnam veterans with posttraumatic stress disorder. *Journal of Consulting and Clinical Psychology, 60,* 916–926.

Jorge, R. E., Robinson, R. G., Moser, D., Tateno, A., Crespo-Facorro, B., & Arndt, S. (2004). Major depression following traumatic brain injury. *Archives of General Psychiatry, 61,* 42–50.

Keane, T. M., Caddell, J. M., & Taylor, K. L. (1988). Mississippi Scale for Combat-

Related Posttraumatic Stress Disorder: Three studies in reliability and validity. *Journal of Consulting and Clinical Psychology, 56,* 85–90.

Kessler, R. C., Chiu, W. T., Demler, O., & Walters, E. E. (2005). Prevalence, severity, and comorbidity of 12–month DSM-IV disorders in the National Comorbidity Survey Replication. *Archives of General Psychiatry, 62,* 617–627.

Kessler, R. C., Sonnega, A., Bromet, E., Hughes, M., & Nelson, C. B. (1995). Posttraumatic stress disorder in the National Comorbidity Survey. *Archives of General Psychiatry, 52,* 1048–1060.

Kilpatrick, D. G., Koenen, K. C., Ruggiero, K. J., Acierno, R., Galea, S., Resnick, H. S., et al. (2007). The serotonin transporter genotype and social support and moderation of posttraumatic stress disorder and depression in hurricane-exposed adults. *American Journal of Psychiatry, 164,* 1693–1699.

Kim, H. K., Viner-Brown, S. I., & Garcia, J. (2007). Children's mental health and family functioning in Rhode Island. *Pediatrics, 119,* S22–S28.

Koenen, K. C. (2007). Genetics of posttraumatic stress disorder: Review and recommendations for future studies. *Journal of Traumatic Stress, 20,* 737–750.

Koenen, K. C., Fu, Q., Ertel, K., Lyons, M. J., Goldberg, J., Eisen, S. A., et al. (2008). Common genetic liability for major depression and posttraumatic stress disorder in men. *Journal of Affective Disorders, 105,* 109–115.

Kulka, R. A., Schlenger, W. E., Fairbank, J. A., Jordan, B. K., Hough, R. L., Marmar, C. R. et al. (1990). *Trauma and the Vietnam war generation: Report of findings from the National Vietnam Veterans Readjustment Study.* New York: Brunner/Mazel.

Mattick, R. P., & Clarke, J. C. (1998). Development and validation of measures of social phobia scrutiny fear and social interaction anxiety. *Behaviour Research and Therapy, 36,* 455–470.

Miller, M. W., Greif, J. L., & Smith, A. A. (2003). Multidimensional personality questionnaire profiles of veterans with traumatic combat exposure: Externalizing and internalizing subtypes. *Psychological Assessment, 15,* 205–215.

Mittal, D., Fortney, J. C., Pyne, J. M., Edlund, M. J., & Wetherell, J. L. (2006). Impact of comorbid anxiety disorders on health-related quality of life among patients with major depressive disorder. *Psychiatric Services, 57,* 1731–1737.

Monson, C. M., Schnurr, P. P., Resick, P. A., Friedman, M. J., Young-Xu, Y., & Stevens, S. P. (2006). Cognitive processing therapy for veterans with military-related posttraumatic stress disorder. *Journal of Consulting and Clinical Psychology, 74,* 898–907.

Najavits, L. M., Ryngala, D., Back, S. E., Bolton, E., Mueser, K. T., & Brady, K. T (2009). Treatment of PTSD and comorbid disorders. In E. B. Foa, T. M. Keane, M. J. Friedman, & J. A. Cohen (Eds.), *Effective treatments for PTSD: Practice guidelines from the International Society for Traumatic Stress Studies* (2nd ed., pp. 508–535). New York: Guilford Press.

Newman, M. G., Holmes, M., Zuellig, A. R., Kachin, K. E., & Behar, E. (2006). The reliability and validity of the Panic Disorder Self-Report: A new diagnostic screening measure of panic disorder. *Psychological Assessment, 18,* 49–61.

Newman, M. G., Zuellig, A. R., Kachin, K. E., Constantino, M. J., Przeworski, A., Erickson, T., et al. (2002). Preliminary reliability and validity of the Generalized Anxiety Disorder Questionnaire–IV: A revised self-report diagnostic measure of generalized anxiety disorder. *Behavior Therapy, 33*, 215–233.

Orsillo, S. M., Weathers, F. W., Litz, B. T., Steinberg, H. R., Huska, J. A., & Keane, T. M. (1996). Current and lifetime psychiatric disorders among veterans with war zone-related posttraumatic stress disorder. *Journal of Nervous and Mental Disease, 184*, 307–313.

O' Toole, B. I., Marshall, R. P., Schureck, R. J., & Dobson, M. (1998). Posttraumatic stress disorder and comorbidity in Australian Vietnam veterans: Risk factors, chronicity, and combat. *Australian and New Zealand Journal of Psychiatry, 32*, 32–42.

Patrick, C. J., Curtin, J. J., & Tellegen, A. (2002). Development and validation of a brief form of the Multidimensional Personality Questionnaire. *Psychological Assessment, 14*, 150–163.

Radloff, L. S. (1977). The CES-D Scale: A self-report depression scale for research in the general population. *Applied Psychological Measurement, 1*, 385–401.

Rauch, S. A. M., Defever, E., Favorite, T., Duroe, A., Garrity, C., Martis, B., et al. (2009). Prolonged exposure for PTSD in a Veterans Health Administration PTSD clinic. *Journal of Traumatic Stress, 22*, 60–64.

Resick, P. A., Galovski, T. E. ., Uhlmansiek, M. O., Scher, C. D., Clum, G. A., & Young-Xu, Y. (2008). A randomized clinical trial to dismantle components of cognitive processing therapy for posttraumatic stress disorder in female victims of interpersonal violence. *Journal of Consulting and Clinical Psychology, 76*, 243–258.

Resick, P. A., Nishith, P., Weaver, T. L., Astin, M. C., & Feuer, C. A. (2002). A comparison of cognitive-processing therapy with prolonged exposure and a waiting condition for the treatment of chronic posttraumatic stress disorder in female rape victims. *Journal of Consulting and Clinical Psychology, 70*, 867–879.

Resick, P. A., & Schnicke, M. K. (1992). Cognitive processing therapy for sexual assault victims. *Journal of Consulting and Clinical Psychology, 60*, 748–756.

Seel, R. T., Kreutzer, J. S., Rosenthal, M., Hammond, F. M., Corrigan, J. D., & Black, K. (2003). Depression and traumatic brain injury: A National Institute on Disability and Rehabilitation Research model systems multicenter investigation. *Archives of Physical Medicine and Rehabilitation, 84*, 177–184.

Stallard, P., Norman, P., Huline-Dickens, S., Salter, E., & Cribb, J. (2004). The effects of parental mental illness upon children: A descriptive study of the views of parents and children. *Clinical Child Psychology and Psychiatry, 9*, 39–52.

Tanelian, T., & Jaycox, L. H. (2008). *Invisible wounds of war: Psychological and cognitive injuries, their consequences, and services to assist recovery.* Santa Monica, CA: RAND.

Tarrier, N., Sommerfield, C., Pilgrim, H., & Faragher, B. (2000). Factors associated with outcome of cognitive-behavioural treatment of chronic posttraumatic stress disorder. *Behaviour Research and Therapy, 38*, 191–202.

Taylor, S., Fedoroff, I. C., Koch, W. J., Thordarson, D. S., Fecteau, G., & Nicki, R. M. (2001). Posttraumatic stress disorder arising after road traffic collisions: Patterns of response to cognitive–behavior therapy. *Journal of Consulting and Clinical Psychology, 69*, 541–551.

Teng, E. J., Bailey, S. D., Chaison, A. D., Petersen, N. J., Hamilton, J. D., & Dunn,

N. J. (2008). Treating comorbid panic disorder in veterans with posttraumatic stress disorder. *Journal of Consulting and Clinical Psychology, 76,* 704–710.

Tuerk, P. W., Grunbaugh, A. L., Hamner, M. B., & Foa, E. B. (2009). Diagnosis and treatment of PTSD-related compulsive checking behaviors in veterans of the Iraq war: The influence of military context on the expression of PTSD symptoms. *American Journal of Psychiatry,166,* 762–767.

van Minnen, A., & Hagenaars, M. (2002). Fear activation and habituation patterns as early process predictors of response to prolonged exposure treatment in PTSD. *Journal of Traumatic Stress, 15,* 359–367.

Weathers, F., Litz, B., Herman, D., Huska, J., & Keane, T. (1993). *The PTSD Checklist (PCL): Reliability, validity, and diagnostic utility.* Paper presented at the annual convention of the International Society for Traumatic Stress Studies, San Antonio, Texas.

Weathers, F. W., Keane, T. M., & Davidson, J. R. T. (2001). Periodical Clinician-Administered PTSD Scale: A review of the first ten years of research. *Depression and Anxiety, 13,* 132–156.

Weiss, D. S., & Marmar, C. R. (1997). The Impact of Event Scale—Revised. In J. P. Wilson & T. M. Keane (Eds.), *Assessing psychological trauma and PTSD* (pp. 399–411). New York: Guilford Press.

Zatzick, D., Jurkovich, G. J., Rivara, F. P., Wang, J., Fan, M., Joesch, J., et al. (2008). A national U.S. study of posttraumatic stress disorder, depression, and work and functional outcomes after hospitalization for traumatic injury. *Annals of Surgery, 248,* 429–437.

CHAPTER 13

Co-Occurring Substance Use Disorders

Marc I. Kruse
Laurie E. Steffen
Nathan A. Kimbrel
Suzy Bird Gulliver

$\mathbf{A}$s clearly detailed throughout the chapters of this book, the prevalence and associated consequences of posttraumatic stress disorder (PTSD) in active-duty service members and military veterans is of significant societal and public health concern. Further, the co-occurrence of substance use disorders (SUDs; i.e., alcohol and/or other drug abuse or dependence) has frequently been identified as a prognosticator of poor physical and psychological health, as well as of poor treatment and functional outcomes, for individuals with PTSD (e.g., Ouimette, Goodwin, & Brown, 2006; Jacobsen, Southwick, & Kosten, 2001). The goals of the current chapter are to (1) provide a brief summary of the evidence of co-occurrence of PTSD and SUDs within military, veteran, and civilian populations; (2) evaluate the gold-standard assessments for substance use and diagnosis of SUD; (3) review published treatment strategies for these co-occurring conditions; and (4) discuss the implications of the co-occurrence of PTSD and SUDs on military service and successful reintegration into the civilian community.

Prevalence of Co-Occurring PTSD and SUDs

The frequent co-occurrence of PTSD and SUDs has been consistently documented over the past several decades within civilian, military, and veteran populations (e.g., McGovern, Xie, Segal, Siembab, & Drake, 2006; Chilcoat & Menard, 2003; Kessler, Sonnega, Bromet, Hughes, & Nelson, 1995; Kofoed, Friedman, & Peck, 1993; McFall, MacKay, & Donovan, 1992; Cottler, Compton, Mager, Spitznagel, & Janca, 1992; Kulka et al., 1990; Druley & Pashko, 1988; Schnitt & Nocks, 1984). Large-scale epidemiological studies conducted in the United States consistently suggest a lifetime prevalence rate for PTSD between 7 and 9% in the general population (e.g., Kessler et al., 2005; Hidalgo & Davidson, 2000; Kessler et al., 1995). Whereas the lifetime prevalence rate of alcohol use disorders in the general population is 13% (Kessler et al., 2005), both men (52%) and women (28%) who have been diagnosed with PTSD are significantly more likely to also meet lifetime diagnostic criteria for alcohol abuse or dependence (Kessler et al., 1995). Similarly high rates of lifetime drug use disorders are observed in men (35%) and women (27%) with a history of PTSD (Kessler et al., 1995) relative to the 8% lifetime prevalence rate observed in the general population (Kessler et al., 2005).

The high rates of co-occurrence between PTSD and SUDs are also apparent within veteran and military populations. For example, approximately one-third of male Vietnam veterans with an alcohol use disorder diagnosis and more than half of those diagnosed with a drug use disorder also meet diagnostic criteria for PTSD (Zatzick et al., 1997). Analyses of data from Operation Enduring Freedom and Operation Iraqi Freedom (OEF/OIF) veterans revealed that 38% of veterans who screen positive for possible PTSD are also at high risk for an alcohol use disorder (data derived from Seal et al., 2008). Similar findings were obtained from a study of more than 13,000 active-duty and National Guard soldiers who served at least one combat tour in Iraq. Of those soldiers who screened positive for either PTSD or depression, approximately 50% also engaged in problematic alcohol use and/or aggressive behavior (Thomas et al., 2010).

Evidence of the high co-occurrence of PTSD and SUDs is also available from an evaluation of patients seeking mental health services for either of these conditions. In a review of the literature, Jacobsen and colleagues (2001) reported prevalence rates between 25 and 42% for current PTSD and 36 and 50% for lifetime PTSD in patients seeking treatment for SUD. Within a sample of cocaine-dependent patients seeking treatment for SUD, 18–24% met current and 45% met lifetime diagnostic criteria for PTSD (Dansky, Byrne, & Brady, 1999; Brady, Dansky, Sonne, & Saladin, 1998). In addition, exposure to traumatic violence (a potential precursor to PTSD) is reported in 30–59% of women with chronic SUDs (Najavits, Weiss, & Shaw, 1997).

As noted by Bernhardt (2009), estimates of the prevalence of PTSD in OEF/OIF veterans seeking services for SUDs are comparable to the rates observed in individuals seeking SUD treatment in the general population (approximately 30%). There is some evidence to suggest, however, that the co-occurrence of SUDs in veterans who seek mental health care for PTSD may be even more pronounced. Specifically, it has been estimated that as many as 60 to 80% of military veterans seeking treatment for PTSD have at least some history of substance abuse (Kofoed et al., 1993).

Proposed Mechanisms of PTSD and SUD Co-Occurrence

Given the substantial evidence documenting consistent associations between an individual's response to traumatic events and his or her substance use, it is perhaps not surprising that a variety of mechanisms have been proposed to explain the high co-occurrence between PTSD and SUDs. In general, these proposed mechanisms can be categorized into one of three causal pathways (the *self-medication hypothesis*, the *high-risk hypothesis*, or the *susceptibility hypothesis*) or a fourth indirect pathway, the *third variable hypothesis*.

The *self-medication hypothesis* (e.g., Khantzian, 1999) asserts that the onset of PTSD following exposure to a traumatic event subsequently increases the risk for the development of SUDs in individuals who use alcohol or drugs as a way to cope with emotional and/or physical distress caused by PTSD symptoms. Proponents of the *high-risk hypothesis* conceptualize behaviors associated with the development of SUDs (e.g., heavy drinking, illicit drug use) as indicative of an individual's general tendency to engage in an overall pattern of high-risk behaviors. From this perspective, it is the frequency with which an individual engages in these other high-risk behaviors (e.g., reckless driving) that determines his or her risk of exposure to potentially traumatic events (e.g., a car accident) and therefore drives the co-occurrence between SUDs and PTSD. Proposed mechanisms associated with the *susceptibility hypothesis* are based on the presumption that the presence of one disorder increases an individual's susceptibility to the development of the other disorder. For example, proposals that suggest that damage to neuroanatomical structures and/or changes in neurotransmitters resulting from heavy alcohol and/or drug use place an individual at greater risk for the development of PTSD are consistent with the susceptibility hypothesis. Finally, proposed mechanisms associated with the *third variable hypothesis* postulate that the co-occurrence between PTSD and SUDs is driven by these disorders' associations with a common third variable, for example shared genetic vulnerability (e.g., Young et al., 2002; Xian et al., 2000), deficits in coping skills (e.g., Brown, Read, & Kahler, 2003), or personality traits (e.g.,

Miller, Vogt, Mozley, Kaloupek, & Keane, 2006; Miller, Greif, & Smith, 2003).

It is important to note that these hypotheses are not mutually exclusive. As an example, data from a longitudinal study examining the association between violent assault victimization and substance use revealed that baseline levels of illicit drug use were associated with increased risk for physical assault (i.e., high-risk hypothesis) and that new incidents of physical assault subsequently increased risk for later drug use (i.e., self-medication hypothesis; Kilpatrick, Acierno, Resnick, Saunders, & Best, 1997). Whereas there are at least some research data to support the validity of proposed mechanisms associated with each of the four categories described earlier, the most compelling evidence tends to support the self-medication hypothesis (e.g., Chilcoat & Breslau, 1998; Breslau, Davis, Peterson, & Schultz, 1997). Specifically, the preponderance of evidence suggests that the onset of PTSD typically precedes the development of SUDs (e.g., Kessler, 2000), that increases in symptoms of PTSD are mirrored by subsequent increases in substance use in veterans (Bremner, Southwick, Darnell, & Charney, 1996), and that reductions in PTSD severity (in particular, reductions in hyperarousal symptoms; Back, Brady, Sonne, & Verduin, 2006) are strongly associated with improvements in SUDs, with minimal evidence that reductions in SUD severity lead to improvements in PTSD symptoms (Hien et al., 2010). In addition, a recent examination of weekly PTSD and SUD symptom levels revealed that PTSD and SUD symptoms covary concurrently and that the transition to a PTSD diagnosis (from subclinical levels) is associated with an increase in the probability of dependence symptoms for alcohol (11%), cocaine (29%), and opioids (94%; Ouimette, Read, Wade, & Tirone, 2010). Although these results are in need of replication with a larger sample size, which would allow for an examination of potential moderators and mediators of these associations, the preliminary findings offer compelling support for the self-medication hypothesis as a causal pathway from PTSD to SUD.

Assessment

As described in detail by Meyer and colleagues (Chapter 12, this volume), the accurate diagnosis of PTSD and assessment of PTSD symptoms is made difficult by symptom overlap and high rates of co-occurrence between PTSD, affective disorders (e.g., major depressive disorder), and other anxiety disorders (e.g., obsessive–compulsive disorder). We concur with their recommendation to focus the assessment of PTSD within a framework that will facilitate differential diagnosis and encourage the reading of Chapter 2 (Castro et al.) and 12 (Meyers et al.) in this volume for thorough reviews of this topic. We now turn our attention to a brief summary of diagnostic criteria for the establishment of a substance use disorder, the gold-standard semistructured clinical interviews for assessing substance use and diagnosing SUDs, and commonly used screening instruments for SUDs.

Diagnostic Criteria for SUDs

Substance Dependence

SUDs (i.e., substance dependence and substance abuse) are defined as a "maladaptive pattern of substance use, leading to clinically significant impairment or distress" (American Psychiatric Association, 2000, p. 197). A diagnosis of substance dependence is based on the endorsement of three or more of the following symptoms occurring at any time during a 12-month period: (1) tolerance; (2) withdrawal; (3) taking the substance in larger amounts or over a longer period of time than was intended; (4) a persistent desire or unsuccessful efforts to cut down or control substance use; (5) a great deal of time spent in activities necessary to obtain, use, or recover from the effects of a substance; (6) reduction or cessation of important social, occupational, or recreational activities because of substance use; and (7) continued substance use in spite of knowledge of having a persistent or recurrent physical or psychological problem that is likely caused or exacerbated by the substance.

Substance Abuse

A diagnosis of substance abuse is determined by the presence of at least one of the following symptoms: (1) recurrent substance use resulting in a failure to fulfill major role obligations at work, school, or home; (2) recurrent substance use in situations in which it is physically hazardous (e.g., driving an automobile); (3) recurrent substance-related legal problems; and (4) continued substance use despite having persistent or recurrent social or interpersonal problems caused or exacerbated by the effects of the substance (American Psychiatric Association, 2000, p. 199). A diagnosis of substance abuse can be assigned only if an individual has never met dependence criteria for the same substance. If criteria for both substance dependence and substance abuse are currently met, the diagnosis of substance dependence is given precedent. As is the case for substance dependence, the diagnostic criteria for substance abuse are the same across substances.

Semistructured Clinical Interviews

Diagnosis of SUDs

Module E of the Structured Clinical Interview for DSM-IV Axis I Disorders (SCID-IV; First, Spitzer, Gibbon, & Williams, 1996) is recognized as the gold standard for the assessment and diagnosis of substance use disorders, according to the diagnostic criteria established in the Diagnostic and Statistical Manual of Mental Disorders (DSM-IV-TR). The SCID-IV provides a semistructured method of assessing each of the diagnostic criteria associated with substance dependence and substance abuse. The SCID-IV contains detailed prompts and inquiries to determine whether each criterion is met and to guide the interviewer through the process of differentiating between dependence and abuse diagnoses and the appropriate application of physiological dependence and course specifiers for diagnoses of substance dependence. The primary limitation of the SCID-IV is the inability to obtain a continuous rating of the severity of substance use disorders, as symptoms are rated as present or absent and not evaluated in terms of frequency or intensity.

Substance Use

The Timeline Follow-Back Interview (TLFB; Sobell & Sobell, 1992) is the gold-standard, episodic-based, semistructured interview for the assessment of substance use. Daily quantities of alcohol and/or drug use are evaluated for each day of the assessment window by using calendars personalized to identify dates of significance (e.g., birthdays, holidays, significant news events) as temporal cues to assist in recall. Typically administered individually, researchers have modified the protocol in order to administer the instrument in group settings with positive results (e.g., Pederson & LaBrie, 2006). Whereas the instrument has been validated for an assessment window up to 2 years (Sobell & Sobell, 1992), consideration should be given to the cognitive abilities and tolerance level of the client or participant in determining the length of the assessment window to be used in clinical or research settings.

Screening Instruments for SUDs

Alcohol Use Disorders Identification Test—Second Edition

The Alcohol Use Disorders Identification Test—Second Edition (AUDIT; Babor, Higgins-Biddle, Saunders, & Monteiro, 2001) was developed by the World Health Organization (WHO) as a simple method of screening for excessive drinking in primary care settings. An additional goal of the instrument is to provide primary care providers with "a framework for intervention to help hazardous and harmful drinkers reduce or cease alcohol consumption and thereby avoid the harmful consequences of their drinking" (Babor et al., 2001, p. 2). The AUDIT contains 10 items that cover the domains of hazardous alcohol use (three items), dependence symptoms (three items), and harmful alcohol use (four items). The potential score for each item ranges from 0 to 4, with higher scores indicative of higher risk for problematic drinking. Interpretation guidelines for the AUDIT suggest that scores between 8 and 15 are appropriate for simple advice geared toward reducing levels of drinking, scores between 16 and 19 are indicative of a need for brief counseling and continued monitoring, and scores between 20 and 40 warrant further diagnostic evaluation for alcohol dependence (Babor et al., 2001).

CAGE

The CAGE (Ewing, 1984) is a brief four-item instrument designed to screen for lifetime prevalence of alcohol use disorders. Positive endorsement of two or more of the items is suggestive of a possible alcohol use disorder. Each letter of the CAGE acronym is associated with one of the four symptoms evaluated:

C: Have you ever felt you should *cut down* on your drinking?
A: Have people *annoyed* you by criticizing your drinking?
G: Have you ever felt bad or *guilty* about your drinking?
E: *Eye-Opener:* Have you ever had a drink first thing in the morning to steady your nerves or to get rid of a hangover?

Michigan Alcohol Screening Test

The Michigan Alcohol Screening Test (MAST; Selzer, 1971) is a 22-item self-report screen designed to evaluate the patient's self-appraisal of the familial, social, and occupational problems associated with his or her heavy drinking. Each answer indicative of problematic drinking receives a score of 1. A total MAST score of 6 or more is suggestive of potentially hazardous drinking and the need for further evaluation for an alcohol use disorder (Selzer, 1971).

Drug Abuse Screening Test

The Drug Abuse Screening Test (DAST; Skinner, 1982) is a 28-item self-report questionnaire designed to screen for problematic drug use in primary care clinics. The content of the DAST items closely mimics that of the MAST items; they evaluate frequency of drug use, as well as familial, social, occupational, and legal consequences of illicit drug use. As is the case with the MAST, responses consistent with illicit drug use and associated consequences receive a score of 1, and a total DAST score of 6 or more is indicative of potentially problematic drug use and cause for further evaluation for a drug use disorder (Skinner, 1982).

Treatment Approaches

Whereas the effectiveness of a variety of treatments for PTSD (e.g., prolonged exposure [PE] and cognitive processing therapy [CPT]) and SUDs (e.g., cognitive-behavioral therapy [CBT], motivational enhancement technique [MET], and 12-step facilitation [TSF]) have been well documented, there is a paucity of research on the effectiveness of treatments for co-occurring PTSD and SUDs. Until quite recently, debate on treatment strategies for individuals with co-occurring PTSD and SUDs had centered on the order in which disorder-specific treatments should be provided sequentially. Many well-intentioned clinicians and researchers argued that treatment for PTSD symptoms in individuals with co-occurring PTSD and SUDs should be initiated only after a period of abstinence had been achieved, echoing concerns articulated by the Substance Abuse and Mental Health Services Administration (SAMHSA) that by "exploring trauma memories, well-intentioned counselors inadvertently may drive a client back to the substance" (Center for Substance Abuse Treatment, 2005, p. 410). On the other side of the debate were equally well-intentioned clinicians and researchers who were concerned that the sudden removal of the presumed primary coping strategy for dealing with PTSD-related distress (substance use) in the absence of formal treatment for PTSD symptoms would result in poor treatment and functional outcomes in these dually diagnosed patients. In addition, the traditional lack of overlap and absence of cross-training (Bernhardt, 2009) between clinicians within the PTSD and substance abuse clinics in the VA Health Care System likely contributed to the divisiveness of this debate between treatment clinics and providers.

As described in detail by Bernhardt (2009), in recent years a number of developments within the VA Health Care System have converged to help bridge this divide. Beginning with a 2004 national directive, OEF/OIF veterans seeking care within the VA system were routinely screened for PTSD, high-risk alcohol use, and depression. In 2007 a memorandum (Deputy Undersecretary of Health for Operations and Management, 2007) prohibited the practice of denying veterans with co-occurring PTSD and SUD admission to inpatient, residential, and specialized treatment programs for PTSD based solely on abstinence status. The VHA's 2008 Uniform Mental Health Service Package (Veterans Health Administration, 2008) dictated that mental health services must be made available to all eligible veterans, required the implementation of empirically supported treatments system-wide for veterans identified as using alcohol in excess (brief motivational counseling) and veterans with PTSD (PE or CPT), and integrated mental health services into all primary care clinics. These changes have been buoyed by an increase in the hiring of psychologists in the VA system, with a particular emphasis placed on the hiring of clinicians with expertise in both

PTSD and substance abuse treatment. Although the zeitgeist regarding the assessment and treatment of co-occurring PTSD and SUDs is clearly shifting within the VA system, state-of-the-art research protocols have failed to keep pace, as evidenced by the small number of treatment outcome studies (including randomized controlled trials) for co-occurring PTSD and SUDs published to date.

What follows is a summary of the findings from a small but representative sample of clinical studies examining treatment outcomes in individuals with co-occurring PTSD and SUD diagnoses. The summary is organized by intervention strategies with "sequential" treatments (in which one condition is treated first, followed by treatment of the second condition) presented first, followed by "concurrent" treatments (in which both conditions are treated at the same time but separately), and then "integrated" treatments (in which both conditions are treated simultaneously by the same provider).

Sequential Treatments

Transcend

The Transcend program is a 12-week partial-hospitalization treatment program designed for Vietnam veterans with co-occurring PTSD and SUDs diagnoses (Donovan, Padin-Rivera, & Kowaliw, 2001). Eligibility for the Transcend program includes the successful completion of a SUD rehabilitation program within the preceding 6 months, as well as abstention from alcohol and drugs for at least 30 days prior to the start of the program. Treatment during the first 6 weeks of Transcend is focused on skill development followed by 6 weeks of trauma processing. In addition to the processing of emotional issues from childhood and military trauma exposure, veterans engage in a variety of strategies, including individual presentations of traumatic events followed by constructive and supportive feedback from peers, a structured nightmare resolution technique, and sand-tray imaging (Donovan et al., 2001). Although SUD-specific treatment technically occurs prior to the start of Transcend, promotion of an addiction-free lifestyle is identified as one of the primary goals of the program, and substance abuse education, relapse prevention training, recovery group discussions, and weekly urine drug tests are part of the standard protocol (Donovan et al., 2001).

Veterans who completed the program showed a statistically significant reduction in PTSD symptoms that was maintained through a 12-month follow-up (Donovan et al., 2001). Further, relative to pre-SUD rehabilitation program levels of substance use, veterans who completed the Transcend program maintained significantly reduced levels of drinking and polysubstance use during the year-long follow-up period (Donovan et al., 2001). Of note, because participants in this study had already received treatment for SUDs and demonstrated a minimum of 30 days of abstinence prior to starting the program, the effectiveness of the Transcend program in reducing rates of substance use in the year following treatment may be better interpreted as signaling a potentially viable method for improving relapse prevention than an effective substance use treatment mechanism per se. That said, the treatment regimen utilized in Transcend may represent one effective strategy for treating co-occurring PTSD and SUDs, particularly if these pilot data can be replicated with other populations (including OEF/OIF veterans) and demonstrated to represent meaningful differences when tested against an appropriate comparison group.

Substance Dependence PTSD Therapy / Assisted Recovery from Trauma and Substances

A second sequential treatment for co-occurring PTSD and SUDs is Substance Dependence PTSD Therapy (SDTP; Triffleman, Carroll, & Kellogg, 1999; also known as Assisted Recovery from Trauma and Substances (ARTS). SDTP/ARTS is a cognitive-behavioral manualized treatment administered twice weekly over a 5-month period to individuals within an outpatient setting. The goal of the first phase of SDTP/ARTS is the initiation of abstinence from substance use. Treatment sessions during the initial phase are focused on psychoeducation and skills training (e.g., anger management, identification of substance use triggers, managing craving, relaxation training), with a particular emphasis placed on the association between PTSD symptoms and substance use. After a patient has maintained abstinence (or a significant reduction in substance use) and developed adequate coping skills (as determined by the clinician), they are transitioned to the second phase of SDTP/ARTS, which is focused on the treatment of PTSD symptoms. During the second phase, symptoms of PTSD are addressed with a combination of Stress Inoculation Training (SIT; e.g., Foa, Rothbaum, Riggs, & Murdock, 1991), Prolonged Exposure (PE; e.g., Foa, Hembree, & Rothbaum, 2007), and graduated *in vivo* exposure to feared situations.

In a small open comparison trial (Triffleman, 2000), 19 participants were assigned to either SDTP/ARTS or twelve-step facilitation (TSF), a standard treatment for SUDs that does not address symptoms of PTSD and is widely available in the community. Participants in both conditions demonstrated improvement in both substance use and PTSD severity, with no statistically significant differences observed between SDTP/ARTS and TSF. Of note, participants in SDTP/ARTS attended more sessions and were able to tolerate the exposure sessions associated with phase 2 of this treatment. A second pilot trial was conducted comparing SDTP/ARTS with Cognitive-Behavioral Coping Skills Therapy (CBCST; Carroll, 1998) in a sample of 36 patients with opiate dependence (Triffleman, unpublished data). Again, no significant differences were observed in reduction of PTSD symptoms, but those who received SDTP/ARTS attended more treatment sessions and had fewer positive toxicology screens.

Concurrent Treatments

Cognitive Behavioral Therapy for PTSD in Addiction Treatment Programs

Designed for individuals with co-occurring PTSD and SUDs, CBT for PTSD in addiction treatment programs (McGovern et al., 2009) is a manualized individual treatment program designed to reduce symptoms of PTSD and substance use. A total of eight modules are administered over 8–12 treatment sessions to provide the patient with (1) psychoeducation about the association between PTSD and substance use, (2) breathing retraining as a behavioral tool for reducing anxiety, and (3) cognitive restructuring geared toward the development of more adaptive cognitions and behaviors (McGovern et al., 2009). Each patient is provided with a client workbook, which is used in conjunction with the therapist manual. Of note, neither imaginal nor *in vivo* exposure components are included in the CBT for PTSD in ATP protocol.

Initial outcome data on the effectiveness of CBT for PTSD in ATP has been reported for a small sample of patients with co-occurring PTSD/SUDs recruited from community-based, intensive outpatient treatment programs for addiction who completed at least 75% of the treatment sessions and provided pre-, post-, and 3-month follow-up data (11 of 23 enrolled; McGovern et al., 2009). Significant reductions in PTSD and SUDs symptom severity were observed between pre- and posttreatment assessments and maintained through the 3-month follow-up. Reductions in frequency of alcohol and/or drug use were also observed but failed to reach the threshold for statistical significance. As noted by the authors, the absence of an appropriate comparison condition precludes a meaningful evaluation of the effectiveness of this program, particularly in light of the fact that the protocol was administered within an intensive outpatient program geared toward the treatment of addiction.

Concurrent Treatment of PTSD and Cocaine Dependence

Concurrent treatment of PTSD and cocaine dependence (CTPCD) is a cognitive-behavioral, manualized treatment program for individuals with co-occurring PTSD and cocaine dependence (Back, Dansky, Carroll, Foa, & Brady, 2001). The CTPCD program comprises sixteen 90-minute individual treatment sessions focused on (1) the provision of psychoeducation regarding the interrelationship between PTSD and cocaine dependence, (2) the initiation and maintenance of cocaine abstinence, and (3) reduction in PTSD symptoms (Back et al., 2001). In addition to a strong reliance on prolonged exposure (PE; Foa et al., 2007) for PTSD and coping skills training (CST; Carroll, 1998) for substance dependence, CTPCD includes modules on coping with craving, managing thoughts about cocaine use; dealing with a lapse in cocaine use; reactions to trauma; anger and negative thinking awareness and management; and assertiveness training (Back et al., 2001). The initial sessions of CTPCD are focused on skills development and promotion of abstinence, followed immediately by sessions geared toward the reduction of PTSD symptoms.

In a preliminary study of CTPCD, clinically significant reductions in both PTSD and SUD (cocaine) symptoms were reported for the subset of patients (40%) who completed treatment (Brady, Dansky, Back, Foa, & Carroll, 2001). Again, the significance of these results should be interpreted with caution given the absence of a control condition. Further, although treatment dropout is a common problem in this population, it was notable that 75% of those who failed to complete the CTPCD protocol dropped out prior to the first exposure session (i.e., the start of PTSD treatment). This finding underscores the intricate balance that researchers and clinicians must negotiate in determining both the course and length of treatment for individuals with co-occurring PTSD and SUDs.

Integrated Treatments

Seeking Safety

To our knowledge, Seeking Safety is the only published manualized CBT program that purports to address both PTSD and SUDs in an integrated fashion. As currently articulated (Najavits, 2002, 2003), the Seeking Safety treatment contains 25 modules centered around the five key principles on which the treatment program is based:

1. The most urgent clinical need is the establishment of safety.
2. Successful treatment of co-occurring PTSD and SUDs necessitates continual integration of these disorders throughout treatment.
3. Restoration of ideals (e.g., honesty, commitment, taking care of oneself) is an important and explicit goal of treatment.
4. Effective treatment addresses the cognitive, behavioral, interpersonal, and case management needs of the patient.
5. Therapist processes are critical to facilitating patient change (including compassion for patients' experience, provision of both positive and negative feedback, use of the treatment's coping skills in the

therapist's personal life, an expectation that the therapist is willing to meet the patient "more than halfway" to achieve meaningful change).

A number of treatment outcome studies examining the effectiveness of Seeking Safety across various modalities in high-risk populations have been published in the literature. An initial report demonstrated significant reductions in both substance use and trauma-related symptoms (among other positive outcomes) in a sample of 17 women with co-occurring PTSD and SUDs who completed group Seeking Safety in an outpatient setting (63% completion rate defined as attending 6 or more of 25 available sessions; Najavits, Weiss, Shaw, & Muenz, 1998). These findings were largely replicated in a sample of dually diagnosed incarcerated women (Zlotnick, Najavits, Rohsenow, & Johnson, 2003), although neither study contained a control group to which comparisons of the effectiveness of Seeking Safety could be made. The effectiveness of individually administered Seeking Safety was evaluated in comparison with a relapse prevention treatment (RPT) in a randomized controlled trial that also included a nonrandomized treatment-as-usual condition (Hien, Cohen, Miele, Litt, & Capstick, 2004). Whereas significant reductions in both PTSD and SUDs outcomes were observed in low-income urban women randomly assigned to either Seeking Safety or RPT when compared with treatment as usual, the effectiveness of these treatments did not differ from one another (Hien et al., 2004).

Several studies have examined the potential additive benefits of Seeking Safety when utilized as an adjunct to standard treatment as usual (Zlotnick, Johnson, & Najavits, 2010; Desai, Harpaz-Rotem, Najavits, & Rosenheck, 2008; Gatz et al., 2007; Najavits, Gallop, & Weiss, 2006; Hien et al., 2004). In two controlled trials (Desai et al., 2008; Gatz et al., 2007) and two randomized controlled trials (Najavits et al., 2006; Hien et al., 2004), patients who received Seeking Safety as an adjunct to standard treatment as usual demonstrated significantly greater improvements than those assigned to treatment as usual alone. In the most recently published randomized controlled trial (Zlotnick et al., 2010), however, there were no significant differences in PTSD or SUDs outcomes in a sample of incarcerated women randomly assigned to receive Seeking Safety as an adjunct to standard treatment as usual. As noted by Zlotnick and colleagues (2010; p. 333), the substantial variability in the "treatment as usual" conditions to which Seeking Safety has been compared to date suggests that some caution is necessary prior to reaching conclusions on the effectiveness of this treatment. For example, in the two randomized controlled trials demonstrating added benefit of Seeking Safety as an adjunct to standard treatment as usual, in one study only 33% of the comparison group received any services as part of "treatment as usual" (Hien et al., 2004), and in the second study it is unclear from the data presented whether all of the participants in the treatment-as-usual condition actually utilized the services available (Najavits et al., 2006). That said, there is evidence to suggest that as an integrated treatment Seeking Safety holds some promise for the treatment of co-occurring PTSD and SUDs, particularly among at-risk female populations. Future research efforts would benefit from an identification of the specific mechanisms of Seeking Safety that are associated with reductions in PTSD and SUDs so that they may be enhanced in order to facilitate greater change in patients with these co-occurring disorders.

Summary and Recommendation

It seems worthy of reiteration that the existing published literature on psychotherapy treatment outcomes for co-occurring PTSD and SUDs is limited, particularly given the well-documented high levels of comorbidity between these disorders. As summarized earlier, many of the peer-reviewed manuscripts published to date report preliminary findings based on small pilot studies designed primarily to test the feasibility of new treatment protocols. Understandably, these pilot projects typically fall short of the gold standard for treatment outcome studies (i.e., randomized controlled trials). The frequent absence of appropriate control conditions in these studies, however, too often precludes a meaningful evaluation of the effectiveness of these treatments due to an inability to account for the benefits that might be anticipated from the base treatment programs to which many of the protocols were added, nonspecific treatment effects (e.g., face-to-face time with a mental health professional, motivation to change in individuals seeking treatment), or merely the passage of time. Even the most well-studied (in terms of number of published studies and scientific methodology) treatment protocol examined thus far, Seeking Safety, has garnered only equivocal support as an effective stand-alone or adjunct treatment capable of producing reliable and significant reductions in PTSD and SUDs symptoms.

Given the absence of compelling data to support widespread training and dissemination of any of the treatment protocols currently available, it is our recommendation that future research efforts should focus explicitly on the identification of specific treatment mechanisms associated with improvement in PTSD and/or SUD symptoms. It is our belief that identification of the specific mechanisms of treatment that account for observed functional changes in PTSD and SUD symptomatology will lead to the greatest possible improvements in the lives of individuals with these co-occurring conditions. Moreover, as the zeitgeist surrounding the treatment of co-occurring PTSD and SUDs has shifted in the face of overwhelming evidence of the interconnectedness of these conditions, we believe that a discernible shift in attitude regarding the appropriateness of using exposure-based treatments of trauma-related symptoms in patients with SUDs has also begun to emerge. Exposure-based treatments, including prolonged exposure (PE; Foa et al., 2007; Rothbaum, Foa, & Hembree, 2007), which is widely recognized as the most effective first-line treatment for PTSD (e.g., Cloitre, 2009; Foa, Davidson, & Frances, 1999), have frequently been viewed unfavorably as a viable treatment strategy for individuals with co-occurring PTSD and SUDs. Concerns regarding the utilization of exposure-based treatments in individuals with co-occurring SUDs have most frequently been expressed as the belief that by reexposing patients to the traumatic experiences precipitating the onset of PTSD, clinicians would increase the likelihood of relapse and/or worsening of substance use (e.g., Pitman et al., 1991). Despite the growing empirical evidence to the contrary (for reviews, see Henslee & Coffey, 2010; Baschnagel, Coffey, & Rash, 2006; Coffey, Schumacher, Brimo, & Brady, 2005; Coffey, Dansky, & Brady, 2003), exposure-based therapies remain largely underutilized with patients with PTSD and SUDs in clinical settings. It is our position that future research and clinical efforts for the treatment of co-occurring PTSD and SUDs strongly consider the inclusion of PE in accordance with the guidelines for its use as recommended by Coffey and colleagues (Coffey et al., 2005; Coffey et al., 2003).

Implications for Military Service and Integration into the Civilian Community

Through the end of 2009, more than 2 million American men and women have been called on to serve in support of the military operations in Afghanistan and Iraq (Defense Manpower Data Center, 2009). For far too many of these servicemen and -women, exposure to traumatic events during military service (e.g., combat; treatment of wounded and dying soldiers, enemy combatants, and civilians; military sexual assault) will result in the development of symptoms associated with posttraumatic stress and substance use disorders. As a result, men and women who develop co-occurring PTSD and SUDs (or either one of these disorders in isolation) are significantly more likely to demonstrate poorer functional outcomes that will negatively atffect both their military service and their reintegration into civilian life.

Whereas the effects of PTSD on military service and reintegration are described in detail elsewhere in this volume, there is an increasing recognition of the impact of substance use and associated negative consequences in active-duty military personnel (e.g., Milliken, Auchterlonie, & Hoge, 2007). A survey of more than 16,000 active-duty military personnel revealed that 43.2% endorsed binge drinking (defined as the consumption of five or more standard drinks in one sitting for men; four or more drinks for women) at least once in the preceding 30 days and that on average service members drank heavily 30 times in the previous year (Stahre, Brewer, Fonseca, & Naimi, 2009). Further, of those who admitted drinking at least once in the previous year, 18.4% reported an adverse effect of drinking on military job performance (Stahre et al., 2009). It is also clear that the negative repercussions associated with problematic substance use typically extend to the lives of those closest to the soldiers. Active-duty service members who endorsed binge drinking were also more than five times as likely to acknowledge interpersonal problems with their significant other, five times as likely to admit that their spouse or live-in partner had threatened to leave or actually did leave the relationship, and almost nine times as likely to report that they were asked to leave by their partner (Stahre et al., 2009). In combination with evidence demonstrating high rates of divorce among veterans with PTSD (e.g., Cook, Riggs, Thompson, Coyne, & Sheikh, 2004), it is apparent that military personnel and veterans with co-occurring PTSD and SUDs may be particularly at risk for experiencing difficulties in interpersonal relationships. Hoge and colleagues (2005) have reported that mental health disorders are the most common reason for early military attrition, and symptoms of PTSD and SUDs (co-occurring and in isolation) are also likely to cause significant impairment in the motivation and ability to successfully obtain and retain work following completion of military service, thereby increasing financial hardship for returning veterans and their families.

Conclusion

Given the prevalence of co-occurring PTSD and SUDs in active-duty military personnel and veterans, as well as the severity and breadth of the negative effects that these disorders have on the ability to effectively function in the military and/or successfully reintegrate into civilian life, it is imperative for healthcare providers in the military, the Veterans Affairs health care system, and civilian practice to explicitly and routinely assess their patients for both PTSD and SUDs. Given the absence of empirically supported treatments for these co-occurring conditions, clinicians and researchers need to work together to identify the specific treatment mechanisms associated with meaningful improvements in both PTSD and SUD symptoms so that these components may be meaningfully combined to provide truly integrated treatment for co-occurring PTSD and SUDs. In turn, these integrated treatments need to be rigorously evaluated through randomized controlled clinical trials. In sum, clinicians and researchers alike must strive to continue to broaden our knowledge base by learning from the expertise of others and moving beyond our comfort zones in order to meaningfully participate in and contribute to the development of best practices for the treatment of co-occurring PTSD and SUDs.

References

American Psychiatric Association. (2000). *Diagnostic and statistical manual of mental disorders* (4th ed., text rev.). Washington, DC: Author.

Babor, T. F., Higgins-Biddle, J. C., Saunders, J. B., & Monteiro, M. G. (2001). *The Alcohol Use Disorders Identification Test: Guidelines for use in primary care* (2nd ed.). World Health Organization, Department of Mental Health and Substance Dependence.

Back, S. E., Brady, K. T., Sonne, S. C., & Verduin, M. L. (2006). Symptom improvement in co-occurring PTSD and alcohol dependence. *Journal of Nervous and Mental Disease, 194*(9), 690–696.

Back, S. E., Dansky, B. S., Carroll, K. M., Foa, E. B., & Brady, K. T. (2001). Exposure therapy in the treatment of PTSD among cocaine-dependent individuals: Description of procedures. *Journal of Substance Abuse Treatment, 21,* 35–45.

Baschnagel, J. S., Coffey, S. F., & Rash, C. J. (2006, December 22). The treatment of co-occurring PTSD and substance use disorders using trauma-focused exposure therapy. Retrieved July 7, 2010, from *www.thefreelibrary.com/The treatment of co-occurring PTSD and substance use disorders using...-a0170157224.*

Bernhardt, A., (2009). Rising to the challenge of treating OEF/OIF Veterans with co-occurring PTSD and substance abuse. *Smith College Studies in Social Work, 79,* 344–367.

Brady, K. T., Dansky, B. S., Back, S. E., Foa, E. B., & Carroll, K. M. (2001). Exposure therapy in the treatment of PTSD among cocaine-dependent individuals: Preliminary findings. *Journal of Substance Abuse Treatment, 21,* 47–54.

Brady, K. T., Dansky, B. S., Sonne, S. C., & Saladin, M. E. (1998). Posttraumatic stress disorder and cocaine dependence: Order of onset. *American Journal on Addictions, 7,* 128–135.

Bremner, J., Southwick, S., Darnell, A., & Charney, D. (1996). Chronic PTSD in Vietnam combat veterans: Course of illness and substance abuse. *American Journal of Psychiatry, 153,* 369–375.

Breslau, N., Davis, G. C., Peterson, E. L., & Schultz, L. (1997). Psychiatric sequelae of posttraumatic stress disorder in women. *Archives of General Psychiatry, 54,* 81–87.

Brown, P. J., Read, J. P., & Kahler, C. W. (2003). Comorbid posttraumatic stress disorder and substance use disorders: Treatment outcome and the role of coping. In P. Ouimette & P. J. Brown (Eds.), *Trauma and substance abuse: Causes, consequences, and treatment of comorbid disorders* (pp. 171–188). Washington, DC: American Psychological Association.

Carroll, K. M. (1998). *Therapy manuals for drug addiction: Manual 1. A cognitive-behavioral approach: Treating cocaine addiction.* Rockville, MD: National Institute on Drug Abuse.

Center for Substance Abuse Treatment. (2005). *Substance abuse treatment for persons with co-occurring disorders, treatment improvement protocol (TIP) Series 42* (DHHS Publication No. [SMA] 05-3992). Rockville, MD: Substance Abuse and Mental Health Services Administration.

Chilcoat, H. D., & Breslau, N. (1998). Investigations of causal pathways between PTSD and drug use disorders. *Addictive Behaviors, 23*(6), 827–840.

Chilcoat, H. D., & Menard, C. (2003). Epidemiological investigations: Comorbidity of posttraumatic stress disorder and substance use disorder. In P. Ouimette & P. J. Brown (Eds.), *Trauma and substance abuse: Causes, consequences, and treatment of comorbid disorders* (pp. 9–28). Washington, DC: American Psychological Association.

Cloitre, M. (2009). Effective psychotherapies for posttraumatic stress disorder: A review and critique. *CNS Spectrums, 14,* 32–43.

Coffey, S. F., Dansky, B. S., & Brady, K. T. (2003). Exposure-based, trauma-focused therapy for comorbid posttraumatic stress disorders–substance use disorder. In P. Ouimette & P. J. Brown (Eds.), *Trauma and substance abuse: Causes, consequences, and treatment of comorbid disorders* (pp. 127–146). Washington, DC: American Psychological Association.

Coffey, S. F., Schumacher, J. A., Brimo, M. L., & Brady, K. T. (2005). Exposure therapy for substance abusers with PTSD: Translating research to practice. *Behavior Modification, 29*(1), 10–38.

Cook, J. M., Riggs, D. S., Thompson, R., Coyne, J. C., & Sheikh, J. L. (2004). Posttraumatic stress disorder and current relationship functioning among World War II ex-prisoners of war. *Journal of Family Psychology, 18,* 36–45.

Cottler, L. B., Compton, W. M., Mager, D., Spitznagel, E. L., & Janca, A. (1992). Posttraumatic stress disorder among substance users from the general population. *American Journal of Psychiatry, 149,* 664–670.

Dansky, B. S., Byrne, C. A., & Brady, K. T. (1999). Intimate violence and posttraumatic stress disorder among individuals with cocaine dependence. *American Journal of Drug and Alcohol Abuse, 25*(2), 257–268.

Defense Manpower Data Center. (2009, December 29). *OEF/OIF deployments since September 11th, 2001 by component, gender, race, marital status, casualty status, deployment count and deployment days.* Seaside, CA: Author.

Deputy Undersecretary of Health for Operations and Management. (2007, November 23). *Memorandum: Management of substance use disorders.* Washington, DC: Department of Veterans Affairs.

Desai, R. A., Harpaz-Rotem, I., Najavits, L. M., & Rosenheck, R. A. (2008). Impact of the Seeking Safety program on clinical outcomes among homeless female veterans with psychiatric disorders. *Psychiatric Services, 59,* 996–1003.

Donovan, B., Padin-Rivera, E., & Kowaliw, S. (2001). "Transcend": Initial outcomes from a posttraumatic stress disorder/substance abuse treatment program. *Journal of Traumatic Stress, 14*(4), 757–772.

Druley, K. A., & Pashko, S. (1988). Posttraumatic stress disorder in World War II and Korean combat veterans with alcohol dependency. *Recent Developments in Alcoholism, 6,* 89–101.

Ewing, J. A. (1984). Detecting alcoholism: The CAGE Questionnaire. *Journal of the American Medical Association, 252,* 1905–1907.

First, M. B., Spitzer, R. L., Gibbon, M., & Williams, J. B. W. (1996). *Structured Clinical Interview for DSM-IV Axis I Disorders.* Washington, DC: American Psychiatric Press.

Foa, E. B., Davidson, J. R., & Frances, A. (1999). The expert consensus guideline series: Treatment of posttraumatic stress disorder. *Journal of Clinical Psychiatry, 60*(Suppl. 16), 3–76.

Foa, E. B., Hembree, E. A., & Rothbaum, B. O. (2007). *Prolonged exposure therapy for PTSD: Emotional processing of traumatic experiences.* New York: Oxford University Press.

Foa, E. B., Rothbaum, B. O., Riggs, D. S., & Murdock, T. B. (1991). Treatment of posttraumatic stress disorder in rape victims: A comparison between cognitive-behavioral procedures and counseling. *Journal of Consulting and Clinical Psychology, 59,* 715–723.

Gatz, M., Brown, V., Hennigan, K., Rechberger, E., O'Keefe, M., Rose, T., et al. (2007). Effectiveness of an integrated trauma-informed approach to treating women with co-occurring disorders and histories of trauma. *Journal of Community Psychology, 35,* 863–878.

Henslee, A. M., & Coffey, S. F. (2010). Exposure therapy for posttraumatic stress disorder in a residential substance use treatment facility. *Professional Psychology: Research and Practice, 41*(1), 34–40.

Hidalgo, R. B., & Davidson, J. R. T. (2000). Posttraumatic stress disorder: Epidemiology and health-related considerations. *Journal of Clinical Psychiatry, 61*(Suppl. 7), S5–S13.

Hien, D. A., Cohen, L. R., Miele, G. M., Litt, L. C., & Capstick, C. (2004). Promising treatments for women with comorbid PTSD and substance use disorders. *American Journal of Psychiatry, 161,* 1426–1432.

Hien, D. A., Jiang, H., Campbell, A. N. C., Hu, M.-C., Miele, G. M., Cohen, L. R., et al. (2010). Do treatment improvements in PTSD severity affect substance use outcomes? A secondary analysis from a randomized clinical trial in NIDA's Clinical Trials Network. *American Journal of Psychiatry, 167*(1), 95–101.

Hoge, C. W., Tobani, H. E., Messer, S. C., Bell, N., Amoroso, P., & Orman, D. T. (2005). The occupational burden of mental disorders in the U.S. military: Psychiatric hospitalizations, involuntary separations, and disability. *American Journal of Psychiatry, 162,* 585–591.

Jacobsen, L., Southwick, S., & Kosten, T. (2001). Substance use disorders in patients with posttraumatic stress disorder: A review of the literature. *American Journal of Psychiatry, 158,* 1184–1190.

Kessler, R. C. (2000). Posttraumatic stress disorder: The burden to the individual and to society. *Journal of Clinical Psychiatry, 61*(Suppl. 5), 4–12.

Kessler, R. C., Berglund, P. A., Demler, O., Jin, R., Merikangas, K. R., & Walters, E. E. (2005). Lifetime prevalence and age-of-onset distributions of DSM-IV disorders in the National Comorbidity Survey Replication (NCS-R). *Archives of General Psychiatry, 62*(6), 593–602.

Kessler, R. C., Sonnega, A., Bromet, E., Hughes, M., & Nelson, C. B. (1995). Posttraumatic stress disorder in the National Comorbidity Survey. *Archives of General Psychiatry, 52,* 1048–1060.

Khantzian, E. J. (1999). *Treating addiction as a human process.* Northvale, NJ: Aronson.

Kilpatrick, D. G., Acierno, R., Resnick, H. S., Saunders, B. E., & Best, C. L. (1997).

A 2–year longitudinal analysis of the relationship between violent assault and substance use in women. *Journal of Consulting and Clinical Psychology, 65,* 834–847.

Kofoed, L., Friedman, M. J., & Peck, R. (1993). Alcoholism and drug abuse in patients with PTSD. *Psychiatric Quarterly, 64,* 151–171.

Kulka, R. A., Schlenger, W. E., Fairbank, J. A., Jordan, B. K., Hough, R. L., Marmar, C. R., et al. (1990). *Trauma and the Vietnam war generation: Report of findings from the National Vietnam Veterans Readjustment Study.* New York: Brunner/Mazel.

McFall, M. E., MacKay, P. W., & Donovan, D. M. (1992). Combat-related posttraumatic stress disorder and severity of substance abuse in Vietnam veterans. *Journal of Studies on Alcohol, 53,* 357–363.

McGovern, M. P., Lambert-Harris, C., Acquilano, S., Xie, H., Alterman, A. I., & Weiss, R. D. (2009). A cognitive behavioral therapy for co-occurring substance use and posttraumatic stress disorders. *Addictive Behaviors, 34,* 892–897.

McGovern, M. P., Xie, H., Segal, S. R., Siembab, L., & Drake, R. E. (2006). Addiction treatment services and co-occurring disorders: Prevalence estimates, treatment practices, and barriers. *Journal of Substance Abuse Treatment, 31,* 267–275.

Miller, M. W., Greif, J. L., & Smith, A. A. (2003). Multidimensional personality questionnaire profiles of veterans with traumatic combat exposure: Externalizing and internalizing subtypes. *Psychological Assessment, 15,* 205–215.

Miller, M. W., Vogt, D. S., Mozley, S. L., Kaloupek, D. G., & Keane, T. M. (2006). PTSD and substance-related problems: The mediating roles of disconstraint and negative emotionality. *Journal of Abnormal Psychology, 115,* 369–379.

Milliken, C. S., Auchterlonie, J. L., & Hoge, C. W. (2007). Longitudinal assessment of mental health among active and reserve component soldiers returning from the Iraq war. *Journal of the American Medical Association, 298*(18), 2141–2148.

Najavits, L. M. (2002). *Seeking Safety: A treatment manual for PTSD and substance abuse.* New York: Guilford Press.

Najavits, L. M. (2003). Comorbid posttraumatic stress disorder and substance use disorders: Treatment outcome and the role of coping. In P. Ouimette & P. J. Brown (Eds.), *Trauma and substance abuse: Causes, consequences, and treatment of comorbid disorders* (pp. 147–169). Washington, DC: American Psychological Association.

Najavits, L. M., Gallop, R. J., & Weiss, R. D. (2006). Seeking Safety therapy for adolescent girls with PTSD and substance use disorders: A randomized controlled trial. *Journal of Behavioral Health Services and Research, 33,* 453–463.

Najavits, L. M., Weiss, R., & Shaw, S. (1997). The link between substance abuse and posttraumatic stress disorder in women. *American Journal on Addictions, 6,* 273–283.

Najavits, L. M., Weiss, R. D., Shaw, S. R., & Muenz, L. (1998). "Seeking Safety": Outcome of a new cognitive-behavioral psychotherapy for women with posttraumatic stress disorder and substance dependence. *Journal of Traumatic Stress, 11,* 437–456.

Ouimette, P., Goodwin, E., & Brown, P. (2006). Health and well-being of substance use disorder patients with and without posttraumatic stress disorder. *Addictive Behaviors, 31*(8), 1415–1423.

Ouimette, P., Read, J. P., Wade, M., & Tirone, V. (2010). Modeling associations between posttraumatic stress disorder and substance use. *Addictive Behaviors, 35,* 64–67.

Pederson, E. R., & LaBrie, J. W. (2006). A within-subjects validation of a group-administered timeline followback for alcohol use. *Journal of Studies on Alcohol, 67*(2), 332–335.

Pitman, R. K., Altman, B., Greenwald, E., Longpre, R. E., Macklin, M. L., Poire, R. E., et al. (1991). Psychiatric complications during flooding therapy for post-traumatic stress disorder. *Journal of Clinical Psychiatry, 52,* 17–20.

Rothbaum, B. O., Foa, E. B., & Hembree, E. A. (2007). *Reclaiming your life from a traumatic experience: Workbook.* New York: Oxford University Press.

Schnitt, J. M., & Nocks, J. J. (1984). Alcoholism treatment of Vietnam veterans with posttraumatic stress disorder. *Journal of Substance Abuse Treatment, 1,* 179–189.

Seal, K. H., Bertenthal, D., Maguen, S., Gima, K., Chu, A., & Marmar, C. R. (2008). Getting beyond "Don't ask; don't tell": An evaluation of U.S. Veterans Administration postdeployment mental health screening of veterans returning from Iraq and Afghanistan. *American Journal of Public Health, 98*(4), 714–720.

Selzer, M. L. (1971). The Michigan Alcoholism Screening Test (MAST): The quest for a new diagnostic instrument. *American Journal of Psychiatry, 127,* 1653–1658.

Skinner, H. A. (1982). The Drug Abuse Screening Test. *Addictive Behaviors, 7*(4), 363–371.

Sobell, L. C., & Sobell, M. B. (1992). Timeline followback: A technique for assessing self-reported alcohol consumption. In R. Z. Litten & J. Allen (Eds.), *Measuring alcohol consumption: Psychosocial and biological methods* (pp. 41–72). Totowa, NJ: Humana Press.

Stahre, M. A., Brewer, R. D., Fonseca, V. P., & Naimi, T. S. (2009). Binge drinking among U. S. active-duty military personnel. *American Journal of Preventive Medicine, 36*(3), 208–217.

Thomas, J. L., Wilk, J. E., Riviere, L. A., McGurk, D., Castro, C. A., & Hoge, C. W. (2010). Prevalence of mental health problems and functional impairment among active component and National Guard soldiers 3 and 12 months following combat. *Archives of General Psychiatry, 67*(6), 614–623.

Triffleman, E. (2000). Gender differences in a controlled pilot study of psychosocial treatments in substance dependent patients with posttraumatic stress disorder. *Alcoholism Treatment Quarterly, 18*(3), 113–126.

Triffleman, E. (unpublished data). *Posttraumatic stress disorder in addictions.* Undated presentation available at *www.csam-asam.org/pdf/misc/Triffleman. ppt.*

Triffleman, E., Carroll, K., & Kellogg, S. (1999). Substance dependence posttraumatic stress disorder therapy: An integrated cognitive-behavioral approach. *Journal of Substance Abuse Treatment, 17*(1–2), 3–14.

Veterans Health Administration (2008). Uniform mental health services in VA medical centers and clinics. In Veterans Health Administration Handbook, 1160.01.

Washington, DC: Department of Veterans Affairs. Available at: *www1.va.gov/ vhapublications/ViewPublication.asp?pub_ID=1762*

Xian, H., Chantarujikapong, S. I., Scherrer, J. F., Eisen, S. A., Lyons, M. J., Goldberg, J., et al. (2000). Genetic and environmental influences on posttraumatic stress disorder, alcohol and drug dependence in twin pairs. *Drug and Alcohol Dependence, 61,* 95–102.

Young, R. M., Lawford, B. R., Noble, E. P., Kann, B., Wilkie, A., Ritchie, T., et al. (2002). Harmful drinking in military veterans with posttraumatic stress disorder: Association with the D2 dopamine receptor A1 allele. *Alcohol and Alcoholism, 37* (5), 451–456.

Zatzick, D. F., Marmur, C. R., Weiss, D. S., Browner, W. S., Metzler, T. Z., Golding, J. M., et al. (1997). Posttraumatic stress disorder and functioning and quality of life outcomes in a nationally represented sample of male Vietnam veterans. *American Journal of Psychiatry, 154,* 1690–1695.

Zlotnick, C., Johnson, J., & Najavits, L. M. (2010). Randomized controlled pilot study of cognitive-behavioral therapy in a sample of incarcerated women with substance use disorder and PTSD. *Behavior Therapy, 40,* 325–336.

Zlotnick, C., Najavits, L. M., Rohsenow, D. J., & Johnson, D. M. (2003). A cognitive-behavioral treatment for incarcerated women with substance use disorder and posttraumatic stress disorder: Findings from a pilot study. *Journal of Substance Abuse Treatment, 25,* 99–105.

CHAPTER 14

Traumatic Brain Injury

Jennifer J. Vasterling
Mieke Verfaellie
Susan M. McGlynn

In addition to being associated with psychological stress, war-zone participation increases risk of physical injury, including traumatic brain injury (TBI). TBI has long been a concern to military healthcare providers, as reflected in such terms as *shell shock* in World War I (Jones, Fear, & Wessely, 2007). More recently, TBI has emerged as a particular concern for those serving in Operation Enduring Freedom (OEF) and Operation Iraqi Freedom (OIF), given the nature of the warfare, which includes exposure to blasts associated with improvised explosive devices (IEDs). Mild TBI (mTBI) and posttraumatic stress disorder (PTSD) are often comorbid (Hoge et al., 2008; Tanielian & Jaycox, 2008) in war veterans, sharing common risk factors (e.g., combat intensity), symptoms (e.g., irritability, sleep disturbance, mild cognitive impairment), and, in some cases, underlying neural substrates (e.g., prefrontal and hippocampal involvement; Stein & McAllister, 2009). Yet mTBI remains poorly understood in terms of how it may complicate psychiatric outcomes, including PTSD and its treatment.

Reflecting the theme of this volume, this chapter addresses TBI from the perspective of PTSD, limiting discussion to milder cases of TBI, which are thought to be the most frequent among returning veterans (Hoge et al., 2008). Subsequent sections address the scope and impact of mTBI in returning veterans, review treatment approaches for mTBI, and discuss potential implications for the treatment of PTSD when associated with mTBI.

mTBI in Military Personnel and Veterans

Definition and Mechanisms of TBI

TBI refers to a physiological disruption of brain function caused by a traumatic mechanical (e.g., direct blow to the head) or biomechanical (e.g., blast injury) force. TBI diagnosis is historical and based on symptoms at the time of injury, such as alteration in mental status (e.g., confusion, amnesia, or loss of consciousness) or focal neurological signs. Most mTBI definitions specify that loss of consciousness cannot exceed 30 minutes and that posttraumatic amnesia (i.e., impaired encoding of new information after the injury) cannot exceed 24 hours. The biomechanics of TBI resulting from direct impact on the brain, as may occur in motor vehicle accidents, point to acceleration–deceleration of the head as the primary cause of injury. However, the biomechanics of blast-induced TBI, which are thought to be the most common source of mTBI among OEF/OIF veterans (Owens et al., 2008), are not as well understood. Animal studies suggest that blast injury is possibly due to direct pressure changes as the blast wave passes through the head and/or there is transfer of kinetic energy to the central nervous system through blood vessels in the chest and abdomen (Cernak & Noble-Haeusslein, 2010). In addition to primary blast effects, brain damage (similar to that seen in nonblast TBI) can result from penetrating injuries due to shrapnel and debris and from direct impact of the head.

Epidemiology of TBI in OIF/OEF Veterans

Because milder deployment-related TBIs may have been undocumented at the time of injury, the prevalence of TBI in nonclinical samples has been difficult to ascertain; estimates range from 12% (Schneiderman, Braver, & Kang, 2008) to 23% (Terrio et al., 2009) in U.S. samples. Differences in prevalence rates across studies may also reflect sample-specific deployment exposures that are not necessarily representative of the deployed forces as a whole, especially as war-zone conditions evolve over time. In a large and possibly more representative sample, the prevalence of TBI was estimated at 19% (Tanielian & Jaycox, 2008).

The comorbidity of TBI and mental health disorders, including PTSD, is likewise high among OEF/OIF veterans. Tanielian and Jaycox (2008) estimated that one-third of combatants with TBI also suffered PTSD or depression. Hoge et al. (2008) similarly found that 44% of service members who reported TBI with loss of consciousness met screening criteria for PTSD, compared with 27% of those who suffered TBI with altered consciousness and 16% of those with non-TBI injuries. Whereas high comorbidity would not be unexpected given common risk factors such as combat intensity, the degree to which reports of TBI are influenced by psychiatric symptoms remains controversial. The results of Hoge et al. (2008), which found that the association between TBI and PTSD remained even after controlling for combat experiences, can alternately be interpreted as mTBI creating additional risk of PTSD or PTSD influencing the reports of mTBI.

Pathophysiological Sequelae

Mild TBI can be associated with persistent changes in brain structure and function. Diffusion tensor imaging studies measure the functional integrity of white matter and have demonstrated abnormalities in long white matter tracts that can be linked to aspects of cognitive dysfunction in individuals with persistent symptoms following mTBI (e.g., Niogi et al., 2008). Alterations in brain metabolism during task performance (McAllister, Flashman, McDonald, & Saykin, 2006) have also been observed in mTBI. A growing body of evidence in animals suggests that primary blast injury can affect the brain (Cernak & Noble-Haeusslein, 2010), but data on the pathophysiology of blast-induced TBI in humans are limited.

Clinical Sequelae

Natural Recovery from mTBI

In civilian samples, the sequelae of mTBI are transient in an overwhelming majority of patients (Carroll et al., 2004). The acute symptoms include physical (e.g., headaches, dizziness, nausea), cognitive (e.g., difficulty concentrating, slowed thinking, memory dysfunction), and emotional (e.g., irritability, anxiety, depression) symptoms. Symptoms typically improve within days or weeks to full recovery, but in a minority of patients they persist at 3 months postinjury. Similar symptoms are also common among individuals with other medical or psychological (e.g., PTSD, depression) conditions. Although postconcussion symptoms are associated with the acute, transient neurological effects of mTBI, it is now generally accepted that psychological, social, and motivational factors may be associated with the maintenance of at least a subset of these symptoms (McCrae, 2008).

Within the first week of injury, measurable impairments in cognitive function are evident on tests that emphasize speed of processing, verbal fluency, and delayed memory (McCrae, 2008). Performance typically returns to baseline by 1–3 months postinjury (Belanger, Curtiss, Demery, Lebowitz, & Vanderploeg, 2005). Despite this generally favorable recovery, patients may continue to show mildly reduced performance on measures of complex attention and working memory years after injury (Vanderploeg, Curtiss, &

Belanger, 2005). Clinically significant neuropsychological impairment may also persist in a small subset of individuals (Pertab, James, & Bigler, 2009). Of potential relevance to war-zone deployments during which service members may experience multiple TBI events, a history of multiple concussions is associated with poorer long-term outcomes in executive functioning and memory (Belanger, Spiegel, & Vanderploeg, 2010).

Comparison with Cognitive and Behavioral PTSD Sequelae

The neurocognitive sequelae of mTBI and PTSD overlap significantly, but the course of recovery differs notably in the two disorders. In contrast to the typically transient symptoms associated with mTBI, PTSD-related emotional and neuropsychological deficits frequently endure years after trauma exposure and may reflect pretrauma vulnerabilities in some cases. As in mTBI, PTSD is associated with relative weaknesses in attention, executive functioning, and memory (Vasterling, Verfaellie, & Sullivan, 2009). Aside from overlap in cognitive symptoms, somatic and emotional symptoms associated with TBI, such as sensitivity to noise, sleep problems, irritability, anxiety, and depression, are also commonly associated with PTSD (Benge, Pastorek, & Thornton, 2009). Moreover, comorbid psychiatric difficulties moderate postconcussion symptoms. In a study of Vietnam-era veterans, the effects of mTBI and PTSD on postconcussion symptoms were additive, but the effects of PTSD were consistently larger than those of mTBI (Vanderploeg, Belanger, & Curtiss, 2009).

Findings in OEF/OIF Military Personnel

The limited extant evidence suggests that the specific mechanism of injury (blast vs. nonblast) does not notably affect neurobehavioral symptoms (Belanger, Kretzmer, Yoash-Gantz, Pickett, & Tupler, 2009) or neuropsychological performance (Belanger, Kretzmer, Vanderploeg, & French, 2009). Several studies have focused on isolating the contribution of mTBI and PTSD to chronic neuropsychological sequelae, but results have been inconsistent, with some studies showing no impact of mTBI (Ivins, Kane, & Schwab, 2009) or PTSD (Brenner et al., 2010; Levin et al., 2010) and others showing poorer performance associated with TBI (Levin et al., 2010) or PTSD (Nelson, Yoash-Gantz, Pickett, & Campbell, 2009). With regard to neurobehavioral symptoms, Hoge et al. (2008) found that all observed variance in physical health and postconcussion symptoms (with the exception of headache) could be accounted for by PTSD and depression. In the same vein, Schneiderman et al. (2008) noted that the strongest factor associated with postconcussion symptoms was PTSD, even when overlapping symptoms between TBI and PTSD were parceled out.

Implications for Assessment

As indicated before, the nonspecific nature of postconcussion symptoms lessens their diagnostic utility. More broadly, however, the failure to observe consistent links between neuropsychological performance and mTBI and PTSD in OEF/OIF veterans challenges the usefulness of attributing complex neuropsychological sequelae to one of two potential diagnoses that share not only significant core features but also underlying neural substrates, including the hippocampus and prefrontal regions (Stein & McAllister, 2009). Rather than attempt to ascribe specific and definitive etiologies to symptoms that may be determined by multiple conditions, a more promising approach may be to focus on better characterization of cognitive, behavioral, and functional problems that manifest postdeployment, regardless of underlying etiology.

Impact of TBI on the Development and Persistence of PTSD

There is now strong evidence that PTSD can develop in the context of mTBI, even following a single incident in which the individual lost consciousness and had no opportunity to encode the event into memory (Harvey, Kopelman, & Brewin, 2005). In the context of military combat, war-zone stress exposures are rarely limited to a single discrete event but more commonly involve a series of repeated or ongoing life-threatening events. Thus, if a specific traumatic event is not remembered, it is still likely embedded in a larger context of psychological trauma. Even when conscious retrieval for a single incident fails completely, implicit encoding of certain aspects of the TBI event, and memory for associated events occurring before or after the TBI event itself, may be responsible for the development of symptoms (Harvey et al., 2005).

Psychologically traumatic events that occur in the context of physical trauma to the brain are more likely to result in PTSD than those not involving brain injury (Bryant et al., 2009; Hoge et al., 2008), although this association is typically limited to the mild end of the TBI spectrum. PTSD can be associated with moderate or severe TBI, but its likelihood is reduced with increased injury severity (Glaesser, Neuner, Lütgehetmann, Schmidt, & Elbert, 2004).

The mechanisms by which mTBI increases the risk of PTSD are likely multifaceted, involving not only the broader context of multiple disabilities and associated psychosocial stressors but also the integrity of neurocognitive processes both during and after the injury (Vasterling et al., 2009). For example, if altered consciousness at the time of the injury leads to a poorly integrated memory of the event or persistent executive dysfunction interferes with memory reconstruction, retrieval of the trauma memory may be difficult to regulate. Such poorly controlled recall of trauma memories may be particularly problematic if intrusive memories lead new contextual elements to be incorporated into the memory, thus creating additional triggers for emotional distress. Brain dysfunction at the time of the injury may also alter affective processing of the trauma event. Diminished cognitive resources can interfere with engagement in adaptive appraisal of the trauma event and active coping strategies that help reduce stress. Reduced cognitive efficiency can also indirectly affect how individuals cope with PTSD through their adverse effects on psychosocial and occupational functioning, leading to additional stress.

Treatment Approaches for mTBI

Treatment interventions for mTBI differ qualitatively from those used with more severe brain injuries and have primarily focused on early education to prevent the development of persistent postconcussion syndrome. However, the smaller group of patients experiencing persisting symptoms may require additional treatment approaches, particularly when there are comorbid conditions that have an impact on recovery and when early intervention is not possible (Howe, 2009). In these cases, a comprehensive neuropsychological assessment can provide critical information about cognitive, emotional, and other noninjury-related factors that may be compromising functioning and can assist in guiding treatment for these patients.

Interventions

A number of evidence-based psychoeducational interventions for mTBI have been developed (Helmick et al., 2010). The Department of Veterans Affairs (DVA)/Department of Defense (DoD) *Clinical Practice Guidelines* (Department of Veterans Affairs, 2009) recommend early education of patients and families with an emphasis on expectation of full recovery within weeks to a few months; symptom management (e.g., headache, pain, anxiety/depression); and a gradual return to normal daily activities as soon as possible postinjury to minimize the risk of developing persisting symptoms. In deployment contexts, early intervention would ideally occur in theater during the acute or subacute period of recovery by providing clear information that accurately describes the expected recovery after mTBI. For veterans and military personnel who have returned from deployment but who experience barriers to in-person treatment, effective psychoeducation and symptom management may also be provided by telephone. Bell et al. (2008)

found that patients who received four to five telephone counseling sessions directed at education and symptom management during the first 3 months after mTBI reported fewer symptoms and reduced impact of symptoms on everyday functioning at 6 months after injury relative to a control group.

There are also potential functional benefits of cognitive rehabilitation, which refers to a range of interventions that retrain prior skills and/or teach compensatory strategies that exploit cognitive strengths to compensate for relative cognitive weaknesses. Cognitive rehabilitation may be domain (e.g., attention) specific or may target multiple types of cognitive and functional impairments simultaneously. However, much of the evidence base for cognitive rehabilitation concerns moderate to severe TBI or nontraumatic brain injury (Rohling, Faust, Beverly, & Demakis, 2009).

Examples of cognitive rehabilitation interventions include attention process training (APT; Sohlberg & Mateer, 1987), an intervention that presents increasingly challenging tasks as patients master each level of difficulty, and goal management training (GMT; Levine et al., 2000). GMT teaches strategies to improve the ability to plan, organize, and achieve goals by following a series of structured steps, including orienting to the current context, selecting appropriate goals, breaking tasks into simpler subtasks, learning and remembering the goals and subgoals, and assessing the usefulness of selected strategies and solutions. Sohlberg, McLaughlin, Pavese, Heidrich, and Posner (2001) found significant improvement in complex attention in postacute patients with mild to severe brain injuries following APT. Likewise, GMT has demonstrated effectiveness for TBI patients with executive dysfunction (Kennedy et al., 2008).

The "burden of adversity" hypothesis (Brenner, Vanderploeg, & Terrio, 2009) suggests that mTBI is just one of a complex constellation of problems affecting recovery of returning veterans and that treating symptoms regardless of etiology reduces the cumulative effects of many contributing problems. Consistent with this perspective, manualized rehabilitation interventions targeting multiple cognitive and functional domains have been developed and/or adapted for use with OEF/OIF veterans who sustained mTBI during deployment and who experience cognitive and functional impairments months or years postinjury due to a variety of possible etiologies. For example, cognitive symptom management and rehabilitation therapy (CogSMART), a 12-week intervention adapted for OEF/OIF veterans from a treatment program initially developed for patients with schizophrenia (Twamley, Savla, Zurhellen, Heaton, & Jeste, 2008), includes psychoeducation, symptom management, and compensatory cognitive components. Preliminary data suggest that, among veterans who were enrolled in supportive employment and had sustained mild to moderate TBI an average of 4 years earlier, those who participated in CogSMART were more likely to find jobs and report fewer postconcussive symptoms than those receiving supportive employment only (Thomas, Williams, Bondi, Dellis, & Twamley, 2010).

Healthcare Delivery Models

Patients with mTBI often have multiple physical and mental health concerns, referred to as "polytrauma" by the VA. Providers reported coordinating the care of patients with polytrauma to be among their most daunting challenges (Sayer et al., 2009), and many questions remain about how to best structure care for these patients. For example, are returning veterans with histories of mTBI and PTSD best treated in specialty clinics (e.g., mental health, neurology), multidisciplinary rehabilitation settings, or primary care? Are treatments best integrated, delivered sequentially, or delivered concurrently? Prototypes of two possible approaches (biopsychosocial and step-care) to healthcare delivery for mTBI follow.

The biopsychosocial approach takes into account the influence of somatic, psychological, social, and motivational factors contributing to persisting symptoms and complaints following mTBI (McCrea et al., 2009). In the military population, chronic pain, sleep disturbance, PTSD, depression, substance abuse, and other psychological disorders all may contribute to the maintenance of symptoms. McCrea (2008) implemented an early multidisciplinary treatment model for civilian TBI that relies on liaison between the emergency department and a team of specialists (neuropsychologist, physiatrist, nurse coordinator) in a TBI clinic during the acute postinjury phase (1–5 days). Based on neuropsychological and medical evaluations, patients are given immediate feedback and recommendations that are often largely psychoeducational, with a follow-up plan if needed. However, most providers caring for OEF/OIF veterans will not see these patients until long after their injuries, when early prevention is no longer an option. Like McCrea's model, the VA polytrauma system of care includes settings that are typically multidisciplinary and consider both physical and psychological issues. Unfortunately, little outcome data are yet available on either model.

Terrio and colleagues (cited in Brenner et al., 2009) proposed a "step-care" treatment model that first provides education and expectation of recovery while simultaneously treating psychiatric symptoms and subsequently addresses somatic complaints and self-care routines. Because cognitive complaints can often be related to poor sleep, chronic pain, and psychological distress, treatment of cognitive symptoms is postponed until the former steps are adequately taken. Adopted in some active-duty military healthcare settings, the step-care approach may decrease unnecessary utilization of medical services. It is also purported to potentially reduce the impact of secondary gain and overuse of disability benefits, which could be framed as a roadblock to recovery during an earlier stage of treatment.

Summary of mTBI Treatment Approaches

Although evidence supports the utility of psychoeducational strategies and cognitive rehabilitation strategies for TBI, less is known about the application of psychoeducation in postacute phases of recovery or of cognitive rehabilitation for milder TBI (Snell, Surgenor, Hay-Smith, & Siegert, 2009). Evidence for the efficacy of post-acute treatment strategies is particularly relevant to military veterans, who may not be diagnosed or treated until months or years after their deployment, when symptoms may have been significantly exacerbated or maintained by a host of other conditions and psychosocial stressors. As important, as veterans return with multiple psychological and physical injuries, questions remain regarding the best models for healthcare delivery and coordination of care.

Treatment of PTSD in Patients with a History of mTBI

We know little about how mTBI may affect PTSD interventions, but the extent to which mTBI affects PTSD treatment outcomes will bear on the clinical management of comorbid PTSD and mTBI. Two core questions pertain to PTSD interventions in patients with history of mTBI and/or persistent cognitive compromise: (1) Are evidenced-based PTSD interventions contraindicated? (2) Is PTSD treatment response attenuated? Unfortunately, empirical evidence addressing these questions is scant. At the writing of this chapter, a VA–DoD Consensus Conference determined only that there was no evidence that evidence-based PTSD interventions would be contraindicated by mTBI (Department of Veterans Affairs PTSD/Mild TBI Consensus Panel, 2009). We focus here on psychosocial interventions for PTSD.

Potential Neurocognitive Mechanisms Affecting PTSD Treatment Response

In considering potential neurocognitive mechanisms affecting PTSD treatment response, we take into account three factors: (1) the nature of the cognitive deficit (e.g., memory, attention, executive); (2) the timeline of the cognitive deficit (i.e., resolved vs. enduring); and (3) the intervention component (e.g., exposure, cognitive reappraisal).

Nonspecific Effects of Neurocognitive Deficits

Neurocognitive compromise may hinder the treatment process in ways nonspecific to particular treatment components. For example, forgetfulness, distractibility, slowed information processing, and difficulties with planning and organization could arguably hamper more general aspects of treatment, such as reliable attendance, follow-through with homework, keeping pace with group discussions, and taking medications as prescribed. Interference of this type implies that deficits are current and, as reviewed earlier, likely affect only a small subset of patients with mTBI.

Deficits Potentially Interfering with Core Elements of Specific Interventions

Cognitive-behavioral therapies (CBTs) with cognitive reappraisal and/or exposure-based components are considered to be among the most empirically supported of any PTSD treatments. These interventions, however, also depend on the successful engagement of cognitive resources that may be impaired following mTBI. At its core, cognitive therapy requires consideration of alternate appraisals of negative or distorted thoughts attached to trauma experiences, with the goal of generating more realistic explanations and thoughts. Such modifications presumably require both sufficiently intact inhibition (of maladaptive thoughts) and cognitive flexibility (to reappraise thoughts and memories) for their success. Exposure-based treatments require controlled retrieval of the trauma memory and the subsequent modification of the memory and associated emotions. Much of the cognitive demand required by cognitive reappraisal, manipulation of trauma memories, and the formation of new associations is dependent on cognitive status at the time of the PTSD intervention and therefore compromised in only a subset of patients. However, even if neurocognitive deficits are resolved at the time of the intervention, neurocognitive impairment at the time of the trauma event potentially influences the encoding of the trauma event, associated affective processing, and the degree to which trauma-related memories and affect can be retrieved in an accessible, controlled manner during therapy.

Effectiveness of Psychosocial PTSD Interventions for Patients with Comorbid mTBI

Virtually no evidence exists addressing the effectiveness of PTSD interventions in patients with history of mTBI, although two small randomized studies of CBT to treat emotional symptoms in patients with mTBI provide some information. In evaluating CBT for the treatment of acute stress disorder following mTBI, Bryant, Moulds, Guthrie, and Nixon (2003) found that CBT reduced the development of PTSD immediately posttreatment and 6 months later. Although CBT was applied to patients with mTBI in the context of acute stress symptoms, it is plausible that it would also successfully reduce more enduring PTSD symptoms in patients with mTBI. In a sample of 20 mild to moderate TBI patients, Tiersky et al. (2005) found that CBT combined with neurorehabilitation reduced anxiety and depression symptoms compared with a wait-list control. Although far from definitive, these studies suggest that CBT can effectively improve emotional outcomes in the context of mTBI.

There is likewise no direct evidence addressing whether PTSD treatment response is attenuated or slowed in patients with mTBI. However, several studies examining normal variation in brain integrity in small non-brain-injured samples suggest that PTSD treatment response may be influenced by neural integrity and/or baseline neurocognitive functioning. Specifically, attenuated CBT response was associated with less proficient pretreatment verbal memory and narrative encoding (Wild & Gur, 2008), smaller rostral anterior cingulate cortex volumes (Bryant, Felmingham, Whitford, et al., 2008), and increased bilateral activation of the amygdala and ventral anterior cingulate (Bryant, Felmingham, Kemp, et al., 2008).

Summary of PTSD Treatment Implications

There is no evidence that current evidence-based PTSD interventions would be contraindicated in patients with history of mTBI, even in cases with persistent mild neurocognitive deficits. Instead, preliminary evidence from randomized trials using small samples suggest that CBT interventions targeting acute stress disorder and other emotional symptoms (anxiety and depression) were successful in preventing PTSD and/or reducing symptoms. As Soo and Tate (2007) suggest, the structure provided by CBT interventions may in itself benefit patients with cognitive deficits. The question remains whether PTSD treatment response is attenuated in mTBI patients, particularly when the mTBI was associated with transient or enduring neurocognitive compromise. If treatment response is attenuated, it may be that PTSD interventions will benefit from augmented strategies (e.g., cognitive rehabilitation) to address neurocognitive deficits or that PTSD interventions will need to be tailored to minimize the impact of the deficits (e.g., additional rehearsal of key treatment concepts, provision of written instructions, removal of distractions in the treatment setting). Until there is more evidence, we recommend using evidence-based PTSD interventions in patients with history of mTBI but with a watchful eye toward monitoring treatment response.

Conclusion

The nature of contemporary warfare has led to increased attention to mTBI among returning veterans. Although we know much about TBI at more severe levels, the factors that determine mTBI outcomes in a military context and the best treatment approaches for mTBI are not as well understood. The introduction of explosive blasts as an etiology has contributed to the many unknowns regarding combat-related mTBI. Moreover, the often prolonged and repetitive psychological stress exposures inherent in combat and consequent development of PTSD and other mental disorders complicate the picture. These unique combat-related factors limit to some degree inferences from the more extensive civilian mTBI literature. Not surprisingly, such ambiguities have fueled controversy surrounding healthcare delivery policies for returning veterans with history of mTBI, particularly in the context of comorbid PTSD. Yet, because of the high rates of mTBI among returning veterans with PTSD, providers caring for OEF/OIF veterans with PTSD regularly confront clinical presentations that include mTBI.

Although there is still much to be learned about mTBI and PTSD, we are able to draw on several basic observations to guide the care of veterans with PTSD and mTBI. First, most people with history of mTBI function relatively well. Psychoeducation, including a clear statement of expectations regarding recovery, currently ranks as the most effective tool in preventing adverse mTBI outcomes. On the other hand, the course of recovery from mTBI is not uniform across individuals, and subtle problems may surface, particularly in contexts of stress (e.g., war-zone participation) or high demand (e.g., transitioning back to civilian life). These seemingly contradictory findings call for a delicate balance of trying not to convey undue alarm or pessimism while nonetheless taking seriously difficulties that veterans may experience. Second, because we know that certain factors may complicate recovery from TBI (e.g., substance abuse, additional TBI), an important component of treatment will be preventing such complications from arising and addressing them, if they do. Finally, because there is no evidence to suggest that current evidence-based PTSD interventions are contraindicated in patients with mTBI, it is critical to continue to use our very best tools to treat PTSD as we await further evidence that addresses whether augmentation or modifications to current treatments may optimize outcomes among patients with mTBI.

References

Belanger, H. G., Curtiss, G., Demery, J. A., Lebowitz, B. K., & Vanderploeg, R. D. (2005). Factors moderating neuropsychological outcomes following mild traumatic brain injury: A meta-analysis. *Journal of the International Neuropsychological Society, 11,* 215–227.

Belanger, H. G., Kretzmer, T., Vanderploeg, R. D., & French, L. M. (2009). Symptom complaints following combat-related traumatic brain injury: Relationship to traumatic brain injury severity and posttraumatic stress disorder. *Journal of the International Neuropsychological Society, 15,* 1–8.

Belanger, H. G., Kretzmer, T., Yoash-Gantz, R., Pickett, T., & Tupler, L. A. (2009). Cognitive sequelae of blast-related versus other mechanisms of brain trauma. *Journal of the International Neuropsychological Society, 15,* 1–8.

Belanger, H. G., Spiegel, E., & Vanderploeg, R. D. (2010). Neuropsychological performance following a history of multiple self-reported concussions: A meta-analysis. *Journal of the International Neuropsychological Society, 16,* 262–267.

Bell, K. R., Hoffman, J. M., Temkin, N. R., Powell, J. M., Fraser, R. T., Esselman, P. C., et al. (2008). The effect of telephone counseling on reducing posttraumatic symptoms after mild traumatic brain injury: A randomized trial. *Journal of Neurology, Neurosurgery, and Psychiatry, 79,* 1275–1281.

Benge, J. F., Pastorek, N. J., & Thornton, G. M. (2009). Postconcussive symptoms in OEF–OIF veterans: Factor structure and impact of posttraumatic stress. *Rehabilitation Psychology, 54,* 270–278.

Brenner, L. A., Terrio, H., Homaifar, B. Y., Gutierrez, P. M., Staves, P. J., Harwood, J. E. F., et al. (2010). Neuropsychological test performance in soldiers with blast-related mild TBI. *Neuropsychology, 24,* 160–167.

Brenner, L. A., Vanderploeg, R. D., & Terrio, H. (2009). Assessment and diagnosis of mild traumatic brain injury, posttraumatic stress disorder, and other polytrauma conditions: Burden of adversity hypothesis. *Rehabilitation Psychology, 54,* 239–246.

Bryant, R. A., Creamer, M., O'Donnell, M., Silove, D., Clark, C. R., & McFarlane, A. C. (2009). Post-traumatic amnesia and the nature of post-traumatic stress disorder after mild traumatic brain injury. *Journal of the International Neuropsychological Society, 15,* 862–867.

Bryant, R. A., Felmingham, K., Kemp, A., Das, P., Hughes, G., Peduto, A., et al. (2008). Amygdala and ventral anterior cingulate activation predicts treatment response to cognitive behaviour therapy for post-traumatic stress disorder. *Psychological Medicine, 38,* 555–561.

Bryant, R. A., Felmingham, K., Whitford, T. J., Kemp, A., Hughes, G., Peduto, A. et al. (2008). Rostral anterior cingulate volume predicts treatment response to cognitive-behavioural therapy for posttraumatic stress disorder. *Journal of Psychiatry Neuroscience, 33,* 142–146.

Bryant, R. A., Moulds, M., Guthrie, R., & Nixon, R. D. (2003). Treating acute stress disorder after traumatic brain injury. *American Journal of Psychiatry, 160,* 585–587.

Carroll, L. J., Cassidy, J. D., Peloso, P. M., Borg, J., von Holst, H., Holm, L., et al. (2004). Prognosis for mild traumatic brain injury: Results of the WHO Collaborating Centre Task Force on Mild Traumatic Brain Injury. *Journal of Rehabilitation Medicine, 43*(Suppl.), 84–105.

Cernak, I., & Noble-Haeusslein, L. J. (2010). Traumatic brain injury: An overview of pathobiology with emphasis on military populations. *Journal of Cerebral Blood Flow and Metabolism, 30,* 255–266.

Department of Veterans Affairs. (2009, March). *VA/DoD clinical practice guideline for management of concussion/mild traumatic brain injury.* Washington, DC: Department of Veterans Affairs.

Department of Veterans Affairs PTSD/Mild TBI Consensus Panel. (2009). *Report of (VA) concensus conference: Practice recommendations for treatment of veterans with comorbid TBI, pain, and PTSD.* Retrieved from *www.ptsd.va.gov/ professional/pages/handouts-pdf/TBI_PTSD_Pain_Practice_Recommend.pdf*

Glaesser, J., Neuner, F., Lütgehetmann, R., Schmidt, R., & Elbert, T. (2004). Posttraumatic stress disorder in patients with traumatic brain injury. *BMC Psychiatry, 9,* 4–5.

Harvey, A. G., Kopelman, M. D., & Brewin, C. R. (2005). PTSD and traumatic brain injury. In J. J. Vasterling & C. R. Brewin (Eds.), *Neuropsychology of PTSD: Biological, cognitive, and clinical perspectives* (pp. 230–246). New York: Guilford Press.

Helmick, K., & Members of Consensus Conference. (2010). Cognitive rehabilitation for military personnel with mild traumatic brain injury and chronic postconcussional disorder: Results of April 2009 consensus conference. *NeuroRehabilitation, 26,* 239–255.

Hoge, C. W., McGurk, D., Thomas, J. L., Cox, A. L., Engel, C. C., & Castro, C. A. (2008). Mild traumatic brain injury in U.S. soldiers returning from Iraq. *New England Journal of Medicine, 358,* 453–463.

Howe, L. L. (2009). Giving context to post-deployment post-concussive-like symptoms: Blast-related potential mild traumatic brain injury and comorbidities. *Clinical Neuropsychologist, 23,* 1315–1337.

Ivins, B. J., Kane, R., & Schwab, K. A. (2009). Performance on the automated neuropsychological assessment metrics in a nonclinical sample of soldiers screened for mild TBI after returning from Iraq and Afghanistan: A descriptive analysis. *Journal of Head Trauma Rehabilitation, 24,* 24–31.

Jones, E., Fear, N.T., & Wessely, S. (2007). Shell shock and mild traumatic brain injury: A historical review. *American Journal of Psychiatry, 164,* 1641–1645.

Kennedy, M. R. T., Coelho, C., Turkstra, L., Ylvisaker, M., Sohlberg, M. M., Yorkston, K., et al. (2008). Intervention for executive functions after traumatic brain injury: A systematic review, meta-analysis and clinical recommendations. *Neuropsychological Rehabilitation,18,* 257–299.

Levin, H. S., Wilde, E., Troyanskaya, M., Petersen, N. J., Scheiber, R., Newsome, M., et al. (2010). Diffusion tensor imaging of mild to moderate blast-related traumatic brain injury and its sequelae. *Journal of Neurotrauma, 27,* 683–694.

Levine, B., Robertson, I. H., Clare, L., Carter, G., Hong, J., Wilson, B. A., et al. (2000). Rehabilitation of executive functioning: An experimental validation of goal management training. *Journal of the International Neuropsychological Society, 6,* 299–312.

McAllister, T. W., Flashman, L. A., McDonald, B. C., & Saykin, A. J. (2006). Mechanisms of working memory dysfunction after mild and moderate TBI: Evidence from functional MRI and neurogenetics. *Journal of Neurotrauma, 23,* 1450–1467.

McCrea, M. A. (2008). *Mild traumatic brain injury and postconcussion syndrome.* New York: Oxford University Press.

McCrea, M. A., Iverson, G. L., McAllister, T. W., Hammeke, T. A., Powell, M. R., Barr, W. B., et al. (2009). An integrated review of recovery after mild traumatic brain injury (MTBI): Implications for clinical management. *Clinical Neuropsychologist, 23,* 1368–1390.

Nelson, L. A., Yoash-Gantz, R. E., Pickett, T., & Campbell, T. A. (2009). Relationship between processing speed and executive functioning performance among OEF/OIF veterans: Implications for postdeployment rehabilitation. *Journal of Head Trauma Rehabilitation, 24*, 32–40.

Niogi, S. M., Mukherjee, P., Ghajar, J., Johnson, C. E., Kolster, R., Lee, H., et al. (2008). Structural dissociation of attentional control and memory in adults with and without mild traumatic brain injury. *Brain, 131*, 3209–3221.

Owens, B. D., Kragh, J. F., Wenke, J. C., Macaitis, J., Wade, C. E., & Holcomb, J. B. (2008). Combat wounds in Operation Iraqi Freedom and Operation Enduring Freedom. *Journal of Trauma, 64*, 295–299.

Pertab, J. L., James, K. M., & Bigler, E. D. (2009). Limitations of mild traumatic brain injury meta-analyses. *Brain Injury, 23*, 498–508.

Rohling, M. L., Faust, M. E., Beverly, B., & Demakis, G. (2009). Effectiveness of cognitive rehabilitation following acquired brain injury: A meta-analytic re-examination of Cicerone et al.'s (2000, 2005) systematic reviews. *Neuropsychology, 23*, 20–39.

Sayer, N. A., Rettmann, N. A., Carlson, K. E., Bernardy, N., Sigford, B .J., Hamblen, J. L., et al. (2009). Veterans with history of mild traumatic brain injury and posttraumatic stress disorder: Challenges from provider perspective. *Journal of Rehabilitation Research and Development, 46*, 703–716.

Schneiderman, A., Braver, E. R., & Kang, H. K. (2008). Understanding sequelae of injury mechanisms and mTBI incurred during the conflicts in Iraq and Afghanistan: Persistent postconcussive symptoms and PTSD. *American Journal of Epidemiology, 167*, 1446–1452.

Snell, D. L., Surgenor, L. J., Hay-Smith, E. J., & Siegert, R. J. (2009). A systematic review of psychological treatments for mild traumatic brain injury: An update on the evidence. *Journal of Clinical and Experimental Neuropsychology, 31*, 20–38.

Sohlberg, M. M., & Mateer, C. A. (1987). Effectiveness of an attention-training program. *Journal of Clinical and Experimental Neuropsychology, 9*, 117–130.

Sohlberg, M. M., McLaughlin, K. A., Pavese, A., Heidrich, A., & Posner, M. (2001). Evaluation of attention process training and brain injury education in persons with acquired brain injury. *Journal of Clinical and Experimental Neuropsychology, 22*, 656–676.

Soo, C., & Tate, R. (2007). Psychological treatment for anxiety in people with TBI. *Cochrane Database of Systematic Reviews, 3*, CD005239.

Stein, M. B., & McAllister, T. W. (2009). Exploring the convergence of posttraumatic stress disorder and mild traumatic brain injury. *American Journal of Psychiatry, 166*, 768–776.

Tanielian, T., & Jaycox, L. H. (2008). *Invisible wounds of war: Psychological and cognitive injuries, their consequences, and services to assist recovery.* Santa Monica, CA: RAND.

Terrio, H., Brenner, L. A., Ivins, B. J., Cho, J. M., Helmick, K., Schwab, K., et al. (2009). Traumatic brain injury screening: Preliminary findings in a U.S. Army brigade combat team. *Journal of Head Trauma Rehabilitation, 24*, 14–23.

Thomas, K. R., Williams, R. E., Bondi, M. W., Dellis, D. C., & Twamley, E. W. (2010). Supported employment plus cognitive training for veterans with traumatic brain injury. *Journal of the International Neuropsychological Society,* *16*(Suppl. 1), 139.

Tiersky, L.A., Anselmi, V., Johnston, M. V., Kurtyka, J., Roosen, E., Schwartz, T., et al. (2005). A trial of neuropsychological rehabilitation in mild-spectrum traumatic brain injury. *Archives of Physical Medicine and Rehabilitation, 86,* 1565–1574.

Twamley, E. W., Savla, G. N., Zurhellen, C. H., Heaton, R. K., & Jeste, D. V. (2008). Development and pilot testing of a novel compensatory cognitive training intervention for people with psychosis. *American Journal of Psychiatric Rehabilitation, 11,* 144–163.

Vanderploeg, R. D., Belanger, H. G., & Curtiss, G. (2009). Mild traumatic brain injury and posttraumatic stress disorder and their associations with health symptoms. *Archives of Physical Medical Rehabilitation, 90,* 1084–1093.

Vanderploeg, R. D., Curtiss, G., & Belanger, H. G. (2005). Long-term neuropsychological outcomes following mild traumatic brain injury. *Journal of the International Neuropsychological Society, 11,* 228–236.

Vasterling, J. J., Verfaellie, M., & Sullivan, K. D. (2009). Mild traumatic brain injury and posttraumatic stress disorder in returning veterans: Perspectives from cognitive neuroscience. *Clinical Psychology Review, 29,* 674–684.

Wild, J., & Gur, R. C. (2008). Verbal memory and treatment response in post-traumatic stress disorder. *British Journal of Psychiatry, 193,* 254–255.

CHAPTER 15

Sexual Assault in the Military

Alina M. Surís
Julia C. Smith

Reticence in acknowledging and addressing the occurrence of sexual harassment and assaults in the military was historically altered in 1991 with the Tailhook Convention scandal in Las Vegas. Over 4,000 Navy and Marine Corps aviation service members (active, reserve, and retired) attended the conference, where reportedly 83 women and 7 men were sexually assaulted ("The Navy Blues," 1993). The resulting congressional hearings highlighted publicly for the first time the issue of sexual misconduct in the military, as well as the latent institutional and cultural attitudes toward women.

The hearings resulted in Public Law 102-585, the Veterans Health Care Act of 1992, which coined the term *military sexual trauma* (MST) and provided the definition that is still used by the VA today. MST is defined as "... psychological trauma, which in the judgment of a mental health professional ... resulted from a physical assault of a sexual nature [or] battery of a sexual nature ... which occurred while the veteran was serving on active duty.... " Sexual harassment is further defined as "repeated, unsolicited verbal or physical contact of a sexual nature which is threatening in character." In 1993, the law was extended by Public Law 103-452, which expanded the program to men and required that the VA screen all veterans for MST and provide services to those who were traumatized by their experiences.

H.R. 3936 §202, the Military Sexual Trauma Counseling Act of 2004, found in Public Law 108-422, the Veterans Health Program Improvement Act of 2004, established permanent provisions for the continued treatment of MST and extends MST counseling and related treatment to active duty for training service members.

Prevalence of MST

The prevalence rates of MST vary significantly depending on multiple factors, including the definition of MST used, the method of obtaining the data (mailed survey, telephone survey, face to face, database), the purpose of the study (descriptive, diagnostic), and the respondent population (treatment seeking, compensation seeking, era of service, veteran status vs. active-duty status). In a review article about prevalence and associated health consequences, Surís and Lind (2008) found that the rates varied from 0.4%—in a sample of Vietnam-era women veterans in which the occurrence of MST was probed with the question, "While serving in and around Vietnam/in the military, were there any ways you were treated unfairly or badly because you were a woman?" (Fontana, Schwartz, & Rosenheck, 1997, p. 170)—to 71% from a compensation-seeking sample of female veterans applying for service connection for PTSD. In the latter study, the definition of MST was presented as "someone had attempted to or successfully forced them to have sex against their will" (Murdoch, Polusny, Hodges, & O'Brien, 2004, p. 393). The large variance is confounded by these methodological issues; thus the actual prevalence of MST is not known. However, most studies report prevalence rates between 20 and 43% (Surís & Lind, 2008).

When MST is defined as sexual assault (leaving out the harassment portion of the definition), the rates are high (Surís & Lind, 2008). The rates of civilian sexual assault average 25% for women (Tjaden & Thoennes, 2000); however, prevalence rates for MST are usually based on a time period of 2–6 years, whereas studies of civilian sexual assault are typically based on lifetime prevalence, suggesting increased risk for sexual assault for active-duty military personnel.

Prevalence of MST at VA

National screening for MST for both men and women began in 2002 throughout the VA system. Through fiscal year 2009, the total number of veterans that have been screened is 6.8 million, including veterans attending appointments at both VA medical centers and community-based outpatient clinics (CBOCs). Specifically for VA medical centers, the rate of veterans endorsing MST was 2.3% (100,095). The rate of endorsement for women was 21.9% (53,295), whereas the rate for males was 1.1% (46,800). These numbers represent 96.8% of all veterans having presented at least once, during fiscal year 2009, for care at VA.

The rates for VA CBOCs are similar, with an overall MST positive rate of 2.1% (47,858). The rates for women were 21.5% (24,454) and for men were 1.1% (23,404), with 97.4% of veterans making at least one visit to the CBOC for screening.

These rates have remained relatively stable over the years for all veterans accessing any VA care (Department of Veterans Affairs, MST Support Team, 2009). Even though the rates for men endorsing MST are significantly lower than the women's rates—because 20 times as many men receive care in the VA system, the actual number of men and women endorsing MST is about equal.

Risk Factors for MST

Recent research has examined the contribution of risk factors present prior to experiencing sexual assault in the military. These risk factors identified as possible precursors to military sexual assault—such as age; history of previous trauma, including physical or sexual assaults; and lower level of education—are generally consistent with recognized risk factors for civilian sexual assault. More specifically, younger age is associated with a greater likelihood of being sexually assaulted in the military, especially for those women who have enlisted at age 19 or younger (Surís & Lind, 2008). Additionally, Sadler, Booth, Cook, and Doebbeling (2003) found that younger women of enlisted rank who also had histories of previous physical or sexual assault were significantly more likely to report being raped during their military service. The young age of some enlisted women may reflect a desire to escape from dysfunctional or abusive family environments. In fact, one study reported that 49% of respondents cited escape from home environment as a primary and purposeful reason for joining the military (Sadler, Booth, Mengeling, & Doebbeling, 2004). Surís and Lind's (2008) comprehensive review of the extant literature found repeated association between preenlistment exposure to violence (including childhood sexual or physical abuse) and sexual assault in the military. Sexual harassment in the military, which can contribute to a hostile and invalidating environment, has also been cited to increase the risk of a woman experiencing sexual assault during active duty (Sadler et al., 2003).

Risk Factors for PTSD from MST

The relationship between civilian sexual assault and the subsequent development of psychiatric disorders such as PTSD and depression has been well examined and documented. Within the last decade, several studies have examined the rates of PTSD resulting from sexual trauma incurred during military service. Surís, Lind, Kashner, Borman, and Petty (2004) assessed the differential impact of military sexual assault, civilian sexual assault, and childhood sexual assault on the likelihood of developing PTSD. Their sample included 270 female veterans seeking care at VA medical centers, with 64.1% having reported a positive history for at least one of the three types of assault: 33% reported MST; 38.9% reported civilian sexual assault; and 27% reported childhood sexual assault. In the sample, 94 women (35%) reported current symptoms that met DSM-IV criteria for PTSD related to their sexual assault. Results also demonstrated that the risk for development of PTSD was nine times higher in those who experienced military sexual assault as compared with those without any history of sexual trauma. After adjustment for demographics and controlling for the additive effect of civilian and childhood sexual assault histories, military sexual assault was still associated with a fourfold increase in PTSD risk. Himmelfarb, Yaeger, and Mintz (2006) examined a sample of 196 female veterans, of which 72% had experienced sexual assault at some point during their lifetimes. In this sample, 80 participants (41%) had experienced MST, of which 48 (60%) met criteria for PTSD. Consistent with previous research (Surís et al., 2004), women who experienced MST demonstrated an increased risk of developing PTSD of almost 2.5 times greater than respondents without MST. Essentially, these results suggest that sexual assault incurred during military service has a stronger association to PTSD than sexual assault experienced as a civilian. Similarly, in a study of 1,381 Gulf War veterans with PTSD, Kang, Dalager, Mahan, and Ishii (2005) examined the impact of reported sexual trauma on postdeployment PTSD risk. Their results demonstrated that both men and women who reported sexual assault in the military experienced more than a fivefold increased risk for developing PTSD. When compared with the PTSD risk from combat exposure, results from this sample indicate that sexual assault is still associated with greater risk, despite combat being classified as a significant stressor.

It has been suggested that elements of the military environment may contribute to this increased PTSD risk. The aspects that can be conceptualized as further risk factors include readily available weapons (which could be used as a means of serious threat), less free time to access appropriate psychiatric and medical care, sexualized work environments, sexual harassment, and close living quarters, as well as perceived support or lack thereof from leadership and superiors (Sadler et al., 2003; Himmelfarb et al., 2006).

Psychological and Physical Consequences and Quality of Life

Sexual assault in the military has been consistently associated with the subsequent development of psychiatric sequelae, poorer quality of life, and a greater number of negative physical health consequences. More specifically, individuals who have experienced MST are 2–3 times more likely than individuals without MST to have a mental health diagnosis, with PTSD being the most common (Kimerling, Gima, Smith, Street, & Frayne, 2007). However, the methods used in this database study do not allow for a causal interpretation between MST and PTSD. When compared with individuals who experienced civilian sexual assault, women veterans with MST demonstrated higher rates of PTSD, depression, and alcohol abuse, along with consistently lower appraisals of physical health and quality of life. Those with MST were more likely to report poorer quality of life in the areas of family relationships, daily activities, and health satisfaction than those who had experienced civilian sexual assault (Surís, Lind, Kashner, & Borman, 2006).

With regard to physical health, MST has been associated with impaired health status, as well as with increased chronicity of health problems. Various studies have reported that MST is associated with increased reporting of pelvic pain, headaches, chronic fatigue, gastrointestinal difficulties, and menstrual problems (Frayne et al., 1999). Additionally, those who experienced MST demonstrated more cardiovascular risk factors, including obesity, smoking, and alcohol use (Surís & Lind, 2008; Sadler et al., 2004). Kimerling et al. (2007) examined the association between MST (in both female and male veterans) and various psychiatric and medical conditions. Their results indicate that liver disease and chronic pulmonary disease had a moderate association with MST, independent of gender. Additionally, they found that obesity and hypothyroidism were found to be significantly related to MST in their sample of women veterans, whereas AIDS was significantly associated with the men who reported MST. Again, readers must be careful not to attribute causation to correlational studies; however, the associations are informative.

Characteristics of the military environment and unique aspects of military service may serve to influence and intensify symptom severity after assault, facilitating poorer physical and psychiatric outcomes. The military work environment differs from civilian work environments in several ways, notably with respect to the victim–perpetrator relationship. In cases of MST, the perpetrator may serve in the role of coworker, supervisor, or higher ranking official vis-à-vis the victim. Additionally, the relationship between the perpetrator and victim may be sustained owing to logistics of duty station and work detail, therefore subjecting the victim to repeated contact over time. Unit cohesion, which is usually considered to be a protective factor in high-stress environments, may facilitate decreased reporting of such assaults for fear of being ostracized for "breaking the code" (Surís & Lind, 2008, p. 16), thus subsequently serving to limit the support the individual receives in the wake of these traumatic situations (Frayne et al, 1999; Surís et al., 2006).

Men with MST

Women currently make up approximately 15% of active-duty forces (Department of Veterans Affairs, Office of Policy & Planning, 2007) and 6% of veterans overall (Department of Defense, 2006), with 20 times more men than women accessing care in the VA system. According to VA data, women are more likely than men to be victimized while on active duty at the approximate rate of 22% versus 1% for men (Department of Veterans Affairs, MST Support Team, 2009). However, it is unclear what part of the cited percentages is due to harassment and what is due to sexual assault. Despite the fact that approximately the same number of men and women report experiencing MST while on active duty, most of the published literature on MST is focused on women. Other than a few VA database studies of VA users that examine prevalence and associations of MST or epidemiological surveys, there are only two peer-reviewed clinical studies that provide a comparison of men and women with MST—O'Brien, Gaher, Pope, and Smily (2008) and Shipherd, Pineles, Gradus, and Resick (2009). Therefore, the following information is based on these studies, as well as anecdotal information from my (A. M. S.) 17 years of clinical experience working with both men and women with MST.

O'Brien et al. (2008) examined the relationship between alexithymia and the persistence of trauma symptoms in 175 participants (17% men, 83% women) enrolled in a residential treatment program for MST. They found that at baseline, men reported significantly more trauma symptoms than women, but there were no differences in alexithymia scores. Although both men and women reported significantly fewer trauma symptoms after 7 weeks of treatment, the effect size was smaller for the men (.53 vs. .74). Additionally, men experienced more persistent sexual problems and more sexual abuse trauma symptoms compared with women. Men and women did not significantly differ on depression, anxiety, dissociation, or sleep disturbance. Regarding alexithymia, it was found to be related to persistence of overall trauma symptoms, sexual abuse trauma symptoms, dissociative symptoms, and anxiety for both genders.

Differences between men and women with MST were also found by Shipard et al (2009) in a group of Marines (91 men and 226 women). MST status and associated sequelae were determined via mailed surveys 21 months after completion of the initial study questionnaire during basic training. The aim of the study was to examine the effects of MST by investigating the relationships between MST, posttraumatic stress symptoms, and perceived physical health. Authors found increased posttraumatic stress symptoms in men compared with women and suggested that the same level of MST was "particularly detrimental to the male participants relative to the women." Regarding perceived physical health, both men and women had declines, but higher frequency of MST was associated with worse perceptions of physical health for men, with lower frequency of MST being associated with worse perceptions for women.

Clinically we have found that male veterans are reluctant to admit to having been victimized, even when directly asked by VA clinicians. When accessing care in the VA, our male MST veterans in treatment tell us that they have often been asked multiple times about sexual assault in the military and report that they denied it many times. They explain that sexual assault is something that is supposed to happen to women, not to men, and admitting that they are victims is difficult for them and challenges their self-views regarding their own masculinity. They often express shame because they were not able to successfully defend themselves against their perpetrator(s), citing that they were well trained not only to defend themselves but also to kill the enemy in basic training. They will often report that they see themselves not only as less than men but also as less than marines or soldiers due to this perceived failure.

Because of the sexual assault in the military, they also express confusion about their sexual orientation, wondering if they were targeted because they are really homosexual, unbeknownst to them. Some men admit to testing this theory, discovering that they are not homosexual, and being left more confused as to why they were targeted. Others become vehemently antihomosexual because they attribute their attacks as being perpetrated by gay men, despite being presented with evidence to the contrary. They become distrustful of homosexual men, and in our experiences, express that they will not come to group treatment if homosexual men with MST are allowed in, despite their own victim status.

Men also struggle with their masculinity and, according to O'Brien et al. (2008), they have issues regarding sexual functioning post-MST assault. Just as women struggle with intimacy after an assault, men do as well. Promiscuity and cheating during committed relationships in an attempt to "prove I am a man" is also common after an assault, according to our MST male patients. Our patients will often express regret at these behaviors and blame their MST for ruining their relationships instead of taking responsibility for their choices.

A discussion of the reasons for male-on-male rape is beyond the scope of this chapter, however; the motive of power and control appears to be the same as in civilian male-on-male rapes. We have noted that our male veterans report that at the time of their assaults, they were typically youngest and lowest ranking and were comparatively slight of frame. Although we were unable to find any information on the sexual orientation of rapists in the military, we assume that, as in the civilian world, most rapists are heterosexual.

Based on the review of the available literature and our clinical experience, men with MST appear to have more deleterious consequences than women, especially regarding mental health issues. Foa, Zinbarg, and Roth-baum (1992) report that unpredictable and uncontrollable stress may lead to worse outcomes. Shipard et al. (2009) hypothesize that because MST for men is unpredictable, the impact on health may be greater. The emphasis on physical prowess and masculinity for men in the military, compounded with the greater social stigma for male victims of sexual assault, most likely not only contributes to a negative impact but also likely affects reporting of the MST. However, much research remains to be done to confirm this hypothesis, as well as to determine the reasons for the differential outcome.

Assessment

As described earlier, Public Law 102-585 defined MST, and Public Law 103-452 mandated that all veterans, male and female, be screened for MST. To this end, MST software and the MST clinical reminder located in the Computerized Patient Record System, the VA's computerized medical records system, were developed to track and monitor the level of national compliance with the standard. The VA clinical reminder reads as follows:

1. When you were in the military, did you ever receive uninvited or unwanted sexual attention (i.e., touching, cornering, pressure for sexual favors or inappropriate verbal remarks, etc. ..)?
2. When you were in the military, did anyone ever use force or threat of force to have sex against your will?

However, Public Law 102-585 defines sexual harassment as "repeated, unsolicited verbal or physical contact of a sexual nature which is threatening in character." This definition is not captured clearly by the VA clinical reminder in that it is missing two crucial descriptors: the words "repeated" and "threatening." Thus any military service member who answered "yes" when asked if an inappropriate sexual remark was directed at him or her technically would qualify as a positive screen for MST if the person doing the screening did not query further to determine whether psychological trauma occurred because of the harassment. Of note, a positive screen for MST does not automatically indicate the need for treatment, as one harassing statement generally will not qualify as psychological trauma requiring treatment.

A second problem with the MST Clinical Reminder is that, as structured, it does not provide an assessment of psychological trauma that is part of the definition of MST (§1720D of Title 38, U.S. Code "Pensions,

Benefits, and Veterans' Relief," under Public Law 102-585). Possibly confounding the accuracy of the screen, there is no unified policy regarding who is to administer the VA MST Clinical Reminder; thus non-mental health professionals in ambulatory care are often doing this one-time screen. If not properly trained, these clinicians could inflate the rates of positive MST screens, because they are not likely to query further regarding psychological trauma as it is not part of the screen. This issue is also pertinent to mental health professionals doing the screen who do not query a positive response further to make an accurate determination that MST occurred by assessing the presence of trauma due to the incident(s). In our opinion, the VA should consider reworking their screen to accurately reflect the law and the directives.

Treatment Approaches

Free treatment of MST is mandated by law and can be found in §1720D of Title 38, U.S. Code ("Pensions"): Veterans can be referred for treatment if the "psychological trauma, which in the judgment of the mental health professional employed by the Department, resulted from a physical assault of a sexual nature, battery of a sexual nature, or sexual harassment which occurred while the veteran was serving on active duty." VHA Directive 2005-015 (Department of Veterans Affairs, Veterans Health Administration, 2005) further mandates that if the VA cannot provide counseling in a timely manner or because of geographical inaccessibility, a qualified mental health professional will be contracted to provide treatment. MST treatment may also be provided for veterans who are otherwise deemed ineligible for VA health services.

Because MST is not a diagnosis but a stressor, treatment is based on individual symptoms and diagnoses resulting from the stressor. As outlined earlier, there are multiple possible psychological sequelae that can result from MST due to sexual assault, with the most common being PTSD. MST that is characterized as sexual harassment alone can also cause distress and even psychological trauma, depending on the nature of the harassment (severe, ongoing, threatening, etc.). However, most veterans do not require treatment for the VA Clinical Reminder's definition of sexual harassment. Relatedly, and as mentioned previously, not all MST events meet the criteria for PTSD because they do not qualify as Criterion A events required to diagnose PTSD: "The person experienced ... an event or events that involved actual or threatened death or serious injury or a threat to the physical integrity of others" (American Psychiatric Association, 2000). Unless severe in nature, sexual harassment does not usually meet this criterion. However, a veteran could feel distressed and upset by harassment and could benefit from counseling provided by the VA.

Regarding treatment for PTSD from MST, the VA's *Uniform Mental Health Services Handbook* (Department of Veterans Affairs, Veterans Health Admimistration, 2008) directs that "all veterans with PTSD must have access to Cognitive Processing Therapy (CPT) or Prolonged Exposure Therapy as designed and shown to be effective" (p. 31). Thus veterans with PTSD from MST should be offered one of these two interventions. If the resultant psychiatric diagnosis from MST is depression or an anxiety disorder, the *Handbook* directs that "all veterans with depression or anxiety disorders must have access to Cognitive Behavioral Therapy (CBT), Acceptance and Commitment Therapy (ACT), or Interpersonal Therapy (IT)" (p. 31).

The VA *Uniform Services Handbook* (2008) also encourages facilities "to provide same sex providers for veterans, men and women, receiving treatment in their facility for conditions related to MST, when clinically indicated" (p. 40). Additionally, treatment for men with MST should be provided separately from treatment for combat-related PTSD due to the need to process sexual trauma separately from the combat trauma (O'Brien et al., 2008).

Because PTSD is the signature diagnosis after sexual assault in the military, we focus on treatment for this diagnosis. The two VA-recommended treatments for PTSD, prolonged exposure therapy (PE) and cognitive processing therapy (CPT) were both originally developed for use with civilian rape survivors (Foa, Rothbaum, Riggs, & Murdock, 1991; Resick, Nishith, Weaver, Astin, & Feuer, 2002). However, research on the effectiveness of these recommended therapies specifically to treat MST sequelae is limited.

The only currently published study of the effectiveness of PE for treating women veterans did not focus exclusively on MST (Schnurr et al., 2007). Of the veterans in the exposure condition, 69.5% reported having military sexual trauma. However, the participants reported an average of 10 traumas, and it is unclear which trauma was addressed in the study. Regardless, this large randomized controlled clinical trial found that participants who received PE had a greater reduction in PTSD symptoms and were more likely to no longer meet the diagnostic criteria for PTSD than participants who received present-centered therapy.

The only currently published randomized wait-list control clinical trial of CPT with veterans with military-related PTSD had 6 females out of 60 participants (Monson et al., 2006). The authors reported that 10 of the 60 participants had a sexual trauma, but the nature of the trauma is unclear other than that it occurred in the military. At the end of treatment, 40% of participants did not meet criteria for PTSD, and 50% had reliable changes in their PTSD symptoms. Authors also report improvements in secondary outcome symptom measures, including co-occurring depression, anxiety, affect functioning, guilt distress, and social adjustment. Regarding PTSD symptoms, emotional numbing improved with CPT, but avoidance and hyperarousal did not differentially improve in the treatment condition relative to the wait-list condition despite a main effect of overall PTSD symptom improvement. The authors attribute this finding as possibly due to improvements in the wait-list condition, as well as inadequate power to detect differences. Also important to note is that, although the study reported positive findings, compared with civilian studies using CPT the effect sizes were smaller.

At the request of the Department of Veterans Affairs, the Institute of Medicine (IOM; 2007) examined the evidence of efficacy of treatments for PTSD. While looking at randomized control trials only, they concluded that "the scientific evidence on treatment modalities for PTSD does not reach the level of certainty that would be desired for such a common and serious condition among veterans." Additionally, they concluded that there is enough evidence for the efficacy of exposure therapies. However, CPT was classified as one of the exposure therapies, which is not entirely accurate, especially in light of a dismantling study that showed that CPT without the exposure techniques was just as effective as traditionally administered CPT, which includes both cognitive and exposure components. (Resick et al., 2008). The IOM also reported that:

- Concluding that evidence is inadequate to determine efficacy is not the same as concluding that a treatment modality is inefficacious.
- There may be difference in civilian and veteran populations in response to treatment and to various types of treatment.
- The returning veterans from Iraq and Afghanistan may be different from other deployed cohorts, so the evidence we have regarding efficacy of treatments may not apply.
- Most PTSD treatment studies do not address high rates of comorbidity among veterans, and this shortcoming affects generalizability.

Many of the studies reviewed by the IOM were conducted on samples of individuals with PTSD from civilian sexual trauma and included CPT and PE. The IOM also noted that there appeared to be a dearth of quality research on PTSD in veterans. In light of their thorough review and recommendations for population-specific randomized controlled trials for treatment of PTSD, combined with the research on MST that indicates worse outcomes for this type of trauma, more research is needed to validate these recommended treatments in veterans generally and in men and women with PTSD from MST.

Foa and Resick, the two prominent researchers in PE and CPT, were asked how many studies examining the efficacy or effectiveness of their

therapies were currently under way with veterans or active-duty populations (Surís, personal communication, 2009). Their answers and a review of
registered clinical trials determined that eight studies of PE and six studies
of CPT are ongoing; our (A. M. S. and J. C. S.) study focuses on treatment
of PTSD from MST. The studies include novel applications (e.g., testing
telemedicine technologies) and novel combinations of these therapies and
medications.

Limitations of Treatments/Treatment Strategies and Gaps in Research

Because DSM-IV-TR (American Psychiatric Association, 2000, p. 467) criterion A events manifest differently in trauma survivors, therapies validated
in one population will not necessarily be as effective in other populations, or
they may need some adjusting to address trauma-specific issues to be applicable and effective. For example, a therapy developed for combat PTSD with
techniques to address guilt and remorse regarding killing may not translate
directly to an MST population in which these issues are less central and others are more important, such as betrayal and sexual identity. This is not to
say that the general concepts, such as examining fear memories or addressing unbalanced cognitions, may not be applicable; however, they should be
specific to population and trauma.

As can be surmised from the summary of treatments for MST, more
controlled trials are needed to examine the effectiveness of therapies for
women and especially men with MST, as to date there are no published
studies with men. Research is also needed to examine the difference of the
impact of MST on men compared with women, as the preliminary information indicates that the psychiatric outcomes may be more severe for men.
Reasons for men not reporting assaults either when they happen or later,
when questioned via the Clinical Reminder System at the VA, can include
feeling humiliated, being accused of homosexuality, being seen as weak, and
fear of a Section 8 discharge (a category of discharge for being "mentally
unfit" no longer used in the military; O'Brien et al., 2008). Experiences of
social stigma, denial, and shame also contribute to lack of reporting and
to failure to seek care, which can have profound impacts on mental health
and quality of life. Understanding their unique experiences with this type of
trauma may help develop methods to increase reporting of MST and therefore increase their access to care.

As noted by the IOM, research on effective treatments for MST should
also take into account comorbid conditions in order to increase the generalizability to the population. Thus, in designing intervention studies, care
should be taken to include veterans with PTSD from MST regardless of

comorbidity, medication status, and attendance in other non-trauma-specific treatments.

Conclusion

MST is an event that can derail a military career if not addressed appropriately, which would include getting adequate and timely medical and mental health care. In the past, our veterans have reported to us that they have had to choose between pursuing justice or pursuing their careers when dealing with reporting perpetrators of assault. Valente and Wight (2007) have noted that characteristics of the military environment can compound the effects of sexual trauma, including fear of stigmatization and possible career repercussions that can, in and of themselves, influence reluctance to report MST.

The impact of MST on veterans is far reaching, often affecting their ability to perform their duties while in service; these difficulties often extend to adjustment after discharge. For example, research has suggested that female veterans who reported sexual harassment or assault in the military reported feeling isolated and lonely during their military experience. These women were twice as likely to report having difficulty adjusting to civilian life after discharge. These adjustment problems were further characterized by difficulty finding employment; increased experience of anxiety, depression, and anger; increased drug and alcohol abuse; and difficulty "settling down" (Skinner et al., 2000, p. 301).

The military has made significant strides in dealing with MST, including establishing procedures for restricted and unrestricted reporting with identified sexual assault response coordinators and victim advocates. The former are responsible for coordinating care and assigning a victim advocate to help service members obtain necessary services and to provide crisis intervention, referral, and ongoing nonclinical support.

References

American Psychiatric Association. (2000). *Diagnostic and statistical manual of mental disorders* (4th ed., text rev.). Washington, DC: Author.

Department of Defense. (2006). *Men and women in active duty by rank and race.* Defense Manpower Data Center. *www.dmdc.usd.mil*

Department of Veterans Affairs, MST Support Team. (2009). Military Sexual Trauma (MST) screening report. Retrieved May 14, 2010, from *vaww.portal. va.gov/sites/mst_community/Lists/MST%20Reports*

Department of Veterans Affairs, Office of Policy & Planning. (2007). Women veterans: Past, present, and future. Retrieved June 14, 2010, from *www1.va.gov/*

VETDATA/docs/SpecialReports/Womenveterans_Past_Present_Future_9–30–07a.pdf.

Department of Veterans Affairs, Veterans Health Administration. (2005). VHA Directive 2005–015, Military Sexual Trauma Counseling. Retrieved May 16, 2010, from *www1.va.gov/vhapublications/ViewPublication.asp?pub_ID=1244*.

Department of Veterans Affairs, Veterans Health Administration. (2008). Uniform mental health services in VA medical centers and clinics. Retrieved June 14, 2010, from *www1.va.gov/vhapublications/ViewPublication.asp*.

Foa, E. B., Rothbaum, B. O., Riggs, D. S., & Murdock, T. B. (1991). Treatment of posttraumatic stress disorder in rape victims: A comparison between cognitive-behavioral procedures and counseling. *Journal of Consulting and Clinical Psychology, 59,* 715–723.

Foa, E. B., Zinbarg, R., & Rothbaum, B. O. (1992). Uncontrollability and unpredictability in posttraumatic stress disorder: An animal model. *Psychological Bulletin, 112,* 218–238.

Fontana, A., Schwartz, L. S., & Rosenheck, R. (1997). Posttraumatic stress disorder among female Vietnam veterans: A causal model of etiology. *American Journal of Public Health, 87,* 169–175.

Frayne, S., Skinner, K., Sullivan, L., Tripp, T., Hankin, C., Kressin, N., et al. (1999). Medical profile of women VA outpatients who report sexual assault while in the military. *Journal of Women's Health, 8,* 835–845.

Himmelfarb, N., Yaeger, D., & Mintz, J. (2006). Posttraumatic Stress Disorder in female veterans with military and civilian sexual trauma. *Journal of Traumatic Stress, 19*(6), 837–846.

Institute of Medicine. (2007). *Treatment of posttraumatic stress disorder: An assessment of the evidence.* Washington, DC: National Academy of Sciences.

Kang, H., Dalager, N., Mahan, C., & Ishii, E. (2005). The role of sexual assault on the risk of PTSD among Gulf War veterans. *Annals of Epidemiology, 15,* 191–195.

Kimerling, R., Gima, K., Smith, M., Street, A., & Frayne, S. (2007). The Veterans Health Administration and military sexual trauma. *Research and Practice, 97*(12), 2160–2166.

Military Sexual Trauma Counseling Act of 2004, H.R. 3936, §202. In Veterans Health Program Improvement Act of 2004, Public Law No. 108-422, 118 Stat. 2385 (2004).

Monson, C. M., Schnurr, P. P., Resick, P. A., Friedman, M. J., Young-Xu, Y., & Stevens, S. P. (2006). A randomized controlled trial of cognitive processing therapy for veterans with military-related posttraumatic stress disorder. *Journal of Consulting and Clinical Psycholology, 74,* 898–907.

Murdoch, M., Polusny, M. A., Hodges, J., & O'Brien, N. (2004). Prevalence of in-service and post-sexual assault among combat and non-combat veterans applying for Department of Veterans Affairs (VA) posttraumatic stress disorder disability benefits. *Military Medicine, 169,* 392–395.

The Navy Blues: Tailhook '91 [Television series episode]. (1993). In *Frontline.* Retrieved June 14, 2010, from *www.pbs.org/wgbh/pages/frontline/shows/navy/tailhook/91.html*.

O'Brien, C. O., Gaher, R. M., Pope, C., & Smily, P. (2008). Difficulty identifying feelings predicts the persistence of trauma symptoms in a sample of veterans who experienced military sexual trauma. *Journal of Nervous and Mental Disease, 196*, 252–255.

Resick, P. A., Galovski, T. A., Uhlmansiek, M. O., Scher, C. D., Clum, G. A., & Young-Xu, Y. (2008). A randomized clinical trial to dismantle components of cognitive processing therapy for posttraumatic stress disorder in female victims of interpersonal violence. *Journal of Consulting and Clinical Psychology, 76*, 243–258.

Resick, P. A., Nishith, P., Weaver, T. L., Astin, M. C., & Feuer, C. A. (2002). A comparison of cognitive-processing therapy with prolonged exposure and a waiting condition for the treatment of chronic posttraumatic stress disorder in female rape victims. *Journal of Consulting and Clinical Psychology, 70*, 867–879.

Sadler, A. G., Booth, B. M., Cook, B. L., & Doebbeling, B. N. (2003). Factors associated with women's risk of rape in the military environment. *American Journal of Industrial Medicine, 43*, 262–273.

Sadler, A. G., Booth, B., Mengeling, M., & Doebbeling, B. (2004). Life span and repeated violence against women during military service: Effects on health status and outpatient utilization. *Journal of Women's Health, 13*, 799–811.

Schnurr, P. P., Friedman, M. J., Engel, C. C., Foa, E. B., Shea, M. T., Chow, B. K., et al. (2007). Cognitive behavioral therapy for posttraumatic stress disorder in women: A randomized controlled trial. *Journal of the American Medical Association, 297*, 820–830.

Shipherd, J. C., Pineles, S. L., Gradus, J. L., & Resick, P. A. (2009). Sexual harassment in the Marines, posttraumatic stress symptoms, and perceived health: Evidence for sex differences. *Journal of Trauma Stress, 22*(1), 3–10.

Skinner, K. M., Kressin, N., Frayne, S., Tripp, T., Hankin, C., Miller, D., et al. (2000). The prevalence of military sexual assault among female Veterans' Administration outpatients. *Journal of Interpersonal Violence, 15*, 291–310.

Surís, A., & Lind, L. (2008). Military sexual trauma: A review of prevalence and associated health consequences in veterans. *Trauma, Violence & Abuse, 9(4)*, 250–269.

Surís, A., Lind, L., Kashner, T. M., & Borman, P. (2006). Mental Health, quality of life, and health functioning in women veterans: Differential outcomes associated with military and civilian sexual assault. *Journal of Interpersonal Violence, 21(12)*, 1–19.

Surís, A., Lind, L., Kashner, T. M., Borman, P., & Petty, F. (2004). Sexual assault in women veterans: An examination of PTSD risk, health care utilization, and cost of care. *Psychosomatic Medicine, 66*, 749–756.

Tjaden, P., & Thoennes, N. (2000). *Full report of the prevalence, incidence and consequences of violence against women: Findings from the National Violence against Women Survey* (Rep. NCJ 183781). Washington DC: National Institute of Justice.

Valente, S., & Wight, C. (2007). Military sexual trauma: Violence and sexual abuse. *Military Medicine, 172*, 259–265.

Pensions, Bonuses, and Veterans Relief, 38 C.F.R. 17 §1720D (1992).

Veterans Health Care Act of 1992, Public Law No. 102-585, 106 Stat. 4943 (1992).

Veterans Health Programs Extension Act of 1994, Pubic Law No. 103-452, 108 Stat. 4783 (1994).

CHAPTER 16

Sleep Disorders

William L. Brim
David S. Riggs

War and sleep are not compatible. This fact is not new, as there is a growing appreciation of the impact not only of combat but also of deployment itself on the sleep health of military members. Until recently the majority of the research in the area of sleep disorders in military personnel has focused on the impact of combat and, more specifically, on combat-related posttraumatic stress disorder (PTSD) and its impact on sleep. We look at more recent studies that suggest that deployment and combat, even in the absence of PTSD symptoms, appear to have an impact on the ability of service members to attain or regain healthy sleep. We then provide an overview of effective assessment and treatment strategies for sleep disorders in general, with a particular focus on insomnia and nightmares. Finally, we explore some of the implications of sleep disturbance on military service and reintegration to civilian life and suggest directions for future research.

Sleep Disturbance

The general term "sleep disturbance" is used to describe a range of sleep problems that range from acute sleep deprivation to insomnia and nightmares. Evidence suggests that sleep disturbance may start early in the deployment phase, with one pilot study showing that 74% of participants rated sleep as significantly worse in the deployed setting within just 2 weeks of beginning deployment (Peterson et al., 2008). The subjects of this study were largely noncombatant medical personnel and civil engineers who reported increases in sleep onset latency, wake after sleep onset, and early awakening shortly after deploying to an Operation Enduring Freedom (OEF) support base in Afghanistan. Loud noises inside the tent, uncomfortable beds, and worry over family back home were the most common factors reported as interfering with sleep. Looking deeper into the deployment phase, the 2008 Mental Health Advisory Team (MHAT-V) found that in the ninth month of their deployment, Army enlisted soldiers, on average, reported regularly getting 1 hour less sleep than they felt they needed and that this lack of sleep limited their ability to do their jobs. Further, the impact of this sleep deprivation rapidly increases as the self-reported duration of the deprivation increases. Twelve percent of soldiers reporting no sleep disturbance scored positive for depression, anxiety, or acute stress, and that number almost doubles to over 23% for those who self reported just two hours of sleep deprivation. While it remains unclear whether sleep problems are a symptom or a precursor of mental health problems (Picchioni, Hope, & Harsh, 2007), it is clear that sleep deprivation is common in a deployed setting and that soldiers who report being sleep deprived are at significant risk of reporting mental health problems.

Sleep disturbances do not appear to resolve on return from deployment, either. Sleep disturbance is the most frequent non-wound- or -injury-related concern reported by active-duty service members on postdeployment assessments. Between December 2009 and November 2010 more than 325,000 active-duty service members had completed the Post-Deployment Health Reassessment (PDHRA) at approximately 6–9 months after leaving the combat theater. Of the PDHRA completers, nearly 30% reported a non-wound- or injury-related health concern associated with their deployment. Forty-seven percent of the respondents with non-wound or injury related health concerns reported a concern related to sleep disturbance.

In addition, over the past 10 years there has been an increase in the number and rate of insomnia diagnosis among active component members of the U.S. military. The crude overall incidence rate was found to be 48.4 cases per 10,000 person, years with the counts and rates of incidence diagnoses of insomnia increasing substantially from 7.2 to 135.8 cases per 10,000 person years between 2000 and 2009. As seen in Figure 16.1, these rate increases were seen across the services; however, the greatest increase by a substantial amount was seen in the Army (Armed Forces Health Surveillance Center, 2010). The Armed Forces Health Surveillance Center epidemiological study also compared incidence rates before Operation Iraqi Freedom (OIF) and Operation Enduring Freedom (OEF) deployment and after OIF or OEF deployment and noted that the Army and the Marine Corps, but not the other armed services, had rates that increased more than twofold from pre- to postdeployment. Additionally, the largest relative increase

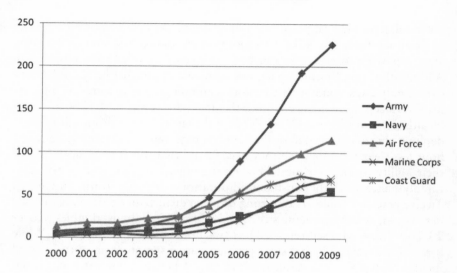

FIGURE 16.1. Annual incidence rates of insomnia, by service and calendar year, active component, U.S. Armed Forces, 2000–2009 (incidence per 10,000 person years).

in rates from pre- to postdeployment were found in service members in combat-specific occupations (i.e., maneuver units). These service members were found to have rates of incidence diagnosis of insomnia that increased more than fourfold from predeployment (12.0 per 10,000 per years) to post deployment (49.1 per 10,000 person years). A recent study analyzing data from the Millennium Cohort Study looking at over 41,000 service members of all ranks found that while 25% of service members who had never deployed reported trouble sleeping, 30.5% of those currently deployed and 27.1% of those previously deployed reported difficulty sleeping, specifically trouble falling or staying asleep (Seelig et al., 2010). Further, those service members who were deployed or had just returned from deployment had significantly shorter sleep duration and increased odds of reporting trouble sleeping compared to those who had not deployed. Additionally, the study found that Cohort members who reported combat exposures had significantly lower sleep duration and were 52% to 74% more likely to report trouble sleeping than other members who were deployed or returning from deployment without combat exposure.

Finally, a recent pilot study by Lewis, Creamer, and Failla (2009) looking at quality of sleep in OIF and OEF veterans suggests that, although there is a clearly demonstrated association between PTSD and quality of sleep in veterans, it may also be true that poor sleep is a more general experience. In addition, all of the veterans in their sample with the diagnosis PTSD ($n = 65$) and 90% of those without the diagnosis of PTSD reported clinically significant sleep disturbance, indicating that serious sleep problems are a concern across the veteran population. It is clear that deployment, regardless of combat exposure, causes sleep disruption and that many service members do not return to predeployment levels of sleep after deployment.

Sleep Disturbance and Nightmares in PTSD

Moving beyond the impact of deployment in general on sleep health, the relationship between PTSD and sleep is clearly documented. Nightmares and sleep disturbances are part of a normal and typical acute response to trauma (Pillar, Malhotra, & Lavie, 2000). In patients not diagnosed with PTSD, these symptoms are transient and generally remit within the first 30 days following a traumatic event. Rates of sleep disruption generally have been found to decline 1–3 months posttrauma in persons who do not develop PTSD. However, sleep disturbances such as difficulty falling asleep and/or difficulty staying asleep are maintained in those who do develop PTSD following trauma (Foa, Riggs, & Gershuny, 1995, Harvey & Bryant, 1998). Although it may be difficult to know whether the sleep disturbances reported by patients with PTSD are specific to the PTSD or are characteristic of psychological disorders in general, at least one study (Inman, Silver, & Doghramji, 1990) found that the sleep disturbances in patients with PTSD were indistinguishable from the sleep disturbances found in clinical patients with primary insomnia related to another cause. Both groups self-reported approximately 2.7 hours of sleep a night. However, the subjects diagnosed with PTSD reported significantly more sleep-related anxiety symptoms, including fear of going to sleep, fear of the dark, disturbing thoughts while lying in bed, yelling during sleep, and waking up confused and disoriented. These findings suggest that PTSD-related sleep disturbance may be different from insomnia related to other clinical causes.

The importance of sleep disturbance in PTSD is clearly indicated by the findings that sleep disturbance has prognostic significance. Harvey and Bryant (1998) found a moderate probability of PTSD diagnosis if sleep symptoms were present soon after a trauma but a high probability of no PTSD diagnosis if no sleep disturbance was evident within 1 month of the trauma. In motor vehicle accident survivors, insomnia at 1 week posttrauma was not predictive of PTSD diagnosis, but sleep complaints at 1 month posttrauma were a significant predictor of PTSD diagnosis at 12 months (Koren, Arnon, Lavie, & Klein, 2002). A recent study of 1,033 traumatically injured patients found clear evidence that sleep disturbance prior to a traumatic event is a risk factor for development of posttraumatic stress disorder (Bryant, Creamer, O'Donnell, Silove, & McFarlane, 2010) which further suggests that service members exposed to combat would be at higher risk for PTSD because of their frequency of sleep disturbance.

Looking specifically at combat-related PTSD, Hoge, Auchterlonie, and Milliken (2006) found that PTSD is prevalent among combat veterans, and other studies have shown that disturbed sleep and nightmares are common symptoms of the disorder with this population (Ross, Ball, Sullivan, & Caroff, 1989) and may in fact predict symptoms of PTSD in U.S. service members returning from deployment (McLay, Klam, & Volkert, 2010). Difficulty falling asleep occurred in 44% of veterans with PTSD and only 5.5 % of veterans without PTSD in one study of Vietnam veterans (Neylan et al., 1998). Difficulty in maintaining sleep occurred among 91% of veterans with PTSD and 63% of veterans without PTSD. Nightmares have been reported in 60 (Kilpatrick et al., 1998) to 71% (Maher, Rego, & Asnis, 2006) of patients with PTSD, and it has been recognized that exposure to combat influences the likelihood of trauma-related nightmares occurring (Neylan et. al., 1998). However, exposure to trauma itself, without the later development of PTSD, does not appear to cause recurrent nightmares. In the Neylan (1998) study of Vietnam veterans, 52% of those with PTSD reported experiencing nightmares, compared with only 5% of veterans without PTSD.

It is important to note that the content of trauma-related nightmares may tend to change over time, from memories directly related to the trauma to more generally anxious dreams along the themes of war and loss of control. However, evidence from a recent study looking at World War II veterans suggests that distressing nightmares will not subside spontaneously if untreated in a veteran population (Scheuder, Kleijn, & Rooijmans, 2000). It has also been noted that PTSD-related sleep disturbances and nightmares are often resistant to typical psychological and pharmacological PTSD treatments, suggesting that these symptoms of PTSD develop into a comorbid disorder quickly and require independent interventions (Zayfert & DeViva, 2004; Spoormaker & Montgomery, 2008).

Another signature injury of OIF/OEF, though largely beyond the scope of this chapter, is that of traumatic brain injury (TBI). Since sleep is regulated by the brain, any damage to the brain has the potential to cause sleep disturbances. In fact, so closely related are sleep and brain injury that sleep improvement may be prognostic for the extent of brain recovery following a TBI (Gassanov, Gitlevich, Lesnyak, & Levin, 1998). One early study (Cohen, Oksenberg, Snir, Stern, & Groswasser, 1992) found that 73% of patients hospitalized with TBI had complaints of sleep problems, with 82% of those complaining of insomnia and 73% complaining of excessive daytime sleepiness. A more recent review (Castriotta & Murthy, 2011) found that approximately 46% of all chronic TBI patients have sleep disorders that require nocturnal polysomnography for diagnosis with assessment finding sleep apnea (23% of patients), hypersomnia (11%), narcolepsy (6%), and periodic limb movements (7%) as the most common medical conditions. While pharmacological interventions remain the most frequent treatment for sleep disturbances related to TBI (Gosselin & Tellier, 2010), Ouellet and Morin (2007) reported that cognitive-behavioral therapy given to TBI patients with insomnia improved sleep efficiency and reduced complaints of physical fatigue. Because problems falling asleep or maintaining sleep can exacerbate other TBI-related problems such as cognitive deficits, fatigue, and irritability and thus interfere with the rehabilitation process, early evaluation and treatment of sleep disturbance must be considered an integral part of the TBI rehabilitation process.

Assessment

Assessment of sleep disturbance can and has filled entire book chapters by itself. This section provides an overview of some self-report, behavioral, and physiological methods that can be used to assess sleep disturbances with a specific focus on insomnia. The reader is also referred to the American Academy of Sleep Medicine's review and practice parameters papers on the assessment of sleep disturbances for further information (see Chesson et al., 2000; Sateia, Doghramji, Hauri, & Morin, 2000).

Of foremost importance is the sleep history portion of a clinical interview. The focus is on obtaining a clear overview of the sleep problem, in particular, the nature and developmental course and impact of the sleep disturbance. It is important to conduct a good functional analysis of the sleep disturbance, gathering information about antecedents, behaviors, and consequences related to the sleep problem and its evolution. The clinician will want to gather detailed information about the current sleep complaint, its pattern, the sleep quality, and the daytime effects of sleep problems. It is often helpful to have the patient describe a typical day and night, including details about eating habits, exercise, stress, napping habits, caffeine, nicotine, alcohol, illicit drug and medication intake, the bedroom environment, bedroom behaviors (such as reading or watching television in bed) and bedtime routines. Information gathered should include the development of the sleep problem over time, any history of sleep disturbances, general health status, and an assessment of any current or past psychological health problems. Finally, a sleep history will address any issues of differential diagnosis with focus on breathing-related disorders, periodic limb movement of sleep (PLMS), restless leg syndrome (RLS), circadian rhythm disorders, parasomnias, and narcolepsy. Several structured or semistructured sleep disturbance interviews are available, such as Spielman and Anderson's (1999) diagnostic interview and Morin's (1993) Insomnia Interview Schedule, which provides a particularly good functional analysis and includes targeted diagnostic questions.

A sleep diary is another cornerstone of sleep assessment. A sleep diary will provide a nightly self-report of sleep pattern and quality that will prove invaluable, not only in assessment but also in treatment of sleep disturbances. A variety of sleep diaries are available that at a minimum gather information on total time in bed (TIB), latency of sleep onset, number and duration of nighttime awakenings, and total sleep time (TST) and allow the clinician to calculate sleep efficiency (a percentage calculated as TST/TIB). Sleep diary applications that can be downloaded to a smart phone are even available. Often sleep diaries will include questions about the quality and restfulness of sleep. The standard is to gather 2 weeks of sleep diary data as part of the assessment phase; however, some interventions, such as sleep restriction, will require sleep diary data during the intervention phase as well.

There are a significant number of questionnaires that can be used in the assessment of sleep disturbance. To gather data about psychiatric problems, the Beck Depression Inventory and Beck Anxiety Inventory are often used. For general health and pain information, the SF-36 Health Survey and the Multidimensional Pain Inventory (MPI) are gold standards. Instruments that are widely used to assess sleep and fatigue are the Pittsburgh Sleep Quality Index (PSQI), which is an excellent assessment of global sleep disturbance; the Insomnia Severity Index (ISI), a global measure of illness severity; and the Epworth Sleepiness Scale (ESS), which is used to measure daytime sleepiness. A combination of these instruments with a thorough sleep history provides a good clinical profile and can suggest whether referral is needed owing to undiagnosed psychiatric issues, unstable medical concerns, or sleep disturbance more effectively addressed by a combination of medical and behavioral interventions, such as obstructive sleep apnea, PLMS/RLS, or narcolepsy. Several measures are available to assess nightmares, including the Nightmare Effects Survey (NES), which assesses impairment associated with nightmares, and the Nightmare Distress Questionnaire (NDQ), which assesses distress associated with nightmares.

Finally, polysomnography (PSG) and actigraphy can be used to assess more complex cases. PSG is typically a laboratory-based procedure (although there are some home-based PSG units) that comprises electroencephalography (EEG), electrooculography (EOG), chin and anterior tibialis electromyography (EMG), electrocardiography (ECG), respiratory effort, airflow, and oximetry. A PSG is the gold standard in diagnostic assessment and provides a wealth of information on the sleeping and waking brain and physiology of the patient. A patient should be referred for a PSG if there is any evidence to suggest obstructive sleep apnea, narcolepsy, or movement disorders such as PLMS, RLS, or REM sleep behavior disorder, among others. Actigraphy provides inexpensive, objective estimates of sleep and uses a small device worn on the wrist to measure body movement, which can be used to distinguish wakefulness from sleep. Actigraphy is particularly useful to assess circadian disorders of sleep over time.

Treatment Approaches

The effectiveness of cognitive-behavioral therapies for insomnia (CBT-I) has been well established (e.g., Morin et al., 2006); however, until recently psychotherapies for sleep disturbance in populations specifically with PTSD have not been widely studied. In recent years we have begun to see published studies that look at the effectiveness of CBT-I and imagery rehearsal therapy (IRT) with this population and even a few studies that look specifically at combat-related PTSD. Some studies examine the use of CBT-I with veterans with medical and psychiatric comorbidities, including PTSD (Edinger, Olsen, Stechuchack, Meansk, Lineberger, et al., 2009; Perlman, Arnedt, Earnheart, Gorman, & Shirley, 2008); however, the impact on nightmares in conjunction with PTSD is not clear from these studies. Psychotherapies that specifically target nightmares do appear to reduce nightmares and improve daytime functioning in civilians with nightmares (Krakow et al., 2001); however, their efficacy does not extend to improving overall sleep quality significantly (Lancee, Spoormaker, Krakow, & van den Bout, 2008). Some studies that include an IRT-based therapy with elements of CBT-I have shown improvements in sleep, dreams, and PTSD symptoms in veteran and civilian samples (Cook, Harb, Ross, Gamble, & Gehrman, 2008; Germain, Shear, Hall & Buysse, 2007). A few recent studies (Nappi, Drummond, Thorp, & McQuaid, 2010, and Swanson, Favonte, Horin, & Arnedt, 2009) looking specifically at the use of IRT with combat veterans suggest that IRT may be an effective short-term treatment to improve sleep and to reduce nightmares, as well as nighttime and daytime PTSD symptoms. In this section we introduce the basic concepts and components of CBT-I and IRT for nightmares.

CBT for Insomnia

Almost all nonpharmacological treatments for sleep disturbance are referred to as cognitive-behavioral therapies, when in fact the underlying theory that governs treatment and the treatments themselves are largely behavioral in nature. The behavioral model of insomnia first articulated by Spielman, Saskin, and Thorpy in 1987 follows a diathesis–stress perspective and takes into account behavioral factors to explain how acute insomnia develops into chronic insomnia and suggests which factors should be targeted for intervention. This three-factor model (Figure 16.2) looks at the role of predisposing factors such as basal hyperarousal levels and tendency to worry, precipitating factors such as medical illness or psychological stress that lead to acute forms of insomnia, and the role of maladaptive behaviors or perpetuating factors such as excessive time in bed and daytime napping in the development of chronic insomnia. Therefore, if chronic insomnia is seen largely as the result of behavioral perpetuating factors, then interventions for chronic insomnia should focus on elimination of those behaviors that exacerbate or maintain the disorder. For chronic insomnia these factors are nonsleep behaviors that occur in the bed or bedroom environment and extensive time in bed when not sleeping. We look first at sleep hygiene education then at the two primary components of CBT-I that address these behaviors: stimulus control therapy (SCT) and sleep restriction therapy (SRT). For a more detailed description of the steps of CBT-I, see Perlis, Jungquist, Smith, and Posner, 2005.

Sleep Hygiene Education

Sleep hygiene education is not considered to be a stand-alone treatment for insomnia but is considered to be an integral part of CBT-I. Sleep hygiene is a psychoeducational intervention that provides the cornerstone for stimulus control and sleep restriction and addresses typical behaviors that may interfere with sleep quality and quantity. These are typically presented to the patient early in treatment, with emphasis placed on areas of concern specific to the patient based on the behavioral assessment of his or her sleep and sleep habits. See Table 16.1 for specific sleep hygiene instructions.

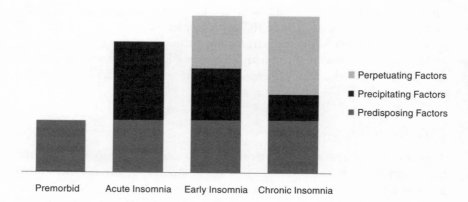

FIGURE 16.2. The nature of insomnia over time (three-factor model). From Spielman, Saskin, and Thorpy (1987). Copyright 1987 by Elsevier, Inc. Reprinted by permission.

TABLE 16.1. Sleep Hygiene Guidelines

- *Sleep only as much as needed to feel refreshed the following day.* Restricting time in bed helps consolidate and deepen sleep. Spending excessive time in bed can lead to fragmented and shallow sleep.

- *Have a routine wake-up time, 7 days a week.* A regular wake-up time in the morning will help set your "biological clock" and lead to regular sleep onset.

- *Your bedroom should be comfortable and free from light and noise.* A comfortable bed and bedroom environment will reduce the likelihood that you will wake up during the night. Excessively warm or cold rooms can disrupt sleep as well. A quiet environment is more sleep promoting than a noisy one. Noises can be masked with background white noise (such as the noise of a fan) or with earplugs. Bedrooms may be darkened with blackout shades, or sleep masks can be worn. Position clocks out of sight, as clock watching can increase anxiety about lack of sleep.

- *Avoid caffeine 4–6 hours before bedtime.* Caffeine disturbs sleep, even in people who do not subjectively experience such an effect. Individuals with insomnia are often more sensitive to mild stimulants than are normal sleepers. Caffeine is found in items such as coffee, tea, soda, chocolate, and many over-the-counter medications (e.g., Excedrin).

- *Avoid nicotine before bedtime.* Although some smokers claim that smoking helps them relax, nicotine is a stimulant. Thus smoking, dipping, or chewing tobacco should be avoided near bedtime and during the night.

- *Avoid alcohol after dinner.* A small amount of alcohol often promotes the onset of sleep, but as alcohol is metabolized sleep becomes disturbed and fragmented. Thus alcohol is a poor sleep aid.

- *Sleep medications are effective only temporarily.* Scientists have shown that sleep medications lose their effectiveness in about 2–4 weeks when taken regularly. Despite advertisements to the contrary, over-the-counter sleeping aids have little impact on sleep beyond the placebo effect. Over time, sleeping pills actually can make sleep problems worse. When sleeping pills have been used for a long period, withdrawal from the medication can lead to an insomnia rebound. Thus many individuals incorrectly conclude that they "need" sleeping pills in order to sleep normally.

- *Avoid vigorous exercise within 2 hours of bedtime.* Regular exercise in the late afternoon or early evening seems to aid sleep, although the positive effect often takes several weeks to become noticeable. Exercising sporadically is not likely to improve sleep, and exercise within 2 hours of bedtime may elevate nervous system activity and interfere with sleep onset. Spending 20 minutes in a tub of hot water an hour or two prior to bedtime may also promote sleep.

- *Avoid daytime napping.* Many individuals with insomnia "pay" for daytime naps with more sleeplessness at night. Thus it is best to avoid daytime napping. If you do nap, be sure to schedule naps before 3:00 P.M.

- *Eating a light snack at bedtime may be sleep promoting.* A light bedtime snack, such as a glass of warm milk, cheese, or a bowl of cereal, can promote sleep. You should avoid the following foods at bedtime: any caffeinated foods (e.g., chocolate), peanuts, beans, most raw fruits and vegetables (as they may cause gas), and high-fat foods such as potato or corn chips. Avoid snacks in the middle of the night as awakening may become associated with hunger.

- *Avoid excessive liquids in the evening.* Reducing liquid intake will decrease the need for nighttime trips to the bathroom.

(continued)

TABLE 16.1. (*continued*)

• *Do not try to fall asleep.* If you are unable to fall sleep within a reasonable time (15–20 minutes) or when you notice that you are beginning to worry about falling asleep, get out of bed. Leave the bedroom and engage in a quiet activity such as reading. Return to bed only when you are sleepy.

• *Don't have worry time in bed.* Plan time earlier in the evening to review the day, plan the next day, or deal with any problems. Worrying in bed can interfere with sleep onset and cause you to have a shallow sleep.

Stimulus Control Therapy

Sleep is a biological necessity, but good sleep is a habit. The "cleaner" the bedroom environment is, the more likely it is to be conducive to sleep. Often patients with chronic insomnia will lie in bed because "at least I am resting" or will report that reading or watching television in the bed allows them to be ready when or if sleep comes. These beliefs and behaviors can be highly reinforcing because they work sometimes; however, in the long run they create an associatiation of the bedroom with activity other than sleeping. For patients with PTSD in particular, the bedroom can become a place of fear where they dread to go. Often we hear complaints that patients can fall asleep elsewhere in the house or during the day but are unable to sleep at night in their beds, as the bedroom becomes associated more with worry and nightmares than with sleep. SCT is considered to be the first-line intervention for chronic insomnia based on its ability to consistently produce good clinical outcomes. The goal of SCT is to strengthen the association between the bedroom environment and sleep by controlling the amount of time spent awake in the bedroom environment and the types of behaviors that occur there. Generally the instructions are to: (1) lie down only when intending to go to sleep and only when sleepy, (2) keep to a regular wake-up time even on the weekends, (3) avoid any behaviors in the bed or bedroom except sleep and sexual activity, (4) get out of the bed and leave the bedroom if awake for more than 15 minutes, and (5) return to bed only when sleepy. Often the last two items will have to be repeated several times over the course of the night. Together with a stable prebedtime routine and basic sleep hygiene adherence, SCT is highly effective at providing a bedroom environment that is conducive to good sleep.

Sleep Restriction Therapy

By spending an increasing amount of time in bed "chasing" sleep, patients are actually achieving a shallower and more fragmented sleep. Sleep restriction therapy requires a patient to limit the amount of time in bed to an amount equal to their average total sleep time. The result will be to consolidate a patient's sleep, reducing sleep latency and waking after sleep onset. Sleep restriction is accomplished by establishing a fixed wake-up time and then decreasing sleep opportunity by limiting time in bed to an amount that is equal to the patient's average total sleep time as derived from his or her sleep diary. The patient's bedtime will be delayed so that the bedroom is not "open" for sleep until a specific time (fixed wake time minus average total sleep time). For example, a patient getting an average of 5 hours total sleep time who has a fixed wake-up time of 6 A.M. would not be allowed to go to bed until 1 A.M. This partial sleep deprivation usually results in a decrease in sleep latency and nighttime awakenings. As sleep efficiency improves to 85–90%, the amount of time in bed is adjusted upward by allowing the patient to go to bed earlier, typically in 15-minute increments.

Cognitive Therapy

The cognitive component of CBT-I is most suitable for patients who are pre-occupied with what they see as the probable consequences of their insomnia and for those who tend to worry or ruminate, especially in bed. Many insomniacs entertain a variety of dysfunctional cognitions that may exacerbate what might have been a transient sleep problem. The cognitive component is designed to correct unrealistic sleep expectations, revising false attributions about the causes of insomnia and reappraising perceptions of its consequences on daytime functioning. Several cognitive factors have been identified as playing a role in insomnia, such as: *faulty appraisal* of transient sleep difficulties, which leads to chronic insomnia; *misattributions* of daytime impairments to poor sleep, which can feed into a self-fulfilling prophecy; *unrealistic expectations* regarding sleep requirements; *excessive ruminations; magnification; catastrophizing; and selective recall.* The cognitive component will often start with psychoeducation about sleep and reemphasize the normal variations that occur in sleep, as well as age-related changes. Standard cognitive therapy approaches are to identify sleep-related thoughts using a thought record, to examine the accuracy of beliefs, and to consider alternative ways of thinking about sleep. For many, bedtime is the first chance to reflect on the day and plan for tomorrow. Setting aside "worry time" can be an effective intervention for patients who worry or ruminate in the bed. Having 15–20 minutes a day for focused planning or worry can help reduce the need to do so in the bed. Several other forms of cognitive therapy for insomnia have been devised, such as using paradoxical intention (Shoham-Salomon & Rosenthal, 1987), distraction, and imagery (Harvey & Payne, 2002). A complete package of CBT-I can range from 4 to 8 sessions and can be provided individually or in groups. It can be delivered via the Internet as well.

IRT for Nightmares

As noted earlier, recurring nightmares have often proven to be resistant to treatment when PTSD is treated with typical psychological and pharmacological treatments; this suggests that chronic nightmares may require a more specifically tailored treatment. Based on these findings, IRT was developed and tested as a short-term treatment specifically for nightmares. The treatment integrates psychoeducation about insomnia, nightmares, and PTSD with relaxation and a cognitive restructuring imagery technique. A recently published retrospective chart review study conducted with veterans from several eras found significant reductions in nightmare frequency, intensity, insomnia severity, and PTSD symptoms following a full course of five sessions (Nappi et al., 2010).

The primary component of IRT has been identified as the "rescripting" of a target nightmare. By developing an alternative and nondistressing version of the dream, it is hypothesized that the patient develops an increased mastery over the nightmare content and experience (Germain et al., 2004) and has a corrective learning experience in the safe, therapeutic environment (Davis & Wright, 2007). IRT is typically conducted over 3–4 sessions.

Session 1 focuses on psychoeducation about sleep, nightmares, imagery, and the theoretical basis for IRT. The goal is to suggest that nightmares may be trauma-induced but that they are also sustained by habit and are therefore no longer helpful in processing the trauma. Patients are provided with pleasant imagery exercises and, in some cases, given a nightmare log in which they document the nightly frequency and intensity of nightmares.

In session 2 patients learn how to use IRT on a single, self-selected nightmare. The therapist will often recommend that the nightmare be one that occurs with the most frequency, but ultimately most IRT interventions allow the patient to choose. The patient writes down the nightmare and is then encouraged to "change it in any way you wish" and then to write out the new dream. Changes could be a new ending, insertion of reminders of the present into the dream, transforming weapons into harmless objects, having the patient develop special powers that allow him or her to escape the nightmare, or using distancing techniques such as imagining viewing the nightmare on television. The patient then uses imagery to rehearse the new dream for 15–20 minutes. Patients are then encouraged to practice the new dream at least twice a day for 10 minutes.

Sessions 3 and 4 are largely for review of treatment progress and a check of compliance with the imagery rehearsal. Any adjustments needed to the new dream script can be made, and barriers to homework completion can be discussed. Often patients are given time to share their experience and ask questions about nightmares, sleep, and PTSD. The session and treatment ends with a review of lessons learned, and relapse prevention issues are discussed.

Several articles describe various IRTs in more detail and provide sample nightmare logs and suggested session content (see Krakow & Zadra, 2006; Thompson, Hamilton, & West 1995; and the Australian Centre for Post-traumatic Mental Health, 2004).

Conclusion

Insomniacs report more health problems, more frequent hospitalization, and more limitations in their work capacity because of sleep problems than good sleepers do. Patients with insomnia report mood and motivational changes, impaired attention and concentration, memory loss for recent events, and variable and slowed responses to tasks. Due to the impact of these consequences, insomnia is a significant public health concern. People with insomnia have been shown to be at increased risk for both on-the-job and motor vehicle accidents (National Institutes of Health, 2005). Within the military the consequences of insomnia can be magnified by the nature and dangerousness of the duties being performed. Failure of routines and impaired task performance, loss of situational awareness, lack of insight into impairment, and failure of verbal communication associated with sleep deprivation can result in mission failure and have been shown to be a primary cause of military aviation mishaps and of "friendly fire" accidents (Caldwell, 2005; Belenky et al., 1994).

Currently there are a limited number of studies looking at sleep disturbance in military members and the treatment of sleep disturbances once they are identified. It would be helpful to have a better understanding of the etiological role of military factors besides combat PTSD, such as deployment in general, on sleep quality. It will be important to see the results of large-scale studies of the use of CBT-I and IRT specifically with military members with deployment-related insomnia. This chapter did not address the use of medications in the treatment of insomnia and nightmares, though there is evidence to support the use of medications on a limited basis in treatment of both conditions (Morin et al., 2009; Raskind et al., 2003), and providers should be aware of these treatment options.

The recognition that deployments and combat have a potential to have a lasting effect on sleep health in military members is growing. Although there are interventions that appear to be efficacious with this population, further study is needed. In the meantime, efforts need to be made to increase the awareness of primary care and behavioral health providers of the need to assess for insomnia and the availability of efficacious behavioral interventions. Behavioral health providers in particular should always assess for sleep disruptions in military members and be trained in basic interventions such as CBT-I and IRT.

References

Armed Forces Health Surveillance Center. (2010). Insomnia, active component, U.S. Armed Forces, January 2000–December 2009. *Medical Surveillance Monthly Report, 17*(5), 12–15.

Australian Centre for Posttraumatic Health. (2004). Imagery rehearsal in the treatment of nightmares in PTSD: Facilitator's treatment manual. (Available from the Australian Centre for Posttraumatic Mental Health, PO Box 5444, Heidelberg West 3081, Australia).

Belenky, G., Penetar, D., Throne, D., Popp, K., Leu, J., Thomas, M., et al. (1994). The effects of sleep deprivation on performance during continuous combat operations. In B. M. Marriot (Ed.), *Food components to enhance performance* (pp. 127–135). Washington, DC: National Academy Press.

Bryant, R. A., Creamer, M., O'Donnell, M., Silove, D., & McFarlane, A. C. (2010). Sleep disturbance immediately prior to trauma predicts subsequent psychiatric disorder. *Sleep, 33*(1), 69–74.

Caldwell, J. A. (2005). Fatigue in aviation. *Travel Medicine and Infectious Disease, 3*(2), 85–96.

Castriotta, R. J., & Murthy, J. N. (2011). Sleep disorders in patients with traumatic brain injury: A review. *CNS Drugs, 25*(3), 175–185.

Chesson, A., Jr., Hartse, K., Anderson, W. M., Davila, D., Johnson, S., Littner, M., et al. (2000). Practice parameter for the evaluation of chronic insomnia. An American Academy of Sleep Medicine report. *Sleep, 23*(2), 237–241.

Cohen, M., Oksenberg, A., Snir, D., Stern, M. J., & Groswasser, Z. (1992). Temporally related changes of sleep complaints in traumatic brain injured patients. *Journal of Neurology, Neurosurgery and Psychiatry, 55*(4), 313–315.

Cook, J., Harb, G., Ross, R., Gamble, G., & Gehrman, P. (2008, November). *Open pilot study of imagery rehearsal with OIF returnees and design of bisite RCT in OEF/OIF veterans.* Paper presented at the annual meeting of the International Society for Traumatic Stress Studies, Chicago, IL.

Davis, J. L., & Wright, D. C. (2007). Randomized clinical trial for treatment of chronic nightmares in trauma-exposed adults. *Journal of Traumatic Stress, 20,* 123–133.

Edinger, J. D., Olsen, M. K., Stechuchak, K. M., Means, M. K., Lineberger, M. D., Kirby, A., et al. (2009). Cognitive behavioral therapy for patients with primary insomnia or insomnia associated predominantly with mixed psychiatric disorders: A randomized clinical trial. *Sleep, 32,* 499–510.

Foa, E. B., Riggs, D. S., & Gershuny, B. S. (1995). Arousal, numbing, and intrusion: Symptom structure of PTSD following assault. *American Journal of Psychiatry, 152*(1), 116–120.

Gasanov, R. L., Gitlevich, T. R., Lesnyak, V. N., & Levin, Y. (1998). Structure of nocturnal sleep in patients with cerebral insult. *Neuroscience and Behavioral Physiology, 28*(3), 325–329.

Germain, A., Krakow, B., Faucher, B., Zadra, A., Nielsen, T., Hollifield, M., et al. (2004). Increased mastery elements associated with imagery rehearsal treatment for nightmares in sexual assault survivors with PTSD. *Dreaming, 14,* 195–206.

Germain, A., Shear, K. M., Hall, M., & Buysse, D. J. (2007). Effects of a brief behavioral treatment for PTSD-related sleep disturbances: A pilot study. *Behaviour Research and Therapy, 45,* 627–632.

Gosselin, N., & Tellier, M. (2010). Patients with traumatic brain injury are at high risk of developing chronic sleep-wake disturbances. *Journal of Neurology, Neurosurgery and Psychiatry, 18*(12), 129–137.

Harvey, A. G. & Bryant, R. A. (1998). The relationship between acute stress disorder and posttraumatic stress disorder: a prospective evaluation of vehicle accident survivors. *Journal of Consulting and Clinical Psychology, 66*(3), 507–512.

Harvey, A. G., & Payne, S. (2002). The management of unwanted pre-sleep thoughts in insomnia: Distraction with imagery versus general distraction. *Behavior Research and Therapy, 40*(3), 267–277.

Hoge, C. W., Auchterlonie, J. L., & Milliken, C. S. (2006). Mental health problems, use of mental health services, and attrition from military service after returning from deployment to Iraq or Afghanistan. *Journal of the American Medical Association, 295*(9), 1023–1032.

Inman, D. J., Silver, S. M., & Doghramji, K. (1990). Sleep disturbance in posttraumatic stress disorder: A comparison with non-PTSD insomnia. *Journal of Traumatic Stress, 3,* 429–437.

Kilpatrick, D. G., Resnick, H. S., Freedy, J. R., Pelcovitz, D., Resick, P. A., Roth, S., et al. (1998). Posttraumatic stress disorder field trial evaluation of the PTSD construct-criteria A through E. In T. A. Frances & H. A. Pincus, R. Ross, M. B. First, W. Davis, & M. Kline (Eds.), *DSM-IV sourcebook* (pp. 803–846). Washington, DC: American Psychiatric Press

Koren, D., Arnon, I., Lavie, P., & Klein, E. (2002). Sleep complaints as early predictors of posttraumatic stress disorder: A 1-year prospective study of injured survivors of motor vehicle accidents. *American Journal of Psychiatry, 159*(5), 85–87.

Krakow, B., Hollifield, M., Johnston, L., Koss, M., Schrader, R., Warner, T. D., et al. (2001). Imagery rehearsal therapy for chronic nightmares in sexual assault survivors with posttraumatic stress disorder: A randomized controlled trial. *Journal of the American Medical Association, 286,* 537–545.

Krakow, B., & Zadra, A. (2006). Clinical management of nightmares: Imagery rehearsal therapy. *Behavioral Sleep Medicine, 4,* 45–70.

Lancee, J., Spoormarker, V. I., Krakow, B., & van den Bout, J. (2008). A systematic review of cognitive-behavioral treatment for nightmares: Toward a well-established treatment. *Journal of Clinical Sleep Medicine, 4,* 475–480.

Lewis, V., Creamer, M., & Failla, S. (2009). Is poor sleep in Veterans a function of post-traumatic stress disorder? *Military Medicine, 174,* 948–951.

Maher, M. J., Rego, S. A., & Asnis, G. M. (2006). Sleep disturbance in patients with posttraumatic stress disorder: Epidemiology, impact and approaches to management. *CNS Drugs, 20*(7), 567–590.

McLay, R. N., Klam, W. P., & Volkert, S. L. (2010). Insomnia is the most commonly reported symptom and predicts other symptoms of posttraumatic stress disorder in U.S. service members returning from military deployments. *Military Medicine, 175,* 759–762.

Mental Health Advisory Team V. (2008) *Operation Iraqi Freedom 06-08: Iraq/ Operation Enduring Freedom 8: Afghanistan.* Washington, DC: Office of the Surgeon General United States Army Medical Command.

Morin, C. M. (1993). *Insomnia: Psychological assessment and management.* New York: Guilford Press.

Morin, C. M., Bootzin, R. R., Buysse, D. J., Edinger, J. D., Espie, C. A., & Lichstein, K. L. (2006). Psychological and behavioral treatment of insomnia: Update of the recent evidence (1998–2004). *Sleep, 29,* 1398–1414.

Morin, C. M., Vallieres, A., Guay, B., Ivers, H., Savard, J., Mérette, C., et al. (2009). Cognitive behavioral therapy, singly and combined with medication, for persistent insomnia: A randomized controlled trial. *Journal of the American Medical Association, 301*(19), 2005–2015.

Nappi, C. M., Drummond, S. P. A., Thorp, S. R., & McQuaid, J. R. (2010). Effectiveness of imagery rehearsal therapy for the treatment of combat-related nightmares in veterans. *Behavior Therapy, 41,* 237–244.

National Institutes of Health. (2005). *NIH state-of-the-science conference statement on manifestations and management of chronic insomnia in adults.* Retrieved June 16, 2010, from consensus *nih.gov/2005/insomniastatement.htm.*

Neylan, T. C., Marmar, C. R., Metzler, T. J., Weiss, D. S., Zatzick, D. F., Delucchi, K. L., et al. (1998). Sleep disturbances in the Vietnam generation: Findings from a nationally representative sample of male Vietnam veterans. *American Journal of Psychiatry, 155,* 929–933.

Ouellet, M.-C., & Morin, C. M. (2007). Efficacy of cognitive-behavioral therapy for insomnia associated with traumatic brain injury: A single-case experimental design. *Archives of Physical Medicine and Rehabilitation, 88,* 1581–1592.

Perlis, M. L., Jungquist, C., Smith, M. T., & Posner, D. (2005). *Cognitive behavioral treatment of insomnia: A session-by-session guide.* New York: Springer.

Perlman, L. M., Arnedt, J. T., Earnheart, K. L., Gorman, A. A., & Shirley, K. G. (2008). Group cognitive-behavioral therapy for insomnia in a VA mental health clinic. *Cognitive and Behavioral Practice, 15,* 426–434.

Peterson, A. L., Goodie, J. L., Satterfield, W. A., & Brim, W. L. (2008). Sleep disturbance during military deployment. *Military Medicine. 173,* 230–235.

Picchioni, D., Hope, C. R., & Harsh, J. R. (2007). A case-control study of environmental risk factors for narcolepsy. *Neuroepidemiology, 29*(3–4) 185–192.

Pillar, G., Malhotra, A., & Lavie P. (2000). Posttraumatic stress disorder and sleep: What a nightmare! *Sleep Medicine Review, 4*(2), 183–200.

Raskind, M. A., Perkind, E. R., Kanter, E. D., Petrie, E. C., Radant, A., Thompson, C. E., et al. (2003). Reduction of nightmares and other PTSD symptoms in combat veterans by prazosin: A placebo-controlled study. *American Journal of Psychiatry, 160*(2), 371–373.

Ross, R. J., Ball, W. A., Sullivan, K. A., & Caroff, S. N. (1989). Sleep disturbance as a hallmark of posttraumatic stress disorder. *American Journal of Psychiatry, 146,* 697–707.

Sateia, M. J., Doghramji, K., Hauri, P. J., & Morin C. M. (2000). Evaluation of chronic insomnia: An American Academy of Sleep Medicine review. *Sleep, 23,* 243–308.

Scheuder, B. J. N., Kleijn, W. C., & Rooijmans, H. G. M. (2000). Nocturnal re-experiencing more than forty years after war trauma. *Journal of Traumatic Stress, 13,* 453–463.

Seelig, A. D., Jackobson, I. G., Smith, B., Hooper, T. I., Boyko, E. J., Gackstetter, G. D., et al. (2010). Sleep patterns before, during and after deployment to Iraq and Afghanistan. *Sleep, 33*(12), 1615–1622.

Shoham-Salomon, V., & Rosenthal, R. (1987). Paradoxical interventions: A meta-analysis. *Journal of Consulting and Clinical Psychology, 55,* 22–28.

Spielman, A. J., & Anderson, M. W. (1999). The clinical interview and treatment planning as a guide to understanding the nature of insomnia: The CCNY Interview for Insomnia. In S. Chokroverty (Eds.) *Sleep disorders medicine: Basic science, technical considerations and clinical aspects* (2nd ed., pp. 385–426). Boston: Butterwork-Heinemann.

Spielman, A. J., Saskin, P., & Thorpy, M. J. (1987). A behavioral perspective on insomnia treatment. *Psychiatric Clinics of North America, 10*(4), 541–553.

Spoormaker, V. I., & Montgomery, P. (2008). Disturbed sleep in posttraumatic stress disorder: Secondary symptom or core feature? *Sleep Medicine Reviews, 12,* 169–184.

Swanson, L. M., Favorite, T. K., Horin, E., & Arnedt, J. T. (2009). A combined group treatment for nightmares and insomnia in combat veterans: A pilot study. *Journal of Traumatic Stress, 22*(6), 639–642.

Thompson, K., Hamilton, M. & West, J. (1995). Group treatment for nightmares in veterans with combat-related PTSD. *National Center for PTSD Clinical Quarterly, 5*(4), 13–17.

Zayfert, C. & DeViva, J. C. (2004). Residual insomnia following cognitive behavioral therapy for PTSD. *Journal of Traumatic Stress, 17*(1), 69–73.

CHAPTER 17

Managing the Service Member
with Suicidal Ideation

Nancy A. Skopp
David D. Luxton
Nigel Bush
M. David Rudd

Posttraumatic stress disorder (PTSD) has been widely associated with suicidal behavior (e.g., Kessler, 2000; Oldham, 2008; see Panagioti, Gooding, & Tarrier, 2009, for a review). Research indicates that suicidal ideation corresponds to subsequent self-harm behaviors, including planned and unplanned suicide attempts (Kessler, Borges, & Walters, 1999). Furthermore, PTSD is a strong predictor of those individuals who move beyond suicidal ideation to suicide attempts (Nock et al., 2009). It is therefore incumbent on military clinicians to understand, assess, and monitor suicidal ideation in the service members under their care. In this chapter we provide an overview of military suicide, suicide risk factors, and theory of suicide, with a focus on the clinical management of suicidal ideation and behaviors, which we define as any self-reported thoughts of engaging in suicide-related behavior (O'Carroll et al., 1996). We provide guidelines and recommendations for the assessment, management, and treatment of suicidal ideation and discuss some of the limitations and gaps in the literature on this topic. We close with a discussion of the implications for military service and integration into the civilian community.

Suicide in the Military

Since the beginning of combat operations in Iraq and Afghanistan (Operation Iraqi Freedom [OIF]/Operation Enduring Freedom [OEF]), military suicides have increased to their highest levels since 1980 when formal documentation of suicide records began (Luxton et al., 2010). Historically, the rates of suicide among military personnel have been lower than in the general U.S. population. Until recently, preenlistment selection or screening for mental and physical health, a structured and cohesive work and social environment, a ubiquitous medical service, and the "healthy worker effect" all have possibly served to mitigate military suicide (Mahon, Tobin, Cusack, Kelleher, & Malone, 2005). However, the 2008 numbers now represent a rate of more than 20 per 100,000, higher than the adjusted civilian rate; in fact, the highest Army suicide rate in nearly three decades (Kang & Bullman, 2009). Numbers for the Marine Corps, Navy, and Air Force also have increased.

PTSD and Suicide Risk

In their review of relations between PTSD and suicidal behavior, Panagioti et al. (2009) concluded that PTSD was associated with suicidal thoughts and behaviors irrespective of the type of trauma experienced. Jakupcak and colleagues (2009) examined suicidal ideation as a risk factor among OIF/ OEF veterans and reported that veterans who screened positive for PTSD were four times as likely to experience suicidal ideation as were veterans not diagnosed with PTSD. Other research suggests that specific symptom clusters may be strongly related to suicide risk among veterans diagnosed with PTSD (Panagioti et al., 2009). Nye and Bell (2007), for example, studied suicidal ideation among Vietnam veterans and found that the reexperiencing symptom cluster was more predictive of suicidal ideation than were the avoidance/numbing and increased arousal clusters. Reexperiencing symptoms such as nightmares, in particular, are also linked to suicidal behavior (Bernert, Joiner, Cukrowicz, Schmidt, & Krakow, 2005). Results of a number of studies also indicate that there is a strong link between combat-related PTSD and suicidal behavior and that comorbid diagnoses further elevate this risk (Panagioti et al., 2009).

Suicide Risk Factors Specific to the Military and U.S. Military Response

Some risk factors are especially pertinent to the military population. Demographically, Army soldiers exhibiting suicidal behavior tend to be male, Caucasian, married, and disproportionately represented by enlisted personnel (Allen, Cross, & Swanner, 2005). Studies within military populations have revealed some additional risk factors related to service. Most obviously, deployments to war zones and exposure to combat, possibly exacerbated over multiple deployments, have been associated with suicidality across a variety of locations, conflicts, and nationalities (Fontana & Rosenheck, 1994; Selby et al., 2010). Other military-specific risk factors may include excessive motivation to excel, the tendency to be autonomous, and the opportunity to access and use firearms as lethal means (Mahon et al., 2005).

In response to the rise in suicide among U.S. service members, substantial efforts have been made by senior leadership to establish suicide research, prevention, and treatment programs. However, the military healthcare system continues to face a significant challenge to addressing mental health issues because of a prevailing cultural barrier among service members. Many service members do not seek mental health services because of a perceived stigma associated with admitting a problem and seeking treatment. Soldiers typically report more discomfort discussing psychological problems than medical problems and are less likely to comply with follow-up psychological referrals (Greene-Shortridge, Britt, & Castro, 2007). Hoge and colleagues (2004) examined perceived barriers to seeking mental health service among Army and Marine Corps personnel after OIF/OEF deployment. Respondents most frequently cited being seen as weak, being treated differently by unit leadership, and fearing a loss of confidence of unit members as obstacles to seeking mental health services. Service members may also be concerned that careers would be harmed or that their leaders would blame them for the problem (Hoge et al., 2004).

It also bears noting that, although suicidal prevention and treatment programs tailored to the military are now increasingly available to active service members, such programs are less available to members of the National Guard and Reserve. Guard and Reserve personnel returning to civilian life after deployment typically seek mental health care from local civilian providers who rarely have experience with or training in the unique demands of postdeployment problems. Consequently, Guard and Reserve veterans may be especially vulnerable to escalations of suicidal behavior because of insufficient and untimely recognition of their symptoms.

Theoretical Underpinnings of Attempted and Completed Suicide in Relation to PTSD

Joiner's (2005) interpersonal–psychological theory of suicide (IPTS) is a leading theory in the field of suicidology. Although this is a relatively new theory, thus far research has supported its validity in predicting suicidal ideation and behavior (see Selby et al., 2010, for a review). IPTS appears to hold particular relevance for suicidality among service members diagnosed with PTSD (Selby et al., 2010). According to IPTS, three conditions must be satisfied for an individual to die by suicide: (1) acquired capacity to enact lethal self-injury (acquired capacity), (2) a sense of being a burden to significant others or society (burdensomeness), and (3) a sense that one does not belong or lacks a connection with a valued group (thwarted belongingness). IPTS posits that all three of the conditions are necessary for completed suicide.

Acquired capacity, in particular, may hold relevance for combat-exposed service members diagnosed with PTSD by virtue of habituation to pain and death encountered in combat zones (Selby et al., 2010). Moreover, service members who are injured as a result of combat exposure are at increased risk of PTSD (Koren, Norman, Cohen, Berman, & Klein, 2005) and suicide (Bullman & Kang, 1996). Chronic pain associated with such injuries may relate to acquired capacity through habituation. The perception of burdensomeness and lack of belongingness may also be particularly relevant among service members diagnosed with PTSD. Military personnel deployed to combat zones may experience survival guilt for having lived through the death of a fellow service member. Such guilt may contribute to feelings of being a burden in service members who feel responsible in some way for not preventing the death, and this may generalize to global feelings of "making things worse" (Selby et al., 2010). Similarly, a service member who has taken another life during combat may experience feelings of isolation and lack of belonging engendered by the sense that they are "different" or "unloveable" (Selby et al., 2010).

Suicide Risk Assessment, Management, and Treatment

Effective assessment and management of suicidal behavior has presented ongoing challenges to the field of suicidology (Jobes, Rudd, Overholser, & Joiner, 2008). These challenges include legal issues, inability to predict suicide, judgments about when hospitalization is warranted, and the life-and-death implications of treatment, to name a few. A single standard of care—defined as the level of care that a reasonably prudent person should exercise in the same or similar circumstances—does not exist for suicide risk and management (Cukrowicz, Wingate, Driscoll, & Joiner, 2004). The American Psychological Association (2003) provides a comprehensive, empirically based document, *Practice Guidelines for the Assessment and Treatment of Patients with Suicidal Behavior*; however, there is a clear need for more succinct clinical guidelines (Bryan & Rudd, 2006). Cukrowicz et al. (2004) proposed a concise set of guidelines for standard of care that can be applied across clinical settings, and several investigators have made recommendations for assessing, managing, and treating suicide risk (e.g., Bryan & Rudd, 2006; Kleespies, Deleppo, Gallagher, & Niles, 1999; Selby et al., 2010; Stellrecht et al., 2006). These guidelines and recommendations are integrated and presented within a military framework here.

Risk Assessment

A central component of suicide risk assessment is inquiry into current suicidal ideation and past self-injurious events (Stellrecht et al., 2006), given research (Kessler et al., 1999) and theory (Joiner, 2005) that indicates that prior self-inflicted injuries or suicide attempts are salient predictors of subsequent attempts and completed suicides. The acquired capacity for self-harm may be particularly relevant for combat-exposed service members diagnosed with PTSD for the aforementioned reasons (e.g., habituation to pain, death). It is important to inquire about the number of previous attempts, as multiple attempters are already at an elevated risk (Cukrowicz et al., 2004). In addition to previous self-harm behavior, Rudd, Joiner, and Rajab (2001) highlight several other factors that have been shown empirically to be crucial to suicide risk assessment. These risk factors, combined with theoretically relevant military specific and PTSD-related risk factors, are summarized in Table 17.1.

The Clinical Interview

A hierarchical approach to questioning about suicide that gradually increases in intensity is useful in collecting relevant information that helps to establish rapport and to reduce anxiety and agitation (Bryan & Rudd, 2006). The reduction of anxiety may also enhance the thoroughness and candor of the service member's report. Hierarchical questioning also can help normalize suicidal ideation within the context of a depressive episode or other mental health problems (Bryan & Rudd, 2006), potentially reducing stigma.

The assessment should begin with an identification of the precipitant (e.g., "Can you tell me about anything that has been particularly stressful?"). Questioning should proceed toward the identification of the symptomatic presentation (e.g., "It sounds like you're feeling depressed. Have you felt anxious and panicky?") and progress toward an assessment of hopelessness (e.g., "It is not unusual for someone feeling that way to think things won't get better. Do you ever feel like that?"). The clinician should next steer the interview toward the nature of the suicidal thoughts (e.g., "When people are feeling hopeless they sometimes think about death and dying. Have you ever thought about killing yourself?"). Bryan and Rudd (2006) also recommend use of a 1-to-10-point rating scale for clarification (e.g., "Could you rate the

TABLE 17.1. Suicide Risk Factors and Relevant Assessment Domains

Suicide risk factors	Relevant assessment domains
General risk factors	
History of self-harm	Previous suicide attempts, methods used, number of attempts
Predisposition to suicidal behaviors	History of abuse, previous trauma, low family support, high family conflict, personal and family history of psychopathology, chaotic family history
Identifiable precipitant or stressors	Significant loss, health problems, relationship instability, legal troubles, interpersonal discord, physical or emotional abuse
Symptomatic presentation	PTSD and depressive symptoms, anxiety, borderline or antisocial traits
Presence of hopelessness	Severity and duration
Nature of suicidal thinking	Frequency, intensity (more than ideation), duration, presence of a plan, preparations, access to and lethality of means, active suicidal behaviors, reasons for living or dying, desire to make a passive suicide attempt (e.g., lethal car accident), desire for active suicide attempt, expected outcome of attempt, presence of deterrents (e.g., children), courage and competence to make attempt
Previous suicidal behavior	Frequency, context, opportunity for rescue or help seeking, preparatory behaviors
Impulsivity and self-control	Subjective and objective (substance abuse, impulsive behaviors, aggression, promiscuous sexual activity), repeated attempts signal a form of intentionality
Protective factors	Social support, problem-solving and coping skills, participation in treatment, hopefulness, children in the home, pregnancy, religious or spiritual commitment, life satisfaction, intact reality testing, fear of social disapproval, fear of suicide and of death, high levels of self-control
Risk factors specific to military and PTSD domains	
Thwarted belongingness	Poor family adjustment, distress over killing others, emotional numbing and disconnection from family, loss of friends to combat, hypervigilance/paranoia, aggression toward spouse or children, feelings of isolation, level of social integration, number and nature of interpersonal relationships
Perceived burdensomeness	Loss of purpose after redeployment, combat-related physical and psychological disability, view of needing help as a "weakness," perceived combat failures, survival guilt
Acquired capacity	Frequent exposure to combat, killing, number and severity of personal injuries, witnessing severe injury and death among friends, reexperiencing combat trauma, habituation to constant anxiety about death, combat training experiences and injuries, training and service-specific habituation—use of guns (Army, Marines), exposure to heights (Air Force), use of rope (Navy)

Note. Adapted from Rudd et al. (2001), Selby et al. (2010), and Cukrowicz et al. (2004).

severity of your hopelessness on a scale of 1 to 10, with 1 being very hopeful and 10 being no hope at all?"). Such anchoring permits comparisons across time as well as symptom monitoring. Additional examples of questions that provide coverage of domains of known risk factors, as outlined by Cukrowicz and colleagues (2004), are presented below:

- "Have you been thinking about suicide recently?"
- "When you think about suicide, what kinds of thoughts do you have?"
- "Have you made any plans for attempting suicide? For example, have you obtained the means necessary to complete suicide, like purchasing a gun or obtaining pills?" (*Note*: The clinician should inquire twice about method because suicidal individuals may not initially report the most accessible or lethal method; see Bryan & Rudd, 2006).
- "Do you have confidence you could complete suicide?"
- "Have you ever attempted suicide previously?"
- "Have you ever harmed yourself intentionally? Cut yourself or swallowed pills?"
- "What are some reasons you would consider attempting suicide?"
- "Tell me about your support system. Do you feel isolated? Are you able to talk to friends and family about your problems?"
- "How do you feel when you think about the future? Are you hopeful that you can do something about your problems?"

Emergency Management

A clinical emergency occurs when there is imminent risk that suicidal behavior will result in death (Kleespies et al., 1999). The clinician should have an established plan of response for the suicidal emergencies. Kleespies et al. (1999) outlined empirically supported recommendations for evaluation and treatment of suicidal emergencies. It is critical that clinicians consider all situations involving suspected suicide risk as possible emergencies until disconfirmed (Kleespies et al., 1999). Foremost, the service member's emotional turmoil must be contained. The first level of response is the creation of a working alliance that conveys empathy and genuineness. When it is not possible to establish a working alliance, more structured means may be necessary (e.g., assistance from another clinician). If there is imminent danger of self-harm, duty of care rises to preventing harm with all available and reasonable means (Kleespies et al., 1999). Mindfulness of the physical safety of all parties is paramount. Bryan and Rudd (2006) provide a suicide risk continuum and indicate responses that incorporate the Sommers-Flanagans' original model (1995; see Table 17.2).

As shown in Table 17.2, there are clear guidelines for managing individuals who exhibit moderate to extreme suicide risk. In situations of severe or extreme risk, immediate inpatient care is indicated; whenever possible, it is desirable to encourage the service member to go voluntarily (Cukrowicz et al., 2004). For individuals falling in the nonexistent and mild risk categories, it is recommended that some variant of the following statement be made at regular intervals during treatment (Joiner, Walker, Rudd, & Jobes, 1999):

> "In the event that you begin to develop suicidal feelings, here's what I want you to do: First, use the strategies for self-control that we will discuss, including seeking social support. Then, if suicidal feelings remain, seek me out or whoever is covering for me. If, for whatever reason, you are unable to get help, or, if you feel that things just won't wait, call or go to the ER—here is the phone number."

Crisis Situations

A crisis is distinguished from an emergency in that hospitalization may not be indicated. The goal of crisis management is to allay distress and regulate emotions prior to beginning treatment or between sessions (Stellrecht et al., 2006). Targeting and challenging distorted thoughts may be a useful way to diffuse such distress and curtail suicidal impulses by shifting attention away from reasons for dying (Stellrecht et al., 2006) to reasons for living. A "crisis card" outlines steps to be taken if an individual becomes suicidal and can directly address relevant concerns, such as burdensomeness and lack of belonging, that may be useful in managing suicidal impulses (Strellrecht et al., 2006). The card might contain a list of activities known to foster connectedness and a sense of self-efficacy and other activities that have proven useful in the past. The card could contain statements challenging distorted thoughts about being a burden to family or others (e.g., "I help my elderly neighbor"; I support other veterans").

Documentation

The clinician should document all services provided, actions taken, content of therapy sessions, recommendations made, and the service member's level of compliance with recommendations (Barnett & Porter, 1998). Such record keeping ensures consistent records and a means of conveying vital information in the case of an emergency.

TABLE 17.2. Suicide Risk Continuum and Indicated Responses

Risk level	Description	Indicated response
Nonexistent	No identifiable suicidal ideation	No particular changes in ongoing treatment
Mild	Frequent suicidal ideation with limited frequency, intensity and duration; no identifiable plans, no intent, mild dysphoria/symptoms, good self-control, few risk factors, and identifiable protective factors	Evaluation of any expressed suicidal ideation to monitor change in risk
Moderate	Frequent suicidal ideation with limited intensity and duration; some specific plans, no intent, good self-control, limited dysphoria/symptoms, some risk factors present, and identifiable risk factors	1. Recurrent evaluation of need for hospitalization 2. Increase frequency or duration of outpatient visits 3. Active involvement of family 4. Frequent reevaluation of treatment plan goals 5. Frequent reevaluation of suicide risk, noting specific changes that reduce or elevate risk 6. 24-hour availability of emergency or crisis services for patient 7. Consideration of medication if symptoms worsen or persist 8. Frequent input from family members with respect to indicators 9. Professional consultation, as indicated
Severe	Frequent, intense, and enduring suicidal ideation; specific plans, not subjective intent but some objective markers of intent (e.g., choice of lethal method[s], available/accessible method, some limited preparatory behavior), evidence of impaired self-control, severe dysphoria/ symptoms, multiple risk factors present and few, if any, protective factors	Immediate evaluation for inpatient hospitalization (voluntary or involuntary, depending on situation)
Extreme	Frequent, intense, and enduring suicidal ideation; specific plans, clear subjective and objective intent, impaired self-control, severe dysphoria/symptoms, many risk factors and no protective factors	

Overview of Treatments for Suicidal Behaviors

The treatment literature on suicidal behaviors is limited (Linehan, 2008), and very little has focused on service members' unique needs and special challenges in military environments. Rudd, Joiner, Jobes, and King (1999) reviewed the empirical literature on the outpatient treatment of suicidality and made the following recommendations:

1. Intensive follow-up treatment following an attempt is appropriate and effective for high-risk patients (i.e., multiple attempts, psychiatric histories, comorbidities).
2. Short-term cognitive-behavioral therapy that integrates problem solving as a core intervention is effective at reducing suicidal ideation, depression, and hopelessness for periods of up to 1 year. Such brief approaches, however, do not appear effective in reducing attempts over enduring time frames.
3. Reducing suicide attempts requires longer term treatment and modalities that target specific skill deficits, such as anger regulation, poor distress tolerance, interpersonal assertiveness, interpersonal relationships, and self-image problems.
4. High-risk cases can be safely treated as outpatients provided acute hospitalization is available and accessible.

Rudd et al. (1999) provide additional outpatient practice recommendations. When risk is high but not imminent and does not dictate hospitalization, outpatient care can be varied in accordance with identified risk factors. This might include scheduling additional appointments and making referrals for concurrent group therapy. Treatment of suicidal ideation and related symptomatology such as depression and anxiety should include a problem-solving component or core intervention. Another important component of outpatient treatment is the development of an explanatory model to identify direct (e.g., suicidal ideation) and indirect (e.g., hopelessness, anger, interpersonal relations, day-to-day functioning at work and home) treatment targets. Outpatient treatment should include standardized follow-up and referral procedures, such as telephone contacts, to enhance compliance and reduce suicidal risk. Finally, the unavailability of data regarding the benefits of one therapeutic approach over another should be reviewed with service members and informed consent must clearly state the limits of confidentiality.

Specific Treatment Approaches

Approaches based on cognitive theory show utility in identifying and managing suicidal thoughts and related behaviors. The cognitive-behavioral analysis system of psychotherapy (CBASP; Driscoll, Cukrowicz, Reardon, & Joiner, 2004) may be particularly suited to the military owing to its portability across clinical settings and relatively simple ease of use. The CBASP involves repeated and highly structured analysis of everyday situations and is designed to teach patients to identify desired outcomes and modify thoughts and behaviors to increase the likelihood of such outcomes. The collaborative assessment and management of suicidality (CAMS; see Jobes, 2006) is a relatively new but promising approach. The cornerstone of this treatment approach is the therapeutic relationship, allowing clinician and patient to "coauthor" their suicide-specific treatment plan (Jobes, 2009). Finally, severe suicidal behaviors such as repeated self-harm have been shown to respond to dialectical behavior therapy (DBT; Linehan et al., 2006).

Limitations of Treatment Strategies and Gaps in Research

One of the primary limitations of current treatment strategies for suicidality is the lack of empirical support and disparateness of interventions (Linehan, 2008). This issue has made it difficult to determine whether one intervention is more effective than another or which combination of interventions encompasses an optimal intervention strategy. Moreover, research findings from one population may not be appropriate for generalization to other populations. It is not clear which populations might benefit from a particular intervention or whether any given strategy should be widely adopted. This issue is particularly true for the military population because of the limited data available on this population compared with the civilian populations.

In addition, there are a number of issues that make the evaluation of suicide treatment strategies a significant challenge. The low base rate of suicide makes this outcome difficult to study in both retrospective and prospective study designs. Further, the causes of suicide are complex and idiosyncratic. Identified risk factors can vary in their degree of effect and can change over time. Most studies on the effectiveness of suicide prevention strategies have used self-harm as an outcome measure. Some of these studies have included randomized controlled trial (RCT) designs that examined cognitive therapy (Brown et al., 2005), DBT (Linehan et al., 2006), and cognitive-behavioral therapy (Slee, Garnefski, van der Leeden, Arensman, & Spinhoven, 2008). Although intentional self-harm is a significant risk factor for suicide, it is not directly comparable to completed suicide or suicidal ideation alone. Intervention strategies that have been shown to be effective in preventing self-harm must also be evaluated for their potential to prevent suicide deaths.

Other research has focused on whether interventions that target psychological disorders result in reductions in suicidal behavior. To date, no published RCTs have shown that such interventions result in significant reductions in suicide attempts or death by suicide (Linehan, 2008). The only treatment ever shown to decrease suicide is the caring letters intervention designed by Motto (1976; Motto & Bostrom, 2001). RCTs are sorely needed to evaluate whether interventions are effective in reducing suicide deaths. The field will also greatly benefit from more research on the combination of psychotherapy and pharmacological interventions (Mann et al., 2005), as well as the comprehensive and longitudinal tracking of suicide risk factors.

Implications for Military Service and Integration into the Civilian Community

As is evident, suicidality is a particularly difficult challenge in the military environment. The military mental health professional needs to be concerned not only about individual safety and performance but also about the larger issue of unit safety and level of functioning. In a combat environment, this issue takes on proportionally more significance, with lives literally in the balance. When suicidality emerges in a military setting, almost immediately the clinician will need to address questions about deployment status, separation from service (and integration into civilian life), performance and safety at the individual and unit levels, and potential risks of repeated exposure to a combat environment.

There is limited but compelling scientific evidence to help answer a few of these questions, though certainly not all of them. Available evidence clearly and convincingly indicates that an individual with a history of multiple suicide attempts most likely will not be able to function effectively in a military environment, particularly in a combat setting (Rudd, Joiner & Rajab, 1996). There are now multiple convergent studies, from adolescence through old age, indicating that multiple-attempt status translates to chronic problems in day-to-day functioning, including dramatically elevated symptoms, greater Axis I and II comorbidity, impaired coping, and markedly greater risk for subsequent suicide attempts and related self-harm acts. It is important to remember that multiple attempters are defined as having made two or more genuine suicide attempts with evidence at the time of the behavior that the intent was to die. The implication for those in a military setting is straightforward; multiple attempters need to be separated from active service.

As is apparent when discussing multiple attempters, some individuals do not reveal their suicidal history when entering the service. However, at the time of the first attempt the history is often revealed, meaning that at the time of the first suicide attempt the military clinician may well find her- or himself having to make a decision about discharge. This situation is routinely coupled with a history of previous trauma, sometimes compounded by combat exposure. The issues of both severity and chronicity of disturbance among multiple attempters should not be underestimated, particularly given concerns about not only individual but also unit safety. The military environment is an inherently stressful one. During a combat deployment the stress level may be magnified many times and compounded by separation from friends and family, among a host of other stressors. Those with a previous history of trauma and suicide attempts are extremely vulnerable in a combat environment.

Although the data regarding chronic disturbance in multiple attempters are straightforward, the implications of suicidal ideation and single-attempt status are more complicated. It is important for the military clinician to keep in mind that under periods of acute stress, nonspecific fleeting suicidal thoughts carry limited risk. Risk elevates in parallel fashion with symptom intensity and complexity, along with the emergence of intent. It is critical to think about both subjective intent (what a patient says) and objective intent (what a patient does, e.g., preparation and rehearsal behaviors). In a combat setting, rapid clinical response to the emergence of fleeting, nonspecific suicidal thinking with no intent can have dramatic impact. It is most likely to occur in response to acute trauma in combat. Providing a contextual understanding to service members, particularly with respect to grieving a personal loss, can prove critical to improved coping and can facilitate a quicker recovery. Deployment is not possible when active intent emerges, regardless of whether it is subjective or objective in nature. In a combat environment service members should be referred for acute care during periods of active suicidality, keeping in mind the high concordance between suicidality and trauma mentioned previously. There certainly are occasions in which a quick response in getting a service member to immediate care allows him or her to be retained in a combat zone (i.e., if there is no prior history of suicidality and no index attempt).

Suicide attempts with lethality in a combat environment likely require evacuation and targeted care. It is important to remember, though, that an individual's response to treatment for single attempters can be effective and enduring, allowing the service members to be retained on active service even if not in a combat environment. The scientific data for single attempters are by no means definitive. There simply are not enough follow-up data to indicate whether continued service in a garrison environment is the best move. Each case needs to be evaluated and tracked individually. There is considerable variability in treatment response with single attempters, with good evidence of treatment effects for cognitive-behavioral therapy (Wenzel, Brown,

& Beck, 2009) and enough evidence to indicate that some single attempters will recover good day-to-day functioning.

When separating a service member from the service, it is critical to recognize that the transition out of the service can be a potentially overwhelming one, even if it is readily embraced by the service member. The military clinician needs to be aware that long-standing identity issues revolving around themes of worthlessness, shame, and guilt are often triggered by the separation process. The transition can be eased if clinical care is available while the service member is still on active duty and also if plans for ongoing care after separation are in place. This often involves familiarizing the service member with resources available from the Department of Veterans Affairs (VA) and/or the local community. It is recommended that the military clinician identify a concrete (and written) transition plan for every service member discharged from active service, incorporating the following elements: (1) a safety and crisis response plan if suicidality should reemerge, (2) VA services available in the local community, (3) targeted referral either through the VA system or the local community.

Conclusion

In this chapter we have provided guidelines for managing suicidal ideation in service members based on theory, the accumulation of clinical knowledge, and the most current findings in the empirical literature. Proper management of suicidal ideation in service members requires judicious symptom evaluation and monitoring, assessment across multiple domains of functioning, knowledge of general and military specific risk factors, and a clear understanding of best practices for responding to a crisis. Given that suicide attempts may in some cases swiftly follow suicidal thoughts (Kessler et al., 1999), the importance of prudent clinical management of suicidal ideation cannot be overstated. We have noted that PTSD may elevate suicide risk. Although there are a number of factors that may increase suicide risk, service members diagnosed with PTSD may require particular attention.

Clearly, much work is needed to more fully comprehend suicide risk among U.S. service members. Some risk may be unique to the military, as we have shown. As more research is conducted on this topic, new findings will supplement the guidelines presented here. It is self-evident that suicide is a highly idiosyncratic act that is extremely difficult to predict; thus it is critical that clinicians regard all indications of possible suicide thinking with the utmost degree of seriousness and attention. Early identification and management of suicidal ideation is crucial to saving lives.

References

Allen, J. P., Cross, G., & Swanner, J. (2005). Suicide in the Army: A review of current information. *Military Medicine, 170,* 580–584.

American Psychological Association. (2003). *Practice guidelines for the assessment and treatment of patients with suicidal behavior.* Washington, DC: Author.

Barnett, J. E., & Porter, J. E. (1998). The suicidal patient: Clinical, ethical, and risk management strategies. In L. VandeCreek, S. Knapp, & T. Jackson (Eds.), *Innovations in clinical practice* (pp. 95–107). Sarasota, FL: Professional Resource Press.

Bernert, R. A., Joiner, T. E., Cukrowicz, K. C., Schmidt, N. B., & Krakow, B. (2005). Suicidality and sleep disturbances. *Sleep, 28,* 1135–1141.

Brown, G., Ten Have, T., Henriques, G., Nie, S., Hollander, J., & Beck, A. (2005). Cognitive therapy for the prevention of suicide attempts: A randomized controlled trial. *Journal of the American Medical Association, 294,* 563–570.

Bryan, C. J., & Rudd, M. D. (2006). Advances in the assessment of suicide risk. *Journal of Clinical Psychology, 62*(2), 185–200.

Bullman, T. A., & Kang, H. K. (1996). The risk of suicide among wounded Vietnam veterans. *American Journal of Public Health, 86,* 662–667.

Cukrowicz, K. C., Wingate, L. R., Driscoll, K. A., & Joiner, T. E. (2004). A standard of care for the assessment of suicide risk and associated treatment: The Florida State University Psychology Clinic as an example. *Journal of Contemporary Psychotherapy, 34,* 87–99.

Driscoll, K. A., Cukrowicz, D. C., Reardon, M. L., & Joiner, T. E., Jr. (2004). *Simple treatment for complex problems: A flexible cognitive behavior analysis system approach to psychotherapy.* Mahwah, NJ: Erlbaum.

Fontana, A., & Rosenheck, R. (1994). Traumatic war stressors and psychiatric symptoms among World War II, Korean, and Vietnam War veterans. *Psychological Aging, 9,* 27–33.

Greene-Shortridge, T. M., Britt, T. W., & Castro, C. A. (2007). The stigma of mental health problems in the military. *Military Medicine, 172,* 157–161.

Hoge, C. W., Castro, C. A., Messer, S. C., McGurk, D., Cotting, D. I., & Koffman, R. L. (2004). Combat duty in Iraq and Afghanistan, mental health problems, and barriers to care. *New England Journal of Medicine, 351,* 13–22.

Jakupcak, M., Cook, J., Imel, Z., Fontana, A., Rosenheck, R., & McFall, M. (2009). Posttraumatic stress disorder as a risk factor for suicidal ideation in Iraq and Afghanistan war veterans. *Journal of Traumatic Stress, 22,* 303–306.

Jobes, D. A. (2006). *Managing suicidal risk: A collaborative approach.* New York: Guilford Press.

Jobes, D. A. (2009). The CAMS approach to suicide risk: Philosophy and clinical procedures. *Suicidology, 14,* 3–7.

Jobes, D. A., Rudd, M. D., Overholser, J. C., & Joiner, T. E. (2008). Ethical and competent care of suicidal patients: Contemporary challenges, new developments, and considerations for clinical practice. *Professional Psycology: Research and Practice, 39,* 405–413.

Joiner, T. E. (2005). *Why people die by suicide*. Cambridge, MA: Harvard University Press.

Joiner, T. E., Walker, R. L., Rudd, M. D., & Jobes, D. A. (1999). Scientizing and routinizing the assessment of suicidality in outpatient practice. *Professional Psychology, Research, and Practice, 30*, 447–453.

Kang, H. K., & Bullman, T. A. (2009). Is there an epidemic of suicides among current and former U. S. military personnel? *Annals of Epidemiology, 19*, 757–760.

Kessler, R. C. (2000). Posttraumatic stress disorder: The burden to the individual and to society. *Journal of Clinical Psychiatry, 61*(Suppl. 5), 4–12.

Kessler, R. C., Borges, G., & Walters, E. E. (1999). Prevalence of and risk factors for lifetime suicide attempts in the National Comorbidity Survey. *Archives of General Psychiatry, 56*, 617–625.

Kleespies, P. M., Deleppo, J. D., Gallagher, P. L., & Niles, B. L. (1999). Managing suicidal emergencies: Recommendations for the practitioner. *Professional Psychology, Research, and Practice, 30*, 454–463.

Koren, D., Norman, D., Cohen, A., Berman, J., & Klein, E. M. (2005). Increased PTSD risk with combat-related injury: A matched comparison study of injured and uninjured soldiers experiencing the same combat events. *American Journal of Psychiatry, 162*(2), 276–282.

Linehan, M., Comtois, K., Murray, A., Brown, M., Gallup, R., Heard, H., et al. (2006). Two-year randomized controlled trial and follow-up of dialectical behavior therapy vs. therapy by experts for suicidal behaviors and borderline personality disorder. *Archives of General Psychiatry, 63*, 757–766.

Linehan, M. M. (2008). Suicide intervention research: A field in desperate need of development. *Suicide and Life-Threatening Behavior, 38*, 483–485.

Luxton, D. D., Skopp, N. A., Kinn, J., Bush, N. E., Reger, M. A., & Gahm, G. A. (2010). DoD Suicide Event Report: Calendar year 2009 annual report. National Center for Telehealth & Technology, Defense Centers of Excellence for Psychological Health and Traumatic Brain Injury, Joint Base Lewis-McChord, WA.

Mahon, M. J., Tobin, J. P., Cusack, D. A., Kelleher, C., & Malone, K. M. (2005). Suicide among regular-duty military personnel: A retrospective case-control study of occupation-specific risk factors for workplace suicide. *American Journal of Psychiatry, 162*, 1688–1696.

Mann, J. J., Apter, A., Bertolote, J., Beautrais, A., Currier, D., Haas, A., et al. (2005) Suicide prevention strategies: A systematic review. Journal of the American Medical Association, 294, 2064–2074.

Motto, J. A. (1976). Suicide prevention for high-risk persons who refuse treatment. *Suicide and Life-Threatening Behavior, 6*(4), 223–230.

Motto, J. A., & Bostrom, A. G. (2001). A randomized controlled trial of postcrisis suicide prevention. *Psychiatric Services, 52*(6), 828–833.

Nock, M. K., Hwang, I., Sampson, N., Kessler, R. C., Angermeyer, M., Beautrais, A., et al. (2009). Cross-sectional prevalence and risk factors for suicidal ideation, plans, and attempts. *British Journal of Psychiatry, 192*, 98–105.

Nye, E. C., & Bell, J. B. (2007). Specific symptoms predict suicidal ideation in Vietnam combat veterans with chronic posttraumatic stress disorder. *Military Medicine, 172*, 1144–1147.

O'Carroll, P., Berman, A., Maris, R., Moscicki, E., Tanney, B., & Silverman, M. (1996). Beyond the Tower of Babel: A nomenclature of suicidology. *Suicide and Life-Threatening Behaviour, 26,* 237–252.

Oldham, J. (2008). PTSD and suicide. *Journal of Psychiatric Practice, 14,* 195.

Panagioti, M., Gooding, P., & Tarrier, N. (2009). Posttraumatic stress disorder and suicidal behavior: A narrative review. *Clinical Psychology Review, 29,* 471–482.

Rudd, D. M., Joiner, T. E., Jobes, D. A., & King, C. A. (1999). The outpatient treatment of suicidality: An integration of science and recognition of its limitations. *Professional Psychology: Research and Practice, 30,* 437–446.

Rudd, M. D., Joiner, T., & Rajab, M. H. (1996). Relationships among suicide ideators, attempters, and multiple attempters in a young-adult sample. *Journal of Abnormal Psychology, 105*(4), 541–550.

Rudd, M. D., Joiner, T., & Rajab, M. H. (2001). *Treating suicidal behavior: An effective, time-limited approach.* New York: Guilford Press.

Selby, E. A., Anestis, M. D., Bender, T. W., Ribeiro, J. D., Nock, M. K., Rudd, M. D., et al. (2010). Overcoming the fear of lethal injury: Evaluating suicidal behavior in the military through the lens of the interpersonal-psychological theory of suicide. *Clinical Psychology Review, 30,* 298–307.

Slee, N., Garnefski, N., van der Leeden, R., Arensman, E., & Spinhoven, P. (2008). Cognitive-behavioural intervention for self-harm: Randomised controlled trial. *British Journal of Psychiatry, 192,* 202–211.

Sommers-Flanagan, J., & Sommers-Flanagan, R. (1995). Intake interviewing with suicidal patients: A systematic approach. *Professional Psychology: Research and Practice, 26,* 41–47.

Stellrecht, N. E., Gordon, K. H., Van Orden, K., Witte, T. K., Wingate, L. R., Cukrowicz, K. C., et al. (2006). Clinical applications of the interpersonal–psychological theory of attempted and completed suicide. *Journal of Clinical Psychology, 62,* 211–222.

Wenzel, A., Beren, G. K., & Beck, A. T. (2009). *Cognitive therapy for suicidal patients: Scientific and clinical applications.* Washington, DC: American Psychological Association.

CHAPTER 18

Anger, Aggression, and Violence

Eric B. Elbogen
Sally C. Johnson
Jean C. Beckham

Anger and aggression are serious problems reported by veterans returning home from combat and are common concerns among those seeking treatment for posttraumatic stress disorder (PTSD). Empirical research demonstrates that a current diagnosis of PTSD is significantly associated with elevated anger and aggression in veterans (Begic & Jokic-Begic, 2001; Carlson, Lauderdale, Hawkins, & Sheikh, 2008; Hartl, Rosen, Drescher, Lee, & Gusman, 2005; Jakupcak et al., 2007; Kulka et al., 1990; Lasko et al., 1994; McFall, Fontana, Raskind, & Rosenheck, 1999). Difficulty managing anger is not only associated with violence perpetration itself (Taft, Street, Marshall, Dowdall, & Riggs, 2007) but is also linked to increased stress (Taylor et al., 2009), low self-esteem (Pekala, Kumar, Maurer, Elliott-Carter, & Moon, 2009), elevated heart rate and blood pressure (Vrana, Hughes, Dennis, Calhoun, & Beckham, 2009), coronary heart disease (Kubzansky, Cole, Kawachi, Vokonas, & Sparrow, 2006), and family and relationship conflict (Murphy, Taft, & Eckhardt, 2007). Anger itself is a PTSD hyperarousal symptom, and recent meta-analyses suggest that effect sizes between PTSD and anger are even larger among samples of veterans with military combat experience compared with samples of civilians who had experienced other types of traumatic events (Orth & Wieland, 2006). Anger experienced by veterans with PTSD is a robust predictor of poorer PTSD treatment efficacy, as well as increased rate of dropout (Forbes et al., 2008). Empirical studies are now reporting aggression as a significant problem in up to one-third of Iraq and Afghanistan War veterans (Jakupcak et al., 2007; Killgore et al., 2008; Sayer et al, 2010; Teten et al., 2010; Thomas et al., 2010). For these reasons, the assessment and treatment of anger and aggression constitute a central component of PTSD treatment among military veterans.

Review of the Literature on Anger, Aggression, and Violence in Military Personnel with PTSD

A review of the literature from 1970 to 2005 in military populations found that prevalence rates of domestic violence (in which the target of violence is an intimate partner) ranged from 13.5% to 58% (Marshall, Panuzio, & Taft, 2005), with higher rates for samples selected on the basis of psychopathology, especially PTSD. Using data from the National Vietnam Veterans Readjustment Study, researchers found that the mean number of acts of family violence committed in the previous year by male combat veterans with PTSD was 4.86, compared with only 1.32 among those male combat veterans without PTSD (Jordan et al., 1992). The link between PTSD and domestic violence seems to be sustained even when accounting for predeployment adjustment and combat experience (Carroll, Rueger, Foy, & Donahoe, 1985). Further, more severe PTSD symptoms are related to a higher frequency of domestic violence (Orcutt, King, & King, 2003). A recent paper confirms that intimate partner violence remains a troubling problem for people diagnosed with PTSD, particularly male veterans (Bell & Orcutt, 2009).

Similar prevalence rates and risk factors have been documented among veterans committing general—as opposed to targeted interpersonal—aggressive acts, as well (Beckham, Moore, & Reynolds, 2000; McFall et al., 1999; Taft, Vogt, Marshall, Panuzio, & Niles, 2007). PTSD among veterans is related to higher incidence of violence, violent thoughts, anger/hostility, and ownership of deadly weapons (Begic & Jokic-Begic, 2001; Carlson et al., 2008; Freeman & Roca, 2001; Hartl et al., 2005; Jakupcak et al., 2007; Lasko et al., 1994; Taft, Vogt, et al., 2007). McFall et al. (1999) found that veterans with PTSD were more likely to destroy property, threaten others without a weapon, become involved in physical fighting, and make violent threats with a weapon than veterans without PTSD. Another study found that veterans with PTSD reported 13–22 acts of interpersonal violence in the preceding year in contrast to 0–3 violent acts among veterans without PTSD (Beckham, Feldman, Kirby, Hertzberg, & Moore, 1997). A recent study of Iraq and Afghanistan veterans showed that 53.2% of those meeting the criteria for PTSD and 52.4% of those with subthreshold PTSD reported at least one act of violence in the preceding 4 months, compared with only 20.3% of those without PTSD (Jakupcak et al., 2007).

It is important to note that the link between PTSD and anger/aggression may be due to the association of PTSD with other factors, such as depression (O'Donnell, Cook, Thompson, Riley, & Neria, 2006; Taft et al., 2005), lack of communication (Carroll et al., 1985), alcohol or drug abuse and dependence, poor marital adjustment, exposure to high levels of atrocities (Taft et al., 2005), and heightened anger reactivity (Taft, Street, et al., 2007). Moreover, certain PTSD symptoms have been shown to be stronger predictors of violent behavior than others; hyperarousal symptoms of PTSD have specifically been related to increased aggression in several analyses (McFall et al., 1999), and aggression itself appears to be exacerbated by alcohol problems (Savarese, Suvak, King, & King, 2001; Taft, Kaloupek, et al., 2007). As a result, there exist a number of clinical and environmental factors that might moderate the relationship between PTSD and anger/aggression that would be critical to consider in the context of clinical care of veterans.

Assessment

For assessment purposes, anger and aggression can be defined by a number of attributes. The attributes of anger include *control* (the extent to which an individual attempts to control outward expression of anger), *expression* (which involves the overt expression of anger toward others), *situation* (indicating high-risk circumstances), or *symptoms* (such as physiological arousal; Saini, 2009). There is also a distinction to make between *state anger* (emotional response to perceived injustice) and *trait anger* (stable pattern of behavior) (Novaco & Chemtob, 2002). Similarly, aggression varies in terms of *frequency, severity, victims, use of weapons,* and *circumstances* in which an individual is at highest risk (Monahan & Steadman, 1994). Scholars also discern between *instrumental* (premeditated and thought out in advance) and *reactive* (impulsive and generally unplanned) violence (Cornell et al., 1996). Each of these categories should be considered by clinicians when attempting to best clarify specifics of anger and aggression problems veterans may present with in treatment.

In terms of formal assessment tools, several have been developed to measure anger in veterans. In the *Iraq War Clinician Guide*, Taft and Niles (2004) review self-report questionnaires for anger and hostility that have demonstrated solid psychometric properties: the Buss–Durkee Hostility Inventory (BDHI) and the State–Trait Anger Expression Inventory (STAXI). The BDHI in its revised form (Aggression Questionaire; Buss & Perry, 1992) has 29 items rated on 5-point Likert scales measuring anger, hostility, verbal aggression, and physical aggression. The STAXI is a more refined instrument for assessment of anger, distinguishing state anger from trait anger as well as the experience of anger from the expression of anger (Castillo, C'De

Baca, Conforti, Qualls, & Fallon, 2002). A more recently developed anger measure for veterans is the Dimension of Angry Reactions (DAR) scale, which is a five-item self-report scale consisting of different facets of anger and hostility (Hawthorne, Mouthaan, Forbes, & Novaco, 2006). Results show the DAR to be unidimensional, reliable, and sensitive to change over time and to have convergent validity with other measures of trait anger (Forbes et al., 2004). Although not captured in these instruments, other factors to assess associated with anger and hostility in veterans include several medical issues, such as headaches (Arena, Bruno, Rozantine, & Meador, 1997), chronic pain (Lombardo, Tan, Jensen, & Anderson, 2005), and sleep problems (Robert et al., 2005).

To our knowledge, there are no formal assessment instruments for aggression and violence among veterans. Research shows that, without such tools clinicians perform only modestly better than chance in assessing risk of violence, a finding replicated in civilian (Mossman, 1994) and veteran (Werner, Rose, Yesavage, & Seeman, 1984) populations. A number of excellent risk assessment tools have been developed over the past decade, including the Violence Risk Appraisal Guide (VRAG; Quinsey, Harris, Rice, & Cormier, 2006), HCR-20 (Douglas, Ogloff, Nicholls, & Grant, 1999; Douglas & Webster, 1999), and Classification of Violence Risk (COVR; Monahan et al., 2005; Snowden, Gray, Taylor, & Fitzgerald, 2009; Steadman et al., 2000). Although these tools have not been validated specifically for veterans, they certainly can be used with the understanding that additional veteran-specific characteristics may need to be considered. Until such screens are developed and validated, it is recommended that clinicians at least be guided by risk factors that have some empirical support (Elbogen et al., 2010).

Research indicates that there are likely other risk factors besides PTSD to consider when assessing anger and aggression in veterans (see Table 18.1). Research in veteran populations has linked anger/aggression to younger age (Fonseca et al., 2006; Forgey & Badger, 2006; McCarroll et al., 1999; McCarroll et al., 2000; McCarroll et al., 2003; Petrik, Rosenberg, & Watson, 1983; Rumm, Cummings, Krauss, Bell, & Rivara, 2000), history of (non-military-related) violence (Begic & Jokic-Begic, 2001; Gondolf & Foster, 1991; Hartl et al., 2005; Yesavage, 1984), combat exposure (Beckham et al., 1997; Gimbel & Booth, 1994; Killgore et al., 2008; Orcutt et al., 2003; Prigerson, Maciejewski, & Rosenheck, 2002), history of childhood abuse or maltreatment (Begic & Jokic-Begic, 2001; Merrill, Hervig, & Milner, 1996; Rosen, Kaminski, Parmley, Knudson, & Fancher, 2003), depressive symptoms (Hartl et al., 2005; Sherman, Sautter, Jackson, Lyons, & Han, 2006; Taft et al., 2005; Teten, Schumacher, Bailey, & Kent, 2009; Taft, Vogt, et al., 2007; Windle & Windle, 1995) and financial status (e.g., being unemployed or having lower income) (Beckham et al., 1997; Begic & Jokic-Begic, 2001; Forgey & Badger, 2006; McCarroll et al., 2003).

TABLE 18.1. Checklist for Treating Anger[a] and Aggression[b] in Veterans with PTSD

Risk factors to consider for assessment	Components to consider for treatment
• Younger age (below 40 years of age)	• Psychoeducation on effects of anger
• History of (nonmilitary) violence	• Medical examination (sleep, pain)
• History of child maltreatment	• Pharmacological intervention
• Combat exposure	• Increasing adherence to medications
• PTSD symptom severity	• Self-monitoring with anger log
• Depressive symptoms	• Relaxation techniques
• Substance abuse	• Substance abuse treatment
• Traumatic brain injury	• Cognitive restructuring
• Financial status	• Referral to domestic violence program

Note. Although more empirical research on risk factors and treatment components is needed to show links with anger and aggression among veterans with PTSD, this list reflects the current state of science and what it recommends clinicians should consider when encountering veterans with PTSD presenting with anger or aggression problems. These risk factors and treatment components should be applied to and tailored for the individual veteran.

[a]Anger can be conceptualized as including the elements of *control* (the extent to which an individual attempts to control outward expression of anger), *expression* (which involves the overt expression of anger toward others), *situation* (indicating high-risk circumstances), or *symptoms* (such as physiological arousal). Clinicians can also make a distinction between *state anger* (emotional response to perceived injustice) and *trait anger* (stable pattern of behavior).

[a]Aggression varies in terms of *frequency, severity, victims, use of weapons,* and *circumstances* in which an individual is at highest risk. Clinicians can additionally discern between *instrumental* (premeditated and thought out in advance) and *reactive* (impulsive and generally unplanned) violence.

Of note, substance abuse is an especially important factor to consider when evaluating risk of violent and aggressive behavior in veterans, particularly those with PTSD (Elbogen, Beckham, Butterfield, Swartz, & Swanson, 2008; Fonseca et al., 2006; Ganzini, Edwards, Surkan, & Drummond, 1995; Jakupcak et al., 2007; McFall et al., 1999; Moss, 1989; Teten et al., 2009). To illustrate the relationships between PTSD, substance abuse, and aggression, one study showed that higher quantity drinking behavior has been related to intimate partner violence in its own right but, combined with the PTSD hyperarousal symptoms, frequent, low-quantity alcohol use may actually lower the veteran's risk of violence (Savarese et al., 2001). Clinical assessment, therefore, should involve examination of different levels of abuse of and dependence on different kinds of substances and how they may interact in ways with different types of PTSD symptoms among veterans. Ongoing assessment for alcohol and drug abuse is thus an important adjunct to treatment of anger and aggression among Veterans with PTSD.

A final assessment issue is related to the overlap of PTSD with traumatic brain injury (TBI). It is estimated that a substantial number of Iraq and

Afghanistan military service members will return from service with combat-related TBI (Hoge, McGurk, Thomas, Cox, Engel, & Castro, 2008).
Research indicates that TBI and PTSD are each associated with cognitive
deficits, including deficits in attention, executive function, and affective and
cognitive control (Vasterling et al., 2006). However, cognitive and affective
sequelae associated with PTSD symptoms are compounded by the presence
of TBI (Nelson, Yoash-Gantz, Pickett, & Campbell, 2009). In particular, it
has been shown that significant frontal lobe dysfunction, particularly disin-
hibition, occurs more often among veterans with both TBI and PTSD than
among Veterans diagnosed with only one of these conditions (Campbell et
al., 2009). Research has suggested that veterans with lesions in their frontal
lobes exhibit more aggression and violence, especially if the lesions are in the
mediofrontal or orbitofrontal regions (Grafman, Schwab, Warden, & Pridgen, 1996). The combination of TBI and PTSD has been linked to increased
risk of violence in military veterans (Elbogen et al., 2008). For these reasons,
examining the roles of TBI, executive dysfunction, and aggression may be
warranted in the context of PTSD treatment for veterans.

Treatment Approaches

There have been a number of reviews of anger management techniques in
civilian populations, most indicating that no one approach is ideal for treating all aspects of anger (Edmondson & Conger, 1996). A comprehensive
literature review (Del Vecchio & O'Leary, 2004) found (1) medium to large
effect sizes across different modalities of counseling and therapy for reducing anger problems; (2) that cognitive-behavioral therapy (CBT) is best for
anger suppression and anger traits; and (3) that relaxation was most effective in reducing state anger. These findings were recently replicated in meta-
analysis of 96 studies and 139 treatment effects for psychological treatment
of anger (Saini, 2009). It is important to note that this literature has been
critiqued on the grounds that CBT techniques may appear to be most effective not because they are most effective but because they are most studied;
other modalities, such as psychodynamic psychotherapy, psychoeducation,
and substance abuse counseling, have largely been unexamined empirically,
and thus little is known about the overall contribution of these approaches
to the reduction of anger in this population (Glancy & Saini, 2005).

Indeed, the majority of empirical research with respect to treatment of
anger and aggression in veterans with PTSD has involved CBT approaches
(Cahill, Rauch, Hembree, Foa, & Taylor, 2004; Chemtob, Novaco, Hamada,
& Gross, 1997; Gerlock, 1994). Gerlock (1994) was one of the first to report
on the effectiveness of a cognitive-behavioral anger management intervention
for veterans, most of whom had been diagnosed with PTSD. This 8-week

anger management intervention used a cognitive-behavioral approach in a class format that included didactic segments on the following topics: (1) physiological, behavioral, and cognitive cues to the anger response, (2) early learning experiences of anger, (3) anger triggers, (4) what makes one vulnerable to anger, (5) short-term anger payoffs versus long-term consequences, and (6) steps to stop abusive anger problems. In between these sessions the veterans would journal in an anger log about anger-inducing situations. The authors found that, whereas most veterans improved, those with past psychological trauma from childhood showed less improvement; thus, the research showed that CBT techniques reduced anger problems for veterans with PTSD but identified moderators of these effects.

To our knowledge, there has been only one randomized trial of CBT specifically aimed at reducing anger among veterans with PTSD (Chemtob et al., 1997). Treatment involved the following components: (1) self-monitoring anger frequency, intensity, and situational triggers; (2) devising a personal anger provocation hierarchy based on self-monitoring; (3) progressive muscle relaxation, breathing-focused relaxation, and guided imagery training to regulate physiological arousal; (4) cognitive restructuring of anger by altering attentional focus, modifying appraisals, and using self-instruction; (5) training in behavioral coping and assertiveness skills; (6) practicing new anger coping skills while visualizing; and (7) role-playing progressively more intense anger arousing scenes from personal hierarchies. The authors found significantly reduced anger scores specifically in the domains of state anger and the ability to control anger, attesting to the therapeutic benefits of using a structured format to address a range of cognitive, behavioral, and affective aspects of anger in veterans with PTSD. However, there was a high exclusion and high dropout rate, suggesting that results did not potentially generalize to most veterans with PTSD.

Other research has involved tailoring CBT techniques to address anger in veterans with PTSD. One approach has been to change the mode of delivery; namely, providing treatment with computer-based technology instead of in a traditional counseling or group format. Specifically, one study helped train veterans in stress inoculation techniques for coping with maladaptive anger using an electronic computer guidance approach (Timmons, Oehlert, Sumerall, & Timmons, 1997). When this was compared with group counseling for stress inoculation, there were no differences in self-reported state anger, trait anger, and anger suppression among veterans. Of note, both computer and group treatment groups endorsed the same level of treatment satisfaction. Another approach has been to tailor CBT for subgroups of veterans with PTSD. To illustrate, one 11-week group-based cognitive behavioral therapy was adapted to veterans with PTSD and schizophrenia or schizoaffective disorder and focused on education, anxiety management therapy, social skills training, and exposure therapy (Frueh et al., 2009).

The researchers found that this format of CBT led to significant improvement in anger control, as well as treatment satisfaction. Finally, a recent randomized trial of anger management for veterans with PTSD found that CBT was as effective in-person as it was via videoteleconferencing for reducing PTSD-related anger problems (Morland et al., 2010).

Although anger has been examined as an outcome in treatment studies, there has been relatively little work devoted to interventions to reduce aggression and violence among veterans with PTSD. One study enrolling veterans with PTSD did measure violence as an outcome measure, examining the role of pretreatment interpersonal relationship functioning in two forms of group CBT (Monson, Rodriguez, & Warner, 2005). Analysis of veterans who completed trauma- or skills-focused CBT showed no overall differences in PTSD symptomatology, alcohol abuse, or violence perpetration at 4 months posttreatment; however, it was found that, for those in the trauma-focused group only, veterans with better pretreatment relationships reported reduced posttreatment violence. As such, the findings suggest that CBT approaches can reduce actual aggression and violence, with the caveat that certain risk and protective factors might moderate outcomes.

Despite some promising initial findings on the effectiveness of CBT approaches in reducing anger and aggression among veterans of PTSD, researchers and clinicians generally agree that there is no current consensus about the best way to treat angry clients (Glancy & Saini, 2005). Still, there is some agreement on components of effective treatment that should, at a minimum, be considered for veterans with PTSD presenting with postdeployment anger and/or aggression problems (see Table 18.1). First, it is important to consider the use of pharmacological interventions (Glancy & Saini, 2005) since these would address psychopathology—especially PTSD and depression—potentially related to anger or aggression in veterans; for example, it has been shown that, by improving sleep disturbances, quetiapine reduced state anger among combat veterans with PTSD (Robert et al., 2005). Second, there are several ways to structure anger treatment for veterans, and the *Iraq War Clinician Guide* recommends including: (1) an overview of the treatment, (2) setting treatment goals and exploring motivation, (3) psychoeducation on anger and PTSD, (4) some type of self-monitoring, (5) assertiveness training, (6) stress management, and (7) communication skills training (Taft & Niles, 2004). Third, the *Veterans and Active Duty Military Psychotherapy Progress Notes Planner* lists additional components for treating veterans with respect to anger management and domestic violence, including: (1) referring a veteran to a domestic violence program; (2) developing a coping card to list strategies, as well as high-risk situations; (3) monitoring medication adherence; (4) referring a veteran for physical examination; and (5) educating the veteran about the impact of anger on his or her body, including heart, brain, and blood pressure (Berghuis & Jongsma,

2010). Overall, the aforementioned components might each be helpful when treating a Veteran with PTSD for anger and aggression, even though it should be noted that more research and empirical support is warranted.

Limitations of Treatment Strategies and Gaps in Research

As can be seen from the preceding review, significant gaps exist in the scientific literature on treatment of anger and aggressiveness among veterans with PTSD. Most empirical research to date has involved Vietnam veterans who were interviewed often decades after service. Even then, only a handful of studies examined anger and aggression in Vietnam veterans in the 1970s (Mikolajczak & Hagen, 1978) and 1980s (Yesavage, 1984). Most were conducted in the 1990s, over 20 years after the Vietnam War ended. The degree to which we can generalize from these studies to the situations of newly returned Iraq and Afghanistan veterans, whose exposure to combat is far more recent, is unknown. Another limitation is that almost every subject in the Vietnam veteran studies is male; however, there are a substantial number of women in the military in the current war on terror who are at risk for PTSD and other factors that might elevate their risk of perpetrating intimate partner violence or general aggression or violence (Owens, Herrera, & Whitesell, 2009). Finally, differences between the draft in the Vietnam War and the voluntary enrollment in the military for Iraq and Afghanistan suggest that the two cohorts are not entirely comparable with respect to predeployment demographic variables that might affect postdeployment anger and aggression.

A second limitation in generalizing from extant research regards the criterion measures used in previous studies. Virtually all the research on risk factors for anger and aggressiveness among veterans is retrospective, correlating past behavior with demographic, clinical, and military service variables. To our knowledge, there have been no studies of veterans that seek to predict hostile and aggressive behaviors prospectively using a longitudinal design. Additionally, to our knowledge, most published studies on veterans and aggressiveness rely solely on self-report. A few studies measure anger and aggression from the veteran and a family member (Beckham et al., 1997; Calhoun et al., 2002; Glenn et al., 2002; Jordan et al., 1992; Panuzio et al., 2006), and no study that we know of has used violence measures obtained from three or more sources. Gathering data from multiple sources is particularly important in this area of scholarship, as social disapproval may lead sources to underreport anger and aggression (Calhoun et al., 2002; Mulvey & Lidz, 1993).

Finally, the literature on risk factors among veterans remains largely disconnected from research on risk reduction. For example, studies on the link between substance abuse and violence committed by veterans are largely ignored in anger treatment or violence prevention efforts. The role of TBI and cognitive rehabilitation will also need to be examined. There have also been no studies examining whether heath services utilization or treatment engagement reduce veterans' violence risk (e.g., does adherence to PTSD treatment reduce risk of posttreatment anger or aggression?). Moreover, the extant literature does not employ an overall methodological framework to link risk factors with risk reduction strategies. Most published research on these interventions has enrolled small sample sizes and involved open trials of interventions examining pre–post data; few have used a randomized design. To our knowledge, only one study has specifically looked at reducing aggression or violence among veterans with PTSD (Monson et al., 2005). Significantly more research is needed to develop evidence-based approaches to assessing and treating anger and aggression among veterans with PTSD.

Implications for Military Service and Integration into the Civilian Community

Although more needs to be learned, the review of the literature suggests several important practical steps for clinicians to take when encountering veterans with PTSD complaining of anger problems. If a veteran with PTSD presents with anger or aggression problems, clinicians should first address potential medical problems in order to rule out physical contributors to anger and aggression. A veteran's problem with sleep or chronic pain may be the most important factor exacerbating his or her anger and/or aggression. Identification of a medical problem with an available treatment intervention should mandate prompt attention to that issue. Similarly, given research showing that pharmacological agents can be effective at treating maladaptive anger (Glancy & Saini, 2005) and that some risk factors for aggression are treatable (e.g., depressive symptoms) by a pharmacological approach, a psychiatric evaluation, with a specific request for a psychopharmacological consultation, is recommended in the early stages of treatment.

Given the varying domains of anger and aggression and the myriad risk factors associated with each, results of this review strongly suggest defining anger in a specific context for each individual veteran and tailoring treatment accordingly. In particular, different sets of variables have been shown to be related to different types of anger in a study of Iraq and Afghanistan veterans (Elbogen et al., 2010), suggesting that clinicians should investigate specific factors such as the following to determine the risk of specific aggressive behaviors:

- A veteran's background involving *violence and aggression*—including whether he or she had experienced high levels of violence in the past (e.g., witnessing family violence) and more recently (e.g., firing a weapon, having a longer deployment in Iraq or Afghanistan)—was significantly related to increased odds of the veteran's reporting problems controlling violent behavior. Clinicians should investigate how past violence affects a veteran's ability to curb current violence.

- A veteran's endorsement of *psychopathology and trauma*—such as family mental illness or history of childhood abuse, as well as currently reexperiencing symptoms (potentially from working in a war zone)—was significantly related to increased odds of the veteran's reporting aggressive impulses or urges. Clinicians should investigate how (or whether) mental health issues are elevating cognitions and emotions related to aggressiveness and more severe anger.

- A veteran's *past and current relationships*—including whether he or she had a chaotic upbringing (e.g., history of parental incarceration), was currently married, or had severe PTSD avoidance symptoms—was significantly associated with the veteran's reporting increased odds of have difficulties managing anger. Clinicians should investigate aspects of the anger as related to relationship conflict, and in what ways a veteran might be expressing anger with his or her spouse, significant other, or family.

It is important to note that it was found that Cluster D hyperarousal symptoms (American Psychiatric Association, 1994) predicted all three types of behaviors just listed. For these reasons, rather than focusing only on PTSD as a diagnosis when assessing anger and aggression, the data indicate the need to focus on specific PTSD symptoms in the context of treatment. Examining links between aggression and specific hyperarousal symptoms may lead to different intervention avenues; for example, cognitive restructuring may be warranted if a veteran's anger is linked to vigilance, whereas increased self-monitoring may be indicated if a veteran's anger is related to difficulty concentrating. Either way, anger and aggression have been shown to be key moderators in the success of PTSD treatment among veterans. Even if a veteran does not present complaining of anger problems, it will still be important for clinicians to gather information about whether and how anger manifests itself in the veteran's life. Several tools exist and can be used to help clarify what kind of anger the veteran with PTSD might be experiencing; such information will ultimately be useful in any treatment of PTSD.

Clinicians should identify situations that contribute to anger and/or aggression, such as financial problems or unemployment. Issues such as whether a veteran is in deep financial debt, was recently laid off, is having difficulty finding a job to match his or her skills, or cannot afford basic needs such as housing, food, clothes, or medical care can contribute to stress, strain, and anger. In this vein, consideration of situational variables is important when veterans in treatment are deciding whether they wish to return to combat or separate from the military. If the veteran has PTSD and is struggling with anger or aggression, clinicians need to examine what factors are contributing to adjustment problems and whether these factors will resume when the veteran returns from combat. Distinct courses of action may be recommended, depending on whether or not the veteran is likely to continue having these problems when deployed. As such, an understanding of how a veteran's social context is exacerbating anger and aggression would be central in this decision-making process.

Specific situational factors have been shown in research to relate to domestic violence in particular and need to be reviewed. Poor marital adjustment (Rosen et al., 2003; Taft et al., 2005) and relationship problems (Byrne & Riggs, 1996) appear to be strong predictors of domestic violence in veterans and service members. Along these lines, effects of recent divorce should be examined in the course of treatment as well. Conversely, newer marriages have been found be more prone to violence (Wasileski, Callaghan-Chaffee, & Chaffee, 1982), especially marriages in which both partners were violent (Forgey & Badger, 2006). Having a child (Campbell et al., 2003; Rumm et al., 2000) or having larger families (three or more children; Campbell et al., 2003) seem also to be related to intimate partner violence among service members currently in active duty. Finally, if a veteran was recently separated from the military, current or recent living circumstances are relevant for assessing domestic violence; specifically, having lived off-post during service has been linked with higher likelihood of postdeployment domestic violence in one study (McCarroll et al., 2003).

After a clinician has (1) investigated medical contributors to anger and aggression, (2) defined these problems individually for a veteran, and (3) explored situational factors that may be contributing, then a plan can be developed to treat anger and aggression for an individual veteran with PTSD. Given that research is still in its infancy, there is no one known best approach to anger management among veterans with PTSD. Review of the literature shows that structured anger management therapies do help reduce anger and aggression among civilians and veterans with PTSD. The science generally attests to the fact that for a veteran with PTSD or experiencing anger problems, enrolling and engaging in treatment could help reduce those problems. Available evidence to date favors CBT over other treatments, but in general it is not clear whether group or individual counseling works best or whether non-cognitive-behavioral techniques are really less effective. What seems most clear is, given the multidimensional nature of anger, ultimately any structured anger treatment needs to accommodate the specific type of anger or aggressiveness experienced by the veteran with

PTSD. Regardless of treatment modality, the need to tailor anger treatments to the individual is crucial.

Review of the components found in effective anger management interventions in civilian populations (Saini, 2009) attests to the potential benefit of including these when treating anger in veteran populations, especially those with PTSD. First, some type of psychoeducation at the onset of treatment about anger and its impact on one's physical and mental health is warranted. Second, skills training is important; for example, if a veteran is having particular difficulty with affect regulation, then stress inoculation, relaxation techniques, and mindfulness training would seem to be in order. Third, having the veteran with PTSD begin to monitor his or her own behavior, collect data on what his or her triggers and high-risk situations are, and make daily logs or journals about success in controlling one's anger are also common exercises in effective anger management programs. Fourth, to the extent that other mental health conditions (e.g., substance abuse, depression, TBI) play a role in a veteran's anger and aggressiveness, this should be addressed in PTSD treatment. Fifth, meta-analyses show that most effective treatments are long term and consist of at least eight sessions of treatment, use manuals to guide treatment, and include fidelity checks to ensure consistency.

Conclusion

In sum, anger and aggression appear related to PTSD among veterans and will likely play a central role in clinical assessment and treatment. In studies enrolling veterans from previous wars, researchers have learned how to assess for anger using valid methods, what factors are empirically related to aggression and violence, and what kinds of cognitive-behavioral techniques seem promising for reducing anger and, by extension, possibly aggression. Despite the need for significantly more research using prospective designs or randomized clinical trials for new veterans returning from Iraq and Afghanistan, the extant research provides some basic guidance for clinicians who encounter veterans complaining of "anger" or "aggression" problems. Table 18.1 provides clinicians with an overview of risk factors and treatment components that are relevant to consider. Ruling out medical causes, identifying high-risk situations, defining anger and aggression for each individual veteran, providing psychoeducation about the effects of anger and its link to PTSD, teaching skills needed to relax and be mindful, encouraging self-monitoring of anger, and engaging veterans in long-term treatment all seem to be critical ingredients in helping veterans reduce postdeployment adjustment problems and in providing clinicians tools to best serve those who have served our country.

References

American Psychiatric Association. (1994). *Diagnostic and statistical manual of mental disorders* (4th ed.). Washington, DC: Author.

Arena, J. G., Bruno, G. M., Rozantine, G. S., & Meador, K. J. (1997). A comparison of tension headache sufferers and nonpain controls on the State–Trait Anger Expression Inventory: An exploratory study with implications for applied psychophysiologists. *Applied Psychophysiology and Biofeedback, 22*(3), 209–214.

Beckham, J. C., Feldman, M. E., Kirby, A. C., Hertzberg, M. A., & Moore, S. D. (1997). Interpersonal violence and its correlates in Vietnam veterans with chronic posttraumatic stress disorder. *Journal of Clinical Psychology, 53*(8), 859–869.

Beckham, J. C., Moore, S. D., & Reynolds, V. (2000). Interpersonal hostility and violence in Vietnam combat veterans with chronic posttraumatic stress disorder: A review of theoretical models and empirical evidence. *Aggression and Violent Behavior, 5*(5), 451–466.

Begic, D., & Jokic-Begic, N. (2001). Aggressive behavior in combat veterans with posttraumatic stress disorder. *Military Medicine, 166*(8), 671–676.

Bell, K. M., & Orcutt, H. K. (2009). Posttraumatic stress disorder and male-perpetrated intimate partner violence. *Journal of the American Medical Association, 302*(5), 562–564.

Berguis, D. J., & Jongsma, A. E. (2010). *The veteran and active duty military psychotherapy progress notes planner.* New Jersey: Wiley.

Buss, A. H., & Perry, M. (1992). The Aggression Questionnaire. *Journal of Personality and Social Psychology, 63*(3), 452–459.

Byrne, C. A., & Riggs, D. S. (1996). The cycle of trauma: Relationship aggression in male Vietnam veterans with symptoms of posttraumatic stress disorder. *Violence and Victims, 11*(3), 213–225.

Cahill, S. P., Rauch, S. A., Hembree, E. A., Foa, E. B., & Taylor, S. (2004). Effect of cognitive-behavioral treatments for PTSD on anger. In S. Taylor (Ed.), *Advances in the treatment of posttraumatic stress disorder: Cognitive-behavioral perspectives* (pp. 175–196). New York: Springer.

Calhoun, P. S., Beckham, J. C., Feldman, M. E., Barefoot, J. C., Haney, T., & Bosworth, H. B. (2002). Partners' ratings of combat veterans' anger. *Journal of Traumatic Stress, 15*(2), 133–136.

Campbell, J. C., Garza, M. A., Gielen, A. C., O'Campo, P., Kub, J., Dienemann, J., et al. (2003). Intimate partner violence and abuse among active duty military women. *Violence Against Women, 9*(9), 1072–1092.

Campbell, T. A., Nelson, L. A., Lumpkin, R., Yoash-Gantz, R. E., Pickett, T. C., & McCormick, C. L. (2009). Neuropsychological measures of processing speed and executive functioning in combat veterans with PTSD, TBI, and comorbid TBI/PTSD. *Psychiatric Annals, 39*(8), 796–803.

Carlson, E. B., Lauderdale, S., Hawkins, J., & Sheikh, J. I. (2008). Posttraumatic stress and aggression among veterans in long-term care. *Journal of Geriatric Psychiatry and Neurology, 21*(1), 61–71.

Carroll, E. M., Rueger, D. B., Foy, D. W., & Donahoe, C. P. (1985). Vietnam combat veterans with posttraumatic stress disorder: Analysis of marital and cohabiting adjustment. *Journal of Abnormal Psychology, 94*(3), 329–337.

Castillo, D. T., C'De Baca, J., Conforti, K., Qualls, C., & Fallon, S. K. (2002). Anger in PTSD: General psychiatric and gender differences on the BDHI. *Journal of Loss and Trauma, 7*(2), 119–128.

Chemtob, C. M., Novaco, R. W., Hamada, R. S., & Gross, D. M. (1997). Cognitive-behavioral treatment for severe anger in posttraumatic stress disorder. *Journal of Consulting and Clinical Psychology, 65*(1), 184–189.

Cornell, D. G., Warren, J., Hawk, G., Stafford, E., Oram, G., & Pine, D. (1996). Psychopathy in instrumental and reactive violent offenders. *Journal of Consulting and Clinical Psychology, 64*(4), 783–790.

Del Vecchio, T., & O'Leary, K. D. (2004). Effectiveness of anger treatments for specific anger problems: A meta-analytic review. *Clinical Psychology Review, 24*(1), 15–34.

Douglas, K. S., Ogloff, J. R., Nicholls, T. L., & Grant, I. (1999). Assessing risk for violence among psychiatric patients: The HCR-20 violence risk assessment scheme and the Psychopathy Checklist: Screening Version. *Journal of Consulting and Clinical Psychology, 67*(6), 917–930.

Douglas, K. S., & Webster, C. D. (1999). The HCR-20 violence risk assessment scheme: Concurrent validity in a sample of incarcerated offenders. *Criminal Justice and Behavior, 26*(1), 3–19.

Edmondson, C. B., & Conger, J. C. (1996). A review of treatment efficacy for individuals with anger problems: Conceptual, assessment, and methodological issues. *Clinical Psychology Review, 16*(3), 251–275.

Elbogen, E. B., Beckham, J. C., Butterfield, M. I., Swartz, M., & Swanson, J. (2008). Assessing risk of violent behavior among veterans with severe mental illness. *Journal of Traumatic Stress, 21*, 113–117.

Elbogen, E. B., Fuller, S., Johnson, S., Brooks, S., Kinneer, P., Calhoun, P., et al. (2010). Improving risk assessment of violence among military veterans: An empirical model for clinical decision-making. *Clinical Psychology Revidw, 30*, 595–607.

Elbogen, E. B., Wagner, H. R., Fuller, S. R., Calhoun, P. S., Kinneer, P. M., Mid-Atlantic Mental Illness Research, Education, and Clinical Center Workgroup, et al. (2010). Correlates of anger and hostility in Iraq and Afghanistan war veterans. *American Journal of Psychiatry, 167*(9), 1051–1058.

Fonseca, C. A., Schmaling, K. B., Stoever, C., Gutierrez, C., Blume, A. W., & Russell, M. L. (2006). Variables associated with intimate partner violence in a deploying military sample. *Military Medicine, 171*(7), 627–631.

Forbes, D., Hawthorne, G., Elliott, P., McHugh, T., Biddle, D., Creamer, M., et al. (2004). A concise measure of anger in combat-related posttraumatic stress disorder. *Journal of Traumatic Stress, 17*(3), 249–256.

Forbes, D., Parslow, R., Creamer, M., Allen, N., McHugh, T., & Hopwood, M. (2008). Mechanisms of anger and treatment outcome in combat veterans with posttraumatic stress disorder. *Journal of Traumatic Stress, 21*(2), 142–149.

Forgey, M. A., & Badger, L. (2006). Patterns of intimate partner violence among married women in the military: Type, level, directionality, and consequences. *Journal of Family Violence, 21*(6), 369–380.

Freeman, T. W., & Roca, V. (2001). Gun use, attitudes toward violence, and aggression among combat veterans with chronic posttraumatic stress disorder. *Journal of Nervous and Mental Disease, 189*(5), 317–320.

Frueh, B. C., Grubaugh, A. L., Cusack, K. J., Kimble, M. O., Elhai, J. D., & Knapp, R. G. (2009). Exposure-based cognitive-behavioral treatment of PTSD in adults with schizophrenia or schizoaffective disorder: A pilot study. *Journal of Anxiety Disorders, 23*(5), 665–675.

Ganzini, L., Edwards, P., Surkan, P. J., & Drummond, D. J. (1995). Characteristics of violent elderly in the emergency department. *International Journal of Geriatric Psychiatry, 10*(11), 945–950.

Gerlock, A. A. (1994). Veterans' responses to anger management intervention. *Issues in Mental Health Nursing, 15*(4), 393–408.

Gimbel, C., & Booth, A. (1994). Why does military combat experience adversely affect marital relations? *Journal of Marriage and the Family, 56*(3), 691–703.

Glancy, G., & Saini, M. A. (2005). An evidenced-based review of psychological treatments of anger and aggression. *Brief Treatment and Crisis Intervention, 5*(2), 229–248.

Glenn, D., Beckham, J. C., Feldman, M. E., Kirby, A. C., Hertzberg, M. A., & Moore, S. D. (2002). Violence and hostility among families of Vietnam veterans with combat-related posttraumatic stress disorder. *Violence and Victims, 17*(4), 473–489.

Gondolf, E. W., & Foster, R. A. (1991). Wife assault among VA alcohol rehabilitation patients. *Hospital and Community Psychiatry, 42*(1), 74–79.

Grafman, J., Schwab, K., Warden, D., & Pridgen, A. (1996). Frontal lobe injuries, violence, and aggression: A report of the Vietnam head injury study. *Neurology, 46*(5), 1231–1238.

Hartl, T. L., Rosen, C., Drescher, K., Lee, T. T., & Gusman, F. (2005). Predicting high-risk behaviors in veterans with posttraumatic stress disorder. *Journal of Nervous and Mental Disease, 193*(7), 464–472.

Hawthorne, G., Mouthaan, J., Forbes, D., & Novaco, R. W. (2006). Response categories and anger measurement: Do fewer categories result in poorer measurement?: Development of the DAR5. *Social Psychiatry and Psychiatric Epidemiology, 41*(2), 164–172.

Hoge, C. W., McGurk, D., Thomas, J. L., Cox, A. L., Engel, C. C., & Castro, C. A. (2008). Mild traumatic brain injury in U.S. soldiers returning from Iraq. *New England Journal of Medicine, 5*, 453–463.

Jakupcak, M., Conybeare, D., Phelps, L., Hunt, S., Holmes, H. A., Felker, B., et al. (2007). Anger, hostility, and aggression among Iraq and Afghanistan war veterans reporting PTSD and subthreshold PTSD. *Journal of Traumatic Stress, 20*(6), 945–954.

Jordan, B., Marmar, C. R., Fairbank, J. A., Schlenger, W. E., & Kulka, R. A. (1992). Problems in families of male Vietnam veterans with posttraumatic stress disorder. *Journal of Consulting and Clinical Psychology, 60*(6), 916–926.

Killgore, W. D. S., Cotting, D. I., Thomas, J. L., Cox, A. L., McGurk, D., Vo, A. H., et al. (2008). Post-combat invincibility: Violent combat experiences are associated with increased risk-taking propensity following deployment. *Journal of Psychiatric Research, 42*(13), 1112–1121.

Kubzansky, L. D., Cole, S. R., Kawachi, I., Vokonas, P., & Sparrow, D. (2006).

Shared and unique contributions of anger, anxiety, and depression to coronary heart disease: A prospective study in the normative aging study. *Annals of Behavioral Medicine, 31*(1), 21–29.

Kulka, R. A., Schlenger, W. E., Fairbank, J. A., Hough, R. L., Jordan, B. K., Marmar, C. R., et al. (1990). *Report of findings from the National Veterans Readjustment Study.* New York: Brunner/Mazel.

Lasko, N. B., Gurvits, T. V., Kuhne, A. A., Orr, S. P., Pittman, R. K., et al. (1994). Aggression and its correlates in Vietnam veterans with and without chronic posttraumatic stress disorder. *Comprehensive Psychiatry, 35*(5), 373–381.

Lombardo, E. R., Tan, G., Jensen, M. P., & Anderson, K. O. (2005). Anger management style and associations with self-efficacy and pain in male veterans. *Journal of Pain, 6*(11), 765–770.

Marshall, A. D., Panuzio, J., & Taft, C. T. (2005). Intimate partner violence among military veterans and active duty servicemen. *Clinical Psychology Review, 25*(7), 862–876.

McCarroll, J. E., Newby, J. H., Thayer, L. E., Norwood, A. E., Fullerton, C. S., & Ursano, R. J. (1999). Reports of spouse abuse in the U.S. Army Central Registry (1989–1997). *Military Medicine, 164*(2), 77–84.

McCarroll, J. E., Ursano, R. J., Liu, X., Thayer, L. E., Newby, J. H., Norwood, A. E., et al. (2000). Deployment and the probability of spousal aggression by U.S. Army soldiers. *Military Medicine, 165*(1), 41–44.

McCarroll, J. E., Ursano, R. J., Newby, J. H., Liu, X., Fullerton, C. S., Norwood, A. E., et al. (2003). Domestic violence and deployment in US Army soldiers. *Journal of Nervous and Mental Disease, 191*(1), 3–9.

McFall, M., Fontana, A., Raskind, M., & Rosenheck, R. (1999). Analysis of violent behavior in Vietnam combat veteran psychiatric inpatients with posttraumatic stress disorder. *Journal of Traumatic Stress, 12*(3), 501–517.

Merrill, L. L., Hervig, L. K., & Milner, J. S. (1996). Childhood parenting experiences, intimate partner conflict resolution, and adult risk for child physical abuse. *Child Abuse and Neglect, 20*(11), 1049–1065.

Mikolajczak, J., & Hagen, D. Q. (1978). Aggression in psychiatric patients in a VA hospital. *Military Medicine, 143*(6), 402–404.

Monahan, J., & Steadman, H. J. (1994). *Violence and mental disorder: Developments in risk assessment.* Chicago: University of Chicago Press.

Monahan, J., Steadman, H. J., Robbins, P. C., Appelbaum, P., Banks, S., Grisso, T., et al. (2005). An actuarial model of violence risk assessment for persons with mental disorders. *Psychiatric Services, 56*(7), 810–815.

Monson, C. M., Rodriguez, B. F., & Warner, R. (2005). Cognitive-behavioral therapy for PTSD in the real world: Do interpersonal relationships make a real difference? *Journal of Clinical Psychology, 61*(6), 751–761.

Morland, L. A., Greene, C. J., Rosen, C., Foy, D., Reilly, P., Shore, J., et al. (2010). Telemedicine for anger management therapy in a rural population of combat veterans with posttraumatic stress disorder: A randomized noninferiority trial. *Journal of Clinical Psychiatry, 71*, 855.

Moss, H. B. (1989). Psychopathy, aggression, and family history in male veteran substance abuse patients: A factor analytic study. *Addictive Behaviors, 14*(5), 565–570.

Mossman, D. (1994). Assessing predictions of violence: Being accurate about accuracy. *Journal of Consulting and Clinical Psychology, 62*(4), 783–792.

Mulvey, E. P., & Lidz, C. W. (1993). Measuring patient violence in dangerousness research. *Law and Human Behavior, 17*(3), 277–288.

Murphy, C. M., Taft, C. T., & Eckhardt, C. I. (2007). Anger problem profiles among partner violent men: Differences in clinical presentation and treatment outcome. *Journal of Counseling Psychology, 54*(2), 189–200.

Nelson, L. A., Yoash-Gantz, R. E., Pickett, T. C., & Campbell, T. A. (2009). Relationship between processing speed and executive functioning performance among OEF/OIF veterans: Implications for postdeployment rehabilitation. *Journal of Head Trauma Rehabilitation, 24*(1), 32–40.

Novaco, R. W., & Chemtob, C. M. (2002). Anger and combat-related posttraumatic stress disorder. *Journal of Traumatic Stress, 15*, 123–132.

O'Donnell, C., Cook, J. M., Thompson, R., Riley, K., & Neria, Y. (2006). Verbal and physical aggression in World War II former prisoners of war: Role of posttraumatic stress disorder and depression. *Journal of Traumatic Stress, 19*(6), 859–866.

Orcutt, H. K., King, L. A., & King, D. W. (2003). Male-perpetrated violence among Vietnam veteran couples: Relationships with veteran's early life characteristics, trauma history, and PTSD symptomatology. *Journal of Traumatic Stress, 16*(4), 381–390.

Orth, U., & Wieland, E. (2006). Anger, hostility, and posttraumatic stress disorder in trauma-exposed adults: A meta-analysis. *Journal of Consulting and Clinical Psychology, 74*(4), 698–706.

Owens, G. P., Herrera, C. J., & Whitesell, A. A. (2009). A preliminary investigation of mental health needs and barriers to mental health care for female veterans of Iraq and Afghanistan. *Traumatology, 15*(2), 31–37.

Panuzio, J., O'Farrell, T., Marshall, A. D., Murphy, C. M., Murphy, M., & Taft, C. T. (2006). Intimate partner aggression reporting concordance and correlates of agreement among men with alcohol use disorders and their female parters. *Assessment, 13*(3), 266–279.

Pekala, R. J., Kumar, V. K., Maurer, R., Elliott-Carter, N. C., & Moon, E. (2009). Self-esteem and its relationship to serenity and anger/impulsivity in an alcohol and other drug-dependent population: Implications for treatment. *Alcoholism Treatment Quarterly, 27*(1), 94–112.

Petrik, N. D., Rosenberg, A. M., & Watson, C. G. (1983). Combat experience and youth: Influences on reported violence against women. *Professional Psychology: Research and Practice, 14*(6), 895–899.

Prigerson, H. G., Maciejewski, P. K., & Rosenheck, R. A. (2002). Population attributable fractions of psychiatric disorders and behavioral outcomes associated with combat exposure among U.S. men. *American Journal of Public Health, 92*(1), 59–63.

Quinsey, V. L., Harris, G. T., Rice, M. E., & Cormier, C. A. (2006). *Violent offenders: Appraising and managing risk* (2nd ed.). Washington, DC: American Psychological Association.

Robert, S., Hamner, M. B., Kose, S., Ulmer, H. G., Deitsch, S. E., & Lorberbaum, J. P. (2005). Quetiapine improves sleep disturbances in combat veterans with

PTSD: Sleep data from a prospective, open-label study. *Journal of Clinical Psychopharmacology, 25*(4), 387–388.

Rosen, L. N., Kaminski, R. J., Parmley, A. M., Knudson, K. H., & Fancher, P. (2003). The effects of peer group climate on intimate partner violence among married male U.S. Army soldiers. *Violence Against Women, 9*(9), 1045–1071.

Rumm, P. D., Cummings, P., Krauss, M. R., Bell, M. A., & Rivara, F. P. (2000). Identified spouse abuse as a risk factor for child abuse. *Child Abuse and Neglect, 24*(11), 1375–1381.

Saini, M. (2009). A meta-analysis of the psychological treatment of anger: Developing guidelines for evidence-based practices. *Journal of the American Academy of Psychiatry and Law, 37*, 473–488.

Savarese, V. W., Suvak, M. K., King, L. A., & King, D. W. (2001). Relationships among alcohol use, hyperarousal, and marital abuse and violence in Vietnam veterans. *Journal of Traumatic Stress, 14*(4), 717–732.

Sayer, N. A., Noorbaloochi, S., Frazier, P., Carlson, K., Gravely, A., & Murdoch, M. (2010). Reintegration problems and treatment interests among Iraq and Afghanistan combat veterans receiving VA medical care. *Psychiatric Services, 61*(6), 589–597.

Sherman, M. D., Sautter, F., Jackson, M. H., Lyons, J. A., & Han, X. (2006). Domestic violence in veterans with posttraumatic stress disorder who seek couples therapy. *Journal of Marital and Family Therapy, 32*(4), 479–490.

Snowden, R. J., Gray, N. S., Taylor, J., & Fitzgerald, S. (2009). Assessing Risk of Future Violence Among Forensic Psychiatric Inpatients With the Classification of Violence Risk (COVR). *Psychiatric Services, 60*(11), 1522–1526.

Steadman, H. J., Silver, E., Monahan, J., Appelbaum, P. S., Clark Robbins, P., Mulvey, E. P., et al. (2000). A classification tree approach to the development of actuarial violence risk assessment tools. *Law and Human Behavior, 24*(1), 83–100.

Taft, C. T., Kaloupek, D. G., Schumm, J. A., Marshall, A. D., Panuzio, J., King, D. W., et al. (2007). Posttraumatic stress disorder symptoms, physiological reactivity, alcohol problems, and aggression among military veterans. *Journal of Abnormal Psychology, 116*(3), 498–507.

Taft, C. T., & Niles, B. L. (2004). Assessment and treatment of anger in combat-related PTSD. In *Iraq War clinician's guide: Second edition* (pp. 70–74). Boston: Department of Veterans Affairs, National Center for PTSD.

Taft, C. T., Pless, A. P., Stalans, L. J., Koenen, K. C., King, L. A., & King, D. W. (2005). Risk factors for partner violence among a national sample of combat veterans. *Journal of Consulting and Clinical Psychology, 73*(1), 151–159.

Taft, C. T., Street, A. E., Marshall, A. D., Dowdall, D. J., & Riggs, D. S. (2007). Posttraumatic stress disorder, anger, and partner abuse among Vietnam combat veterans. *Journal of Family Psychology, 21*(2), 270–277.

Taft, C. T., Vogt, D. S., Marshall, A. D., Panuzio, J., & Niles, B. L. (2007). Aggression among combat veterans: Relationships with combat exposure and symptoms of posttraumatic stress disorder, dysphoria, and anxiety. *Journal of Traumatic Stress, 20*(2), 135–145.

Taylor, M. K., Mujica-Parodi, L. R., Potterat, E. G., Momen, N., Dial Ward, M. D.,

Padilla, G. A., et al. (2009). Anger expression and stress responses in military men. *Aviation, Space, and Environmental Medicine, 80*(11), 962–967.

Teten, A. L., Schumacher, J. A., Bailey, S. D., Kent, T. A. (2009). Male-to-female sexual aggression among Iraq, Afghanistan, and Vietnam veterans: Co-occurring substance abuse and intimate partner aggression. *Journal of Traumatic Stress, 22*(4), 307–311.

Thomas, J. L., Wilk, J. E., Riviere, L. A., McGurk, D., Castro, C. A., & Hoge, C. W. (2010). Prevalence of mental health problems and functional impairment among Active Component and National Guard soldiers 3 and 12 months following combat in Iraq. *Archives of General Psychiatry, 67*(6), 614–623.

Timmons, P. L., Oehlert, M. E., Sumerall, S. W., & Timmons, C. W. (1997). Stress inoculation training for maladaptive anger: Comparison of group counseling versus computer guidance. *Computers in Human Behavior, 13*(1), 51–64.

Vasterling, J. J., Proctor, S. P., Amoroso, P., Kane, R., Heeren, T., & White, R. F. (2006). Neuropsychological outcomes of army personnel following deployment to the Iraq war. *Journal of the American Medical Association, 296*(5), 519–529.

Vrana, S. R., Hughes, J. W., Dennis, M. F., Calhoun, P. S., & Beckham, J. C. (2009). Effects of posttraumatic stress disorder status and covert hostility on cardiovascular responses to relived anger in women with and without PTSD. *Biological Psychology, 82*(3), 274–280.

Wasileski, M., Callaghan-Chaffee, M. E., & Chaffee, R. B. (1982). Spousal violence in military homes: An initial survey. *Military Medicine, 147*(9), 761–765.

Werner, P. D., Rose, T. L., Yesavage, J. A., & Seeman, K. (1984). Psychiatrists' judgments of dangerousness in patients on an acute care unit. *American Journal of Psychiatry, 141*(2), 263–266.

Windle, R. C., & Windle, M. (1995). Longitudinal patterns of physical aggression: Associations with adult social, psychiatric, and personality functioning and testosterone levels. *Development and Psychopathology, 7*(3), 563–585.

Yesavage, J. A. (1984). Correlates of dangerous behavior by schizophrenics in hospital. *Journal of Psychiatric Research, 18*(3), 225–231.

CHAPTER 19

Resiliency Building as a Means to Prevent PTSD and Related Adjustment Problems in Military Personnel

Donald Meichenbaum

Recently, the Public Broadcasting System program *Frontline* presented a documentary, "The Wounded Platoon," which told the story of the men of the Third Platoon, Charlie Company, who recently returned to Fort Carson, Colorado (see *PBS.org* to view this documentary). This 1-hour 26-minute film highlighted the tragic story of the incidence of some 20 suicides and 12 homicidal violent acts by returning soldiers. The intended message is that this is the aftermath that soldiers experience as a result of combat exposure. "This is a normal reaction to an abnormal situation," as one counselor tells a distressed soldier. One has to wait 1 hour and 18 minutes to hear "the rest of the story." At this point in the moving and dramatic account, nine returning soldiers attend the funeral of their squad leader, who died in combat. As the narrator comments in passing, these soldiers are "living productive lives," pursuing their educations, happily married, raising families; some are still working with the military as instructors. In fact, the PBS website has included pictures of all members of the Third Platoon. One can click on the many faces and learn of their current level of adjustment and resilience.

Their courage, sense of honor, and loyalty is a story that is worth telling and is one that has been supported repeatedly by the research literature. An examination of Table 19.1, which summarizes illustrative research findings on resilience in returning warriors, raises a challenging question: What distinguishes those soldiers who develop posttraumatic stress disorder (PTSD) and related postdeployment adjustment problems (anxiety, depression, substance abuse, aggressive behaviors toward themselves and others, moral injuries, and the like) from those who evidence resilience? Moreover, what are the implications for both preventative resiliency training programs and treatment interventions?

In this chapter, I:

1. Consider the concept of resilience.
2. Examine the research findings on resilient soldiers who endured combat exposure, were prisoners of war, and had war-related experiences and consider the lessons learned.
3. Provide an algorithm or formula for what returning warriors have *to do* and *not do* in order to develop chronic PTSD and related adjustment difficulties and consider the implications for interventions.
4. Consider the efforts to train and bolster resilience in soldiers and their family members.
5. Explore what needs to be included in such well-intended intervention efforts if they are going to prove successful and reduce PTSD and related adjustment difficulties.

This chapter is about "the rest of the story" that the media often do *not* highlight. It is both a riveting and an uplifting tale.

What Is Resilience?

Resilience has numerous definitions and meanings. It is more than the absence of symptoms. Resilience generally refers to a pattern of adaptation in the context of risk adversity. Resilience has been characterized as the ability to "bounce back" from adversities, "bend, but not break" under extreme stress, handle setbacks, and perservere in spite of ongoing stresses and even when things go awry.[1] Resilience has been characterized as a set of good

---

[1]This concept of resilience was originally used in material science to refer to the ability of certain materials, such as rubber, to withstand compression or expansion and return to their original shape or position.

TABLE 19.1. Illustrative Data of Resilience in Returning Warriors

- Research has continually shown that from the time of World War I, veterans as a group resume normal lives, are less likely to be incarcerated, have higher education ,and generally achieve more success upon return to the civilian world than do their nonserving peers (Grossman & Christensen, 2007; Reich et al., 2010).

- Following combat exposure, somewhere between 10 and 20% of soldiers may evidence PTSD, depression, anxiety, and related problems. But the majority (> 80%) do not (Hoge at al., 2004; Litz, 2007; Tanielian & Jaycox, 2008).

- The majority of Vietnam veterans (70%) appraised the impact of their service on their present lives as "mainly positive." Over 40% of the veterans felt that the war's influence was still highly important in their lives (Dohrenwend et al., 2004; Elder & Clipp, 1989; Fontana & Rosenheck, 1998).

- The vast majority of Vietnam veterans were as well adjusted as or even more successful than their nonserving civilian peers (Burkett & Whitely, 1998; Dohrenwend et al., 2006).

- Studies of enlisted service members in Vietnam indicated that 10–15% used narcotics, but follow-up assessments back home indicated only an incidence of 1% of continual addictive behaviors (Robins, Davis, & Nurco, 1974; Burkett & Whitely, 1998).

- In fact, many soldiers report experiencing "combat flow" and enhanced meaning and comradeship ("band of brothers") as a result of their combat experience. They report feeling an energized focus, full involvement ("in the zone, or groove"; "on the ball"), heightened pride and patriotism as a result of their military experience (Harari, 2008; Schok, Kleber, Elands, & Weerts, 2008).

- A study of soldiers and families in Operation Desert Storm found that 62–73% of respondents felt that they had readjusted to family life within 1 month after return home; 17–21% had readjusted after several months; and only 8–17% were still adjusting 2 years after return (single parents being the largest group; Caliber Associates, 2007).

- A survey of army spouses indicated that some 58% believed that deployment had strengthened their marriages, that 31% believed it had no effect, and that only 10% felt it had weakened their marriages (Caliber Associates, 2007; Henderson, 2006).

- Although deployment can be quite stressful, many families report that outcomes of these deployments have included the development of new skills and competencies, as well as a sense of independence and self-reliance (Caliber Associates, 2007; Hall, 2008).

- Children in military families are typically resilient even after experiencing significant trauma and family deaths (Morgillo-Freeman et al. 2009).

outcomes that occur in spite of serious threats to adaptation or development and as specific coping skills that are marshalled when faced with challenging situations.

The concept of resilience is often linked with the notion of sustainability, which refers to the ability to continue forward and maintain equilibrium in the face of chronic adversity. Resilience is tied to the ability to learn to live with ongoing fear and uncertainty and the ability to adapt to difficult and challenging life experiences.

Following the exposure to traumatic events, most people readjust successfully. Resilience is more the rule than the exception, more common than rare. Moveover, resilience is *not* a sign of exceptional strength but a fundamental feature of normal coping skills, or what Masten (2001) characterizes as "ordinary magic."

Research has indicated that resilience develops over time and that its expression may be a slow developmental process. An individual may be resilient with respect to some kinds of stressors but not others; in one context or in one area of life but not in others; at one time in life but not at other times (Mancini & Bonanno, 2010; Meichenbaum, 2009a). It is also important to recognize that positive and negative emotions may co-occur, operating side-by-side, following exposure to traumatic events (Lyubomirsky & Della Porta, 2010; Moskowitz, 2010). There are multiple pathways to resilience, with no single dominant factor, or "magic bullet," that determines it. Rather, resilience-engendering activities need to be "practiced" and "replenished" on a daily basis, like a set of muscles that has to be exercised regularly, so that such coping responses become automatic and incorporated into one's repertoire (Muraven & Baumeister, 2000).

The evidence for resilience following trauma exposure is evident in civilian populations as well. Antonovsky (1987), Bonanno (2004), Helgeson, Reynolds, and Tomich(2006), Johnson and Thompson (2008), Mancini and Bonnano (2010), Ryff and Singer (2003), and Sawyer, Ayers, and Field (2010) review data from Holocaust survivors, bereaved individuals, cancer and HIV/AIDS survivors, torture victims, victims of sexual abuse or rape, and survivors of terrorist attacks and natural disasters who evidence remarkable resilience. As time passes, some individuals report in retrospect that their lives are somehow improved because of their exposure to a traumatic event. Their resultant outcomes have been characterized as "posttraumatic growth" (Calhoun & Tedeschi, 2006). They report that they have benefited and been transformed by their struggle with adversities. They report such benefits as the development of self-discipline, increasing their stress tolerance and self-confidence, broadening their perspective on life, change in life priorities, improved relationships, and an increased sense of spirituality.

Two prominent examples highlight the widespread incidence of resilience following trauma exposure. Some 50–60% of adults in the United States are exposed to traumatic events, but only 5–10% develop PTSD and related clinical problems (Kessler, Davis, & Kendler, 1997). Following the September 11 terrorist attacks in New York City, only 7.5% of Manhattan residents evidenced clinical problems, and this rate dropped to less than 1% at 6 months (Bonanno, 2004). A similar pattern of resilience was evident in residents in London, England, following the subway terrorist attack of July 7, 2005. Less than 1% of those who were directly affected sought professional help. Most people, following such attacks, were able to turn to natural social supports and to their faith for comfort, support, and growth (Charuvastra & Cloitre, 2008; Pargament & Cummings, 2010). As Levin (2006, p. 20) observes "Resilience, rather than pathology, should become the standard expectation in the aftermath of trauma."

What Characterizes Resilient Individuals?

Much research has been conducted to identify the characteristics of resilient individuals who have experienced combat or who have been prisoners of war (Bartone, 1999; Benotsch, 2000; Burkett & Whitley, 1998; Erbes et al., 2005; Hunter, 1993; King, King, Fairbank, Keane, & Adams, 1998; Litz, 2007; Satel, 2005; Sharkansky et al., 2000; Southwick, Vythilingam, & Charney, 2005, Sutker, Davis, Uddo, & Ditta, 1995; Waysman, Schwarzwald, & Solomon, 2001; Zakin, Solomon, & Neria, 2003).

The search for mediating and moderating factors and processes that have contributed to resilience has ranged from the biological heritable underpinnings of resilience (Haglund, Nestadt, Cooper, Southwick, & Charney, 2007; Reich, Zautran, & Hall, 2010) to the broader social domain (Morgillo-Freeman, Moore, & Freeman, 2009). The need to incorporate the social context is highlighted by the observation that resilience rests fundamentally on relationships, both the perceived and actually received amount and quality of social supports (Charuvastra & Cloitre, 2008; Masten, 2001). The degree of social capital and resources available is a critical contributor to the development of resilience and sustainability (Hobfoll, 2002). Thus the concept of resilience needs to be extended to include resilient families (Hall, 2008; Henderson, 2006), resilient organizations (Denhardt & Denhardt, 2010), and resilient communities (Kretzmann, 2010). The intervention implications of this ecological conceptualization of resilience are considered later.

A favorite pastime for mental health workers is to generate a checklist of behaviors or essential skills that promote natural recovery following trauma exposure and that bolster resilience (e.g., Kent & Davis, 2010; Milne, 2007; Reivich & Shatte, 2002; and see such websites as *www.asu.edu/resilience*).

Table 19.2 provides a composite summary of the psychological characteristics or qualities of resilient individuals.

TABLE 19.2. Psychological Characteristics of Resilient Individuals

- *Experience of positive emotions and regulation of strong negative emotions.* Being realistically optimistic, hopeful, able to laugh at oneself; having humor, courage; able to face one's fears and manage emotions. Positive expectations about the future. Positive self-image. Build on existing strengths, talents, and social supports.

- *Adaptive task-oriented coping style.* Able to match one's coping skills—namely direct-action present-focused and emotionally palliative—acceptance with the demands of the situation. Able to actively seek help and garner social supports. Having a resilient role model, even a heroic figure who can act as a mentor. Having self-efficacy and a belief that one can control one's environment effectively. Self-confidence. Seeking out new and challenging experiences out of one's "comfort zone" and evidence "grit," or the perserverance and passion to pursue long-term goals.

- *Cognitive flexibility.* Able to reframe, redefine, restory, find benefits, engage in social problem solving and alternative thinking to adaptively meet changing demands and handle transitional stressors.

- *Meaning making.* Able to create meaning and a purpose in life; survivor's mission. Using one's faith, spirituality, and values as a "moral compass." Being altruistic and making a "gift" of one's experience. Sharing one's story. Having a general sense of trust in others.

- *Keeping fit and safe.* Exercise, follow a routine, reduce risks, avoid unsafe high-risk behaviors (substance abuse, chasing "adrenaline rush" activities).

Behaviors That Contribute to the Development of Chronic PTSD and Related Adjustment Problems

PTSD has been characterized as a "disorder of nonrecovery," as most individuals recover from the aftermath of trauma exposure over time. If 80% or more of returning soldiers evidence resilience and lead productive lives, what factors account for the other 20% evidencing chronic clinical problems (Hoge et al., 2004; Tanielian, & Jaycox, 2008), as well as the alarming rate of suicidal behavior (Brenner, Gutierrez, & Cornette, 2008; Scoville, Gubata, & Potter, 2007; Staal & Hughes, 2002)? The answer to this challenging question is complex, because it involves premilitary factors (e.g., previous vulnerabilities, prior psychopathology, experience of prior trauma events), combat factors (e.g., multiple deployments, poor combat leadership, absence of unit cohesion, injuries with comorbid disorders), and postdeployment factors (e.g., posttrauma additional stressful life events, homecoming stress, absence of social supports). Elsewhere, I have discussed how these various factors can be incorporated into a case conceptualization model that informs both assessment and treatment decision making (Meichenbaum, 2009b).

Presently, the focus is on what returning soldiers and significant others in their lives have *to do* and *not do* in order to develop and maintain chronic

TABLE 19.3. "How to" Develop Persistent PTSD and Related Adjustment Problems

At the cognitive level

Engage in self-focused, "mental defeating" type of thinking. Perceive that one has lost autonomy as a human being, lost the will to exert control and maintain identity, lost the belief that one has a "free will." See self as a "victim," controlled by uninvited thoughts, feelings, and circumstances, continually vulnerable, unlovable, undesirable, unworthy. Use dramatic metaphors that reinforce this style of thinking; "I am a prisoner of the past," "entrapped," "contaminated," "damaged goods," "a doormat," "a pariah." A form of mental exhaustion, mental weariness.

Hold erroneous beliefs that changes are permanent, the world is unsafe and unpredictable, and that people are untrustworthy. Hold a negative, foreshortened view of the future and the belief that life has lost its meaning.

Engage in self-berating, self-condemnation, self-derogatory "storytelling" to oneself and to others (i.e., self blame, guilt-engendering hindsight, biased thinking; anger-engendering thoughts, viewing provocations as being done "on purpose").

Engage in upward social comparisons, so one compares poorly in one's coping abilities. Be preoccupied with what others think of oneself. Engage in comparison of self versus others; before versus now; now versus what might have been.

Ruminate repeatedly; dwell on, focus on, brood, pine over losses, "near miss" experiences. Replay over and over one's concerns about the causes, consequences, and symptoms related to negative affect and losses. Use repetitive thinking cycles ("loss spiral").

Engage in contrafactual thinking, repeating "If only," statements and asking "Why me" questions for which there are no satisfactory answers.

Engage in avoidant thinking processes of deliberately suppressing thoughts, using distracting behaviors, using substances; avoidant coping behaviors and dissociation.

Have an overgeneralized memory and recall style that intensifies hopelessness and impairs problem solving. Have difficulty remembering specific positive experiences. Memories are fragmented and sensory driven and fail to integrate traumatic events into autobiographical memory or narrative.

Engage in "thinking traps"; for example, tunnel vision as evident in the failure to believe anything positive could result from trauma experience; confirmatory bias as evident in the failure to retrieve anything positive about one's self-identity or recall any positive coping memories of what one did to survive or what one is still able to accomplish "in spite of" victimization; mind reading, overgeneralizing, personalizing, jumping to conclusions, catastrophizing; "sweating the small stuff"; and emotional reasoning, such as viewing failures and lapses as "end points."

Evidence "stuckness" in one's thinking processes and behavior. Respond to new situations in postdeployment settings "as if" one were still in combat (misperceive threats).

At the emotional level

Engage in emotional avoidance strategies ("pine over losses," deny your feelings and the possible consequences).

Intensify your fears and anger.

(continued)

TABLE 19.3. (continued)

Experience guilt (hindsight bias), shame, complicated grief, demoralization.

Fail to engage in grief work that honors and memorializes loved ones or buddies who were lost.

Fail to share or disclose feelings, process traumatic memories. Focus on "hot spots" and "stuck points."

At the behavioral level

Engage in avoidant behaviors of trauma-related feelings, thoughts, reminders, activities and situations; dissociating behaviors.

Be continually hypervigilant, overestimating the likelihood and severity of danger.

Engage in safety behaviors that interfere with the disconfirmation of emotional beliefs and the processing ("restorying") of trauma-related memories and beliefs.

Engage in delay-seeking behaviors. Avoid seeking help. Keep secrets and "clam up."

Engage in high risk-taking behaviors; chasing the "adrenaline rush" in an unsafe fashion; put oneself at risk for revictimization.

Engage in health-compromising behaviors (smoking, substance abuse as a form of self-medication, lack of exercise, sleep disturbance that goes untreated, poor diet, dependence on energy drinks, abandonment of healthy behavioral routines).

Engage in self-handicapping behaviors ("excuse-making"), failure-avoidance behaviors.

Use passive, disengaged coping behaviors, social withdrawal, resigned acceptance, wishful thinking, and emotional distancing.

At the social level

Withdraw, isolate oneself, detach from others.

Perceive oneself as being unwanted, a "burden"; thwarted belongingness, distrusting others ("no one cares"; "no one understands"; "no one can be trusted").

Associate with peers and family members who reinforce and support maladaptive behaviors. Put oneself in high-risk situations.

Experience an unsupportive and indifferent social environment (i.e., critical, intrusive, unsympathetic—offering "moving on" statements).

Fail to seek social support or help, such as peer-related groups, chaplain services, or professional assistance.

At the spiritual level

Fail to use one's faith or religion as a means of coping.

Have a "spiritual struggle" and view God as having punished and abandoned one.

Use negative spiritual coping responses. Relinquish actions to a higher power, plead for miracles or divine intervention; become angry with God; demanding.

Experience "moral injuries" that compromise values. Lose one's "moral compass" and "shatterproof beliefs"; experience a "soul wound."

Avoid contact with members of religious orders.

adjustment problems. I then consider the implications for resiliency training programs. The list of self-sustaining factors and processes identified in Table 19.3 is informed by research findings of Ebert and Dyck (2004), Ehlers and Clark (2000), Folkman and Moskowitz (2000), Harvey and Tummala-Narra (2007), Helgeson et al. (2006), King et al. (1998), Maeraker and Zoellner (2004), Pargament and Cummings (2010); Park and Folkman (1997); Smith and Alloy (2009), and Watkins (2008).

Just as there is no one pathway to resilience, there is no particular algorithm that contributes to the persistence of chronic PTSD and related problems. It is the combination of cognitive, emotional, behavioral, social, and spiritual processes that contribute to chronic PTSD and accompanying adjustment problems.

Addressing the Psychological Needs of Service Members

The U.S. military has a long and successful tradition of implementing programs designed to identify, treat, and prevent war-related stress reactions. Since World War I, the military has implemented the doctrine of combat stress control. At that time, the U.S. Army attached a psychiatrist to each division, with the role of advising command on the prevention of stress casualties and increasing the likelihood of return of soldiers to duty whenever possible.

In this tradition a number of predeployment, deployment, and postdeployment training programs, informational resources, and support agencies have been established (for example, see Military One Source and the Marine Corps website, *www.manpower.usmc.mil.com*). The Veterans Administration has also developed websites for returning soldiers and their family members designed to facilitate the transition to civilian life (*www.mentalhealth.va.gov*) and the RE-SET program (*harold.kudler@va.gov*). Penk and Ainspan (2009) provide an extensive list of military and community-based programs and resources designed to address stress-related reactions in soldiers and their family members.

The most recent major effort in this tradition is the preventative program Battlemind, developed by the Walter Reed Army Institute of Research led by Colonel Carl Castro (Castro, 2006; *www.battlemind.army.mil*). This program is designed to boost resilience before deployment and to help soldiers and their family members adjust to life back home. The warrior is taught that Battlemind is an inner strength for facing fear and adversity in combat and for applying these skills in the transition to civilian life with courage and adaptability. The program includes self-development in four key areas of emotional, social, spiritual, and family well-being. There is a set of training modules implemented at 3 and 6 months following deployment,

TABLE 19.4. BATTLEMIND

- Buddies (cohesion) versus withdrawal
- Accountability versus controlling
- Targeted aggression versus inappropriate aggression
- Tactical awareness versus hypervigilance
- Lethally armed versus "locked and loaded"
- Emotional control versus anger/detachment
- Mission operational security versus secretiveness
- Individual responsibility versus guilt
- Nondefensive (combat) driving versus aggressive driving
- Discipline versus conflict

Note. From a Battlemind training brochure.

after the "honeymoon" homecoming period has ended. There has also been a parallel Battlemind set of resilience-enhancing modules for spouses and family members.

BATTLEMIND is an acronym, in which each letter stands for a different set of coping skills that would help soldiers survive in combat but could prove problematic when carried over to life at home. Table 19.4 provides a description of the 10 specific mental skills and how these strengths in combat could represent a "stuckness" problem when maintained in a civilian setting. The sentence "Battlemind skills helped you survive in combat, but they can cause you problems if *not* adapted when you get home" (from a Battlemind training brochure) is an example of what is called "negative transfer." In working with members of the National Guard, we have identified what aspects of military life could be "positively transferred" back to civilian life. Table 19.5 summarizes the acronym H-SLIDER, which reflects the character traits and mind-set that soldiers bring home from combat. We have asked returning soldiers to share examples of these characteristics, "strengths," and lessons learned that can be posted on a website (*www. warfighterdiaries.com*) that soldiers can download to an iPod. There is an effort to make this website interactive so that soldiers and family members can submit their examples of "signs of resilience." This is an example of the "rest of the story," being told by returning soldiers.

The Battlemind and H-SLIDER programs focus on soldiers relearning adaptive civilian habits that facilitate transition while retaining the discipline, safety habits, and mental focus that characterized them in combat. Moreover, returning soldiers could make a "gift" of their ennobling experiences to civilians.

TABLE 19.5. H-SLIDER: Warriors' Character Traits and Mindset Brought Home from Combat

H—**Honor,** hard work, honesty, hardiness

S—**Selfless service,** sacrifice, subordinate self to the group; commitment and accountability to one's comrades, which is more powerful than self-preservation; one's "warriorhood."

L—**Loyalty,** brotherhood, closeness, commitment to one's unit, "band of brothers"; values and traditions of warriorhood; identification with group, service, and country.

I—**Integrity,** "grit," leadership, commitment to a higher cause, patriotism.

D—**Duty,** dedication, discipline, sense of responsibility to others, commitment to mission accomplishment, mental focus and learned safety habits; ability to be clear-minded, strategic, and alert.

E—**Courage,** bravery, confidence, controlled aggression, pride, adaptability, valor, knowledge of how precious and fragile life is.

R—**Respect,** readiness, responsibility, robustness, and resilience.

Although the initial results of the Battlemind program have been encouraging, more comprehensive evaluations are warranted. These evaluations have included interventions that compare large- and small-group Battlemind training versus stress education classes (Adler, Bliese, McGurk, Hoge, & Castro, 2009).

Most recently, the urgency for preventative resiliency training has been highlighted by the high incidence of suicides in the military (Brenner et al., 2008; Scoville et al., 2007; Selby, Anestis, & Bender, 2010). Army Chief of Staff General George Casey Jr. has initiated a "comprehensive soldier fitness program" with a budget of $120 million. This program is designed to address physical, emotional, social, spiritual, and family needs. This program addresses bringing "mental fitness" up to the level of effort for developing physical fitness and provides soldiers and family members with the skills and attitudes they need to be more resilient (Mash, Krantz, Stein, Westphal, & Litz, 2011).

What have we learned from the literature reviewed in this chapter that can be applied to improving resiliency training programs and reducing PTSD and related adjustment problems?

Intervention Implications for Resiliency Training Programs

Space limits my full discussion of each of these training implications, so they are enumerated in a training checklist manner.

1. Because resilience develops gradually and varies across response domains and contexts, resiliency training programs need to be implemented across the entire deployment cycle, from predeployment through redeployment. Each phase has its own unique set of task demands that require distinct resilience skills. Anticipatory problem solving, proactive coping efforts, and stress inoculation skills training procedures can be built into the training regimen (Meichenbaum, 2006, 2007).

2. Because the basic building block of resilience is social relationships, family members need to be included from the outset of any training program, and "rear guard" interventions need to be maintained throughout the entire deployment cycle and tailored to whether one is dealing with the family members of active-duty or National Guard members. Israeli studies found that the strongest factor that distinguished between soldiers who were decorated for heroic acts and soldiers who were battle casualties was how many and how well they handled home-front stressors (e.g., "Dear John" letters, sick parent or child, bad debts). Worrying about what was going on back home distracted soldiers from focusing on the demands of combat (Solomon, Wayoman, Neria, Orly, Schwarzwald, et al., 1999; Zakin et al., 2003).

3. Because the deployment of resilience is so contextually and ecologically influenced, there needs to be an equal emphasis on creating resilience-engendering organizations and communities. Any attempts by the military to bolster soldiers' psychological and mental fitness needs to focus on organizational issues such as removing barriers to and stigma about help-seeking behaviors, reduction of sexual harassment and abuse, provision of support services, adequate time periods between deployments, reduction of the number of multiple deployments, improved combat leadership, increased level of unit cohesion, and the like.

The Mental Health Advisory Team (2008) reported that "positive leadership may be the panacea or silver bullet for sustaining the mental health and well-being of the deployed forces" (p. 79). Soldiers who became casualties of war were more often committed to battle with strangers, whereas those who proved to be "heroes" fought alongside unit members they knew well, trained with, and felt responsible for and in whom they took special pride and depended upon. High unit cohesion and good leadership that elicits confidence, provides good communication, and instills a belief in the objectives of the mission have been found to nurture resilience. The Marine Corps website provides multiple examples of such organizational features that contribute to resilience, even going back to Julius Caesar's famous and elite Tenth Unit, which wore the Golden Eagle standard insignia. What keeps soldiers in battle and willing to face the fear of death and injury is, above all else, their loyalty to their fellow soldiers. Once again, it is personal bonding that is the backbone of resilience training. Any resiliency training program needs to be focused on the various levels of the organization, from the top down (Nash, Krantz, Stein, Westphal, & Litz, 2011). Just teaching frontline soldiers a variety of coping skills without changing the organizational supports will have limited benefits. Moreover, community networks of former veterans and others can help returning service members with readjustment.

4. Because soldiers enter the service with varied preexisting vulnerabilities and specific needs (e.g., dual military families, single parents, prior psychopathology, trauma exposure, and the like), there is a need to be able to tailor and individualize resiliency training programs. Research has indicated that soldiers with low levels of psychological health prior to combat had 2–3 times the risk of developing PTSD after deployment compared to those with higher baseline mental health behaviors (King et al., 1998; Southwick et al., 2005).

5. Because research indicates the variety of risk and protective factors and the mechanisms that distinguish resilient individuals (80%) from those (20%) who become combat casualties, there is a need to educate and incorporate these factors into training and treatment and to change the social norm and expectations about the outcome of military service. There is an urgent need to educate the media so that they do not "sensationalize" combat casualties. Perhaps in the future PBS *Frontline* will tell "the rest of the story" about resilience. This educational information about resilience can also be built into assessment and training programs. For example, when soldiers return from combat, they presently are assessed routinely on the Post-Deployment Health Assessment (PDHA) and the Post-Deployment Health Reassessment (PDHRA). I am presently working with the National Guard in developing a computer-based self-assessment checklist of resiliency-enhancing activities in the physical, interpersonal, emotional, cognitive, behavioral and spiritual areas, each accompanied by modeling films of soldiers discussing and demonstrating these coping skills in action. There is a need to build practical measures of resiliency into the military assessment routine. As the adage goes, "What gets measured, gets implemented." The inclusion of such tools conveys an expectation that resilience is the norm.

6. Because the incidence of PTSD, suicidality, and related adjustment problems persists despite the innumerable intervention programs and advice books for returning soldiers and their family members, there is a need for a careful analysis of why these programs are not more effective (e.g., see programs and books by Armstrong, Best, & Domenici, 2006; Drescher & Ramirez, 2004; Drescher et al., 2009; Fava, 1994; Frankl, 1984; Hall, 2008; Lepore & Smyth, 2006; Litz, Engel, Bryant, & Papa, 2007; Litz & Schlenger, 2009; Lyubomirsky, 2008; Maddi, 1999; Matthews, 2009; Moore & Kennedy, 2010; Reivich & Shatte, 2002; Seligman, Steen, Park,

& Peterson, 2005; Skovholt, 2001; Slone & Friedman, 2008; Taylor, 2009; Tick, 2005; and many others). The question is, Why aren't these multiple resources more effective in reaching those who are most high risk? There is a need to make this useful information more accessible and user-friendly. There is a need to conduct a barrier analysis of what gets in the way of implementing resilience-enhancing skills. Research on predictors of combat casualties indicates that it is *not* the personality characteristics of the individual soldiers, but rather the social contextual factors that undermine their implementation (Reich et al. 2010). Moreover, when such resiliency training programs are conducted, there is an explicit need not to just "train and hope" for generalization and maintenance of treatment effects but to explicitly build into the training regimen explicit guidelines to enhance the likelihood of transfer (see *www.melissainstitute.org* for an enumeration of ways to conduct such training programs).

Finally, when we consider one of the more effective means of treating soldiers with PTSD, namely, cognitive-behavioral therapy (CBT), it is worth concluding with the observation offered by Brewin and Holmes (2003). They propose that CBT interventions do *not* directly modify negative information in memory; rather, they influence the *relative retrievability* of the different meanings in memory. It is the strengthening of positive representations that are in retrieval competition with negative representations that is the major target of cognitive-behavioral interventions. In short, CBT challenges, cajoles, assists, and nurtures the recall and implementation of a different narrative of resilience, of strength, courage, and adaptability that is the norm following trauma exposure. This is the story that PBS *Frontline* needs to tell and retell.

References

Adler, A. B., Bliese, P. D., McGurk, D., Hoge, C. W., & Castro, C. A. (2009). Battlemind debriefing and Battlemind training as early interventions with soldiers returning from Iraq: Randomization by platoon. *Journal of Consulting and Clinical Psychology, 77*, 928–940.

Antonovsky, A. (1987). *Unravelling the mystery of health: How people manage stress and stay well*. San Francisco: Jossey-Bass.

Armstrong, K., Best, S., & Domenici, P. (2006). *Courage after fire*. Berkeley, CA: Ulysses Press.

Bartone, P. T. (1999). Hardiness protects against war-related stress in Army reserve forces. *Consulting Psychology Journal: Practice and Research, 51*, 72–82.

Benotsch, E. G., Brailey, K., Vasterling, J. J., Uddo, M., Constans, J. I., & Sutker, P. B. (2000). War zone stress, personal and environmental resources and PTSD symptoms in Gulf war veterans: A longitudinal study. *Journal of Abnormal Psychology, 109*, 205–213.

Bonanno, G. A. (2004). Loss, trauma and human resilience: Have we underestimated the human capacity to thrive after extremely aversive events. *American Psychologist, 59*, 20–28.

Brenner, R. A., Gutierrez, P. M., & Cornette, M. M. (2008). A qualitative study of potential suicide risk factors in returning combat veterans. *Journal of Mental Health Counselling, 30*, 211–225.

Brewin, C. R., & Holmes, E. A. (2003). Psychological theories of posttraumatic stress disorder. *Clinical Psychology Review, 23*, 339–376.

Burkett, B. G., & Whitley, G. (1998). *Stolen valour: How the Vietnam generation was robbed of its heroes and its history*. Dallas, TX: Verity Press.

Calhoun, L. G., & Tedeschi, R. G. (Eds.). (2006). *Handbook of posttraumatic growth: Research and practice*. Mahwah, NJ: Erlbaum.

Caliber Associates. (2007). *What we know about Army families* (Prepared for the Family and Morale, Welfare, Recreation Command). Fairfax, VA: Author.

Castro, C. (2006). *Battlemind*. Washington, DC: Walter Reed Army Medical Center, WRAIR Land Combat Study Team.

Charuvastra, A., & Cloitre, M. (2008). Social support and posttraumatic stress disorder. *Annual Review of Psychology, 59*, 301–328.

Denhardt, J., & Denhardt, R. (2010). Building organizational resilience and adaptive management. In J. W. Reich, A. J. Zautra, & J. S. Hall (Eds.), *Handbook of adult resilience* (pp. 333–349). New York: Guilford Press.

Dohrenwend, B. P., Turner, J. B., Turk, N. A., Adams, B., Koenen, K. C., & Marshall, R. D. (2006). The psychological risks of Vietnam for U. S. veterans: A revisit with new data and methods. *Science, 313*, 979–982.

Dohrenwend, B. P., Neria, Y., Turner, J. B., Turse, N., Marshall, R., & Lewis-Fernandez, R. (2004). Positive tertiary appraisals and post-traumatic stress disorder in U. S. male veterans of the war in Vietnam: The roles of positive affirmation, positive reformulation and defensive denial. *Journal of Consulting and Clinical Psychology, 3*, 417–433.

Drescher, K. D., Burgoyne, M., Curran, E., Lovato, L., Carran, E., Pivar, I., et al. (2009). Issues of grief, loss, honor and remembrance: Spirituality and work with military personnel and their families. In S. Morgillo Freeman, B. A. Moore, & A. Freeman (Eds.). *Living and surviving in harm's way: A psychological treatment for pre- and post-deployment of military personnel* (pp. 437–465). New York: Routledge.

Drescher, K. D., & Ramirez, G. (2004). Spirituality and trauma. Development of a group therapy module. *Group Journal, 28*, 71–87.

Ebert, A., & Dyck, M. (2004). The experience of mental death: The core feature of complex posttraumatic stress disorder. *Clinical Psychology Review, 24*, 617–636.

Ehlers, A., & Clark, D. M. (2000). A cognitive model of posttraumatic stress disorder. *Behaviour Research and Therapy, 38*, 319–345.

Elder, G. H., Jr., & Clipp, E. C. (1989). Combat experience and emotional health: Impairment and resilience in later life. *Journal of Personality, 57*, 310–341.

Erbes, C., Eberly, R., Dikel, T., Johnsen, E., Harris, I., & Enghdahl, B. (2005). Posttraumatic growth among American former prisoners of war. *Traumatology, 11*, 285–295.

Fava, G. A. (1994). Well-being therapy: Conceptual and technical issues. *Psychotherapy and Psychosomatics, 68*, 171–179.

Folkman, S., & Moskowitz, J. T. (2000). Positive affect and the other side of coping. *American Psychologist, 55*, 647–654.

Fontana, A., & Rosenheck, R. (1998). Psychological benefits and liabilities of traumatic exposure in the war zone. *Journal of Traumatic Stress, 3*, 485–503.

Frankl, V. E. (1984). *Man's search for meaning: An introduction to logotherapy* (3rd ed.). New York: Touchstone.

Grossman, D., & Christensen, B. W. (2007). *On combat: The psychology and physiology of deadly conflict in war and peace* (2nd ed.). Bellville, IL: PPCT Research.

Haglund, M. E., Nestadt, J. S., Cooper, P. S., Southwick, S. M., & Charney, D. S. (2007). Psychobiological mechanisms of resilience: Relevance to prevention and treatment of stress-related psychopathology. *Development and Psychopathology, 19*, 889–920.

Hall, L. K. (2008). *Counseling military families.* New York: Routledge.

Harari, J. N. (2008). Combat flow: Military, political and ethical dimensions of subjective well-being in war. *Review of General Psychology, 12*, 253–263.

Harvey, M. R., & Tummala-Narra, P. (Eds.). (2007). *Sources and expressions of resiliency in trauma survivors: Ecological theory, multicultural practices.* Binghamton, NY: Harvarth Press.

Helgeson, V. S., Reynolds, K. A., & Tomich, P. I. (2006). A meta-analytical review of benefit findings and growth. Journal of Conducting and Clinical Psychology, 74, 797–816.

Henderson, K. (2006). *While they're at war: The true story of American families on the home front.* New York: Houghton Mofflin.

Hobfoll, S. E. (2002). Social and psychological resources and adaptation. *Review of General Psychology, 6*, 307–324.

Hoge, C. W., Castro, C., Messer, S., McGurk, D., Cotting, D. I., & Koffman, R. L. (2004). Combat duty in Iraq and Afghanistan, mental health problems and barriers to care. *New England Journal of Medicine, 357*, 13–22.

Hunter, E. J. (1993). The Vietnam prisoner of war experience. In J. P. Wilson & B. Raphael (Eds.), *International handbook of traumatic stress syndromes* (pp. 297–303). New York: Plenum Press.

Johnson, H., & Thompson, A. (2008). The development and maintenance of posttraumatic stress disorder (PTSD) in civilian adult survivors of war trauma and torture: A review. *Clinical Psychology Review, 28*, 36–47.

Kent, M., & Davis, M. C. (2010). Resilience interventions: The emergence of capacity building programs and models. In J. W. Reich, A. J. Zautra, & J. S. Hall (Eds.), *Handbook of adult resilience* (pp. 427–449). New York: Guilford Press.

Kessler, R. C., Davis, C. G., & Kendler, K. S. (1997). Childhood adversity and adult psychiatric disorder in the U. S. National Comorbidity Survey. *Psychological Medicine, 27*, 1101–1119.

King, I. A., King, D. W., Fairbank, J. A., Keane, T. M., & Adams, G. A. (1998). Resilience–recovery factors in posttraumatic stress disorder among female and male Vietnam veterans: Hardiness, postwar social support, and additional stressful life events. *Journal of Personality and Social Psychology, 74*, 420–434.

Kretzmann, J. P. (2010). Asset-based strategies for building resilient communities. In J. W. Reich, A. J. Zautra, & J. S. Hall (Eds.), *Handbook of adult resilience* (pp. 484–495). New York: Guilford Press.

Lepore, S. J., & Smyth, J. M. (Eds.). (2006). *The writing cure: How expressive writing promotes health and emotional well-being.* Washington, DC: American Psychological Association.

Litz, B. T. (2005). Has resilience to severe trauma been underestimated? *American Psychologist, 60,* 202.

Litz, B. T. (2007). Research on the impact of military trauma: Current status and future directions. *Military Psychology, 19,* 217–238.

Litz, B. T., Engel, C. C., Bryant, R. A., & Papa, A. (2007). A randomized, controlled proof-of-concept trial of on Internet-based, therapist-assisted self-management for posttraumatic stress disorder. *American Journal of Psychiatry, 164,* 1676–1683.

Litz, B. T., & Schlenger, W. E. (2009). PTSD in service members and new veterans of the Iraq and Afghanistan wars: A bibliography and critique. *PTSD Research Quarterly, 20,* 2–8.

Lyubomirsky, S. (2008). *The how of happiness: A scientific approach to getting the life you want.* New York: Penguin Press.

Lyubomirsky, S., & Della Porta, M. D. (2010). Boosting happiness, buttressing resilience: Results from cognitive and behavioral interventions. In J. W. Reich, A. J. Zautra, & J. S. Hall (Eds.), *Handbook of adult resilience* (pp. 450–464). New York: Guilford Press.

Maddi, S. R. (1999). The personality construct of hardness: Effects on experiences, coping and stress. *Consulting Psychology Journal, Practice and Research, 51,* 83–94.

Maeraker, A., & Zoellner, T. (2004). The Janus face of self-perceived growth: Toward a two-component model of posttraumatic growth. *Psychological Inquiry, 15,* 41–48.

Mancini, A. D., & Bonanno, G. A. (2010). Resilience to potential trauma: Toward a lifespan approach. In J. Reich, A. J. Zautra, & J. S. Hall (Eds.), *Handbook of adult resilience* (pp. 258–280). New York: Guilford Press.

Mash, W. P., Krantz, L., Stein, N., Westphal, R. J., & Litz, B. (2011). Comprehensive soldier fitness, battlemind and the stress continuum model: Military organizational approaches to prevention. In J. I. Ruzek, P. P. Schnurr, J. J. Vasterling, & M. J. Friedman (Eds.). *Caring for veterans with deployment-related stress disorders: Iraq, Afghanistan and beyond* (pp. 193–214). Washington, DC: American Psychological Association.

Masten, A. S. (2001). Ordinary magic: Resilience processes in development. *American Psychologist, 56,* 227–238.

Matthews, M. D. (2009). The soldier's mind: Motivation, mindset, and attitude. In S. Morgillo Freeman, B. Moore, & A. Freeman (Eds.), *Living and surviving in harm's way: A psychological treatment for pre- and post-deployment of military personnel* (pp. 9–26). New York: Routledge.

Meichenbaum, D. (2006). Resilience and posttraumatic growth: A constructive narrative perspective. In L. G. Calhoun & R. G. Tedeschi (Eds.), *Handbook of posttraumatic growth* (pp. 355–368). Mahwah, NJ: Erlbaum.

Meichenbaum, D. (2007). Stress inoculation training: A preventative and treatment approach. In P. M. Lehrer, R. L. Woolfolk, & W. E. Sime (Eds.), *Principles and practice of stress management* (3rd ed., pp. 497–518). New York: Guilford Press.

Meichenbaum, D. (2009a). Bolstering resilience: Benefitting from lessons learned. In D. Brom, R. Pat-Horenczyk, & J. D. Ford (Eds.), *Treating traumatized children: Risk, resilience and recovery* (pp. 183–192). New York: Routledge.

Meichenbaum, D. (2009b). Core psychotherapeutic tasks with returning soldiers: A case conceptualization approach. In S. Morgillo Freeman, B. A. Moore, & A. Freeman (Eds.), *Living and surviving in harm's way: A psychological treatment for pre- and post-deployment of military personnel* (pp. 193–210). New York: Routledge.

Mental Health Advisory Team. (2008). Mental Health Advisory Team (MHATV). Operations Iraqi Freedom and Operation Enduring Freedom 06-08.

Milne, D. (2007). People can learn markers on the road to resilience. *Psychiatry News, 42*, 57.

Moore, B. A., & Kennedy, C. H. (2010). *Wheels down: Adjusting to life after deployment*. Washington, DC: American Psychological Association.

Morgillo Freeman, S., Moore, B. A., & Freeman, A. (Eds.). (2009). *Living and surviving in harm's way*. New York: Routledge.

Moskowitz, J. T. (2010). Positive affect at the onset of chronic illness: Planting the seeds of resilience. In J. W. Reich, A. J. Zautra, & J. S. Hall (Eds.), *Handbook of adult resilience* (pp. 465–483). New York: Guilford Press.

Muraven, M., & Baumeister, R. F. (2000). Self-regulation and depletion of limited resources: Does self-control resemble a muscle? *Psychological Bulletin, 126*, 247–259.

Nash, W. P., Krantz, L., Stein, N., Westphal, R. J., & Litz, B. (2011). Comprehensive soldier fitness, Battlemind and the Stress Continuum Model: Military organizational approaches to prevention. In J. I. Ruzek, P. P. Schnurr, J. J. Vasterling, & M. J. Friedman (Eds.), *Caring for veterans with deployment-related stress disorders: Iraq, Afghanistan and beyond* (pp. 193–214). Washington, DC: American Psychological Association.

Pargament, K. T., & Cummings, J. (2010). Anchored by faith: Religion as a resilience factor. In J. W. Reich, A. J. Zautra, & J. S. Hall (Eds.), *Handbook of adult resilience* (pp. 193–210). New York: Guilford Press.

Park, C. L., & Folkman, S. (1997). Meaning in the context of stress and coping. *Review of General Psychology, 1*, 115–144.

Penk, W., & Ainspan, D. (2009). Community response to returning military. In S. Morgillo Freeman, B. A. Moore, & A. Freeman (Eds.), *Living and surviving in harm's way: A psychological treatment for pre- and post-deployment of military personnel* (pp 417–435). New York: Routledge.

Reich, J. W., Zautra, A. J., & Hall, J. S. (Eds.). (2010). *Handbook of adult resilience*. New York: Guilford Press.

Reivich, K., & Shatte, A. (2002). *The resilience factor*. New York: Random House.

Robins, L. N., Davis, D. H., & Nurco, D. N. (1974). How permanent was Vietnam drug addiction? *American Journal of Public Health, 64*, 38–43.

Ryff, C. D., & Singer, B. (2003). Flourishing under fire: Resilience as a prototype of challenged thriving. In C. L. Keyes & J. Haidt (Eds.), *Flourishing: Positive psychology and the life well-lived* (pp. 15–36). Washington, DC: American Psychological Association.

Satel, S. L. (2005). The mental health crisis that wasn't. *Psychiatric Services, 64,* 1571.

Sawyer, A., Ayers, S., & Field, A. P. (2010). Posttraumatic growth and adjustment among individuals with cancer or HIV/AIDS: A meta-analysis. *Clinical Psychology Review, 30,* 436–447.

Schok, M. L., Kleber, R. J., Elands, M., & Weerts, J. M. (2008). Meaning as a mission: A review of empirical studies on appraisals of war and peacekeeping experiences. *Clinical Psychology Review, 28,* 357–365.

Scoville, S. L., Gubata, M. E., & Potter, R. N. (2007). Deaths attributed to suicide among enlisted U. S. armed forces. *Military Medicine, 172,* 1024–1031.

Selby, E. A., Anestis, M. D., & Bender, T. W. (2010). Overcoming the fear of lethal injury: Evaluating suicidal behavior in the military through the lens of the interpersonal–psychological theory of suicide. *Clinical Psychology Review, 28,* 357–356.

Seligman, M. E., Steen, T. A., Park, N., & Peterson, G. (2005). Positive psychology: Empirical validation of interventions. *American Psychologist, 60,* 410–421.

Sharkansky, E. J., King, D. W., King, L. A., Wolfe, J., Erickson, D. J., & Stokes, L. R. (2000). Coping with Gulf War combat stress: Mediating and moderating effects. *Journal of Abnormal Psychology, 109,* 188–197.

Skovholt, T. M. (2001). *The resilient practitioner.* Boston: Allyn & Boston.

Slone, L. B., & Friedman, M. J. (2008). *After the war zone.* Philadelphia: De Capo Press.

Smith, J. M., & Alloy, L. B. (2009). A roadmap to rumination: A review of the definition, assessment and conceptualization of this multifaceted construct. *Clinical Psychology Review, 29,* 116–128.

Solomon, Z., Waysman, M. A., Neria, Y., Orly, A., Schwarzwald, J., & Wiener, M. (1999). Positive and negative changes in the lives of Israeli former prisoners of war. *Journal of Social and Clinical Psychology, 18,* 419–435.

Southwick, S. M., Vythilingam, M., & Charney, D. S. (2005). The psychobiology of depression and resilience to stress: Implications for prevention and treatment. *Annual Review of Clinical Psychology, 1,* 255–291.

Staal, M. A., & Hughes, T. G. (2002). Suicide predictions in the U. S. Air Force: Implications for practice. *Professional Psychology: Research and Practice, 33,* 190–196.

Sutker, P. B., Davis, J. M., Uddo, M., & Ditta, S. R. (1995). War zone stress, personal resources, and PTSD in Persian Gulf War returnees. *Journal of Abnormal Psychology, 104,* 444–453.

Tanielian, T., & Jaycox, L. H. (Eds.). (2008). *Invisible wounds of war: Psychological and cognitive injuries, their consequences, and services to assist recovery.* Santa Monica, CA: RAND Center for Military Health Policy.

Taylor, J. B. (2009). *My stroke of insight.* New York: Penguin.

Tick, E. (2005). *War and the soul.* Wheaton, IL: Quest Books.

Watkins, E. (2008). Constructive and unconstructive repetitive thoughts. *Psychological Bulletin, 143,* 163–206.

Waysman, M., Schwarzwald, J., & Solomon, Z. (2001). Hardiness: An examination of its relationship with positive and negative long term changes following trauma. *Journal of Traumatic Stress, 14*, 531–548.

Zakin, G., Solomon, Z., & Neria, Y. (2003). Hardiness, attachment style and long-term psychological distress among Israeli POWs and combat veterans. *Personality and Individual Differences, 34*, 819–829.

Recommendations for Gaining Military Cultural and Clinical Competence

Training Opportunities

Training opportunities with various military organizations and programs are available. Programs and workshops may not deal specifically with military culture; it is often a peripheral topic. Yet it is still invaluable to the nonmilitary clinician. Following are representative examples of helpful organizations and programs.

Center for Deployment Psychology
www.deploymentpsych.org

The Center for Deployment Psychology trains military and civilian behavioral health professionals to provide high-quality deployment-related behavioral health services to military personnel and their families.

National Center for PTSD
www.ptsd.va.gov

The National Center for PTSD aims to help U.S. veterans and others through research, education, and training on trauma and PTSD.

National Center for Telehealth and Technology
t2health.org

The National Center for Telehealth and Technology researches, develops, evaluates, and deploys new and existing technologies for psychological health and traumatic brain injury across the Department of Defense.

Partial list compiled by Kenneth S. Pope, PhD, ABPP. A current and more comprehensive list of references can be found at *www.kspope.com*.

Warrior Resiliency Program (Training Division)
bamcwrp@amedd.army.mil

The Warrior Resiliency Program focuses on the prevention and treatment of combat- and deployment-related problems affecting service members and their families.

Publications

The clinician unfamiliar with military culture may find reviewing various publications helpful, including books, military regulations, and journal articles. Following are some of the more relevant ones.

Books

Ainspan, N. D., & Penk, W. E. (2008). *Returning wars' wounded, injured, and ill.* Westport, CT: Praeger.

Cantrell, B., & Dean, C. (2006). *Down range: To Iraq and Back.* Bellingham, WA: Hearts Toward Home International.

Dalessandro, R. J. (2009). *Army officer's guide.* Mechanicsburg, PA: Stackpole Books.

Department of the Army. (2007). *The soldier's guide: The complete guide to U.S. army traditions, training, duties, and responsibilities.* New York: Skyhorse.

Finley, J., & Moore, B. A. (2011). *The veterans and active duty military homework planner.* New York: Wiley.

Jones, F. D., Sparacino, L. R., Wilcox, V. L., Rothberg, J. M., & Stokes, J. W. (1995). *War psychiatry.* Washington, DC: Department of the Army.

Hall, L. (2008). *Counseling military families: What mental health professionals need to know.* New York: Routledge/Taylor & Francis Group.

Helmus, T., & Glenn, R. (2005). *Steeling the mind: Combat stress reactions and their implications for urban warfare.* Washington, DC: RAND.

Henderson, K. (2006). *While they're at war: The true story of American families on the homefront.* New York: Houghton Mifflin.

Higbee, D. (2010). *Military culture and education.* Surrey, UK: Ashgate.

Kennedy, C. H., & Moore, J. (2010). *Military neuropsychology.* New York: Springer.

Kennedy, C. H., & Williams, T. J. (2010). *Ethical practice in operational psychology: Military and national intelligence applications.* Washington, DC: American Psychological Association.

Kennedy, C. H., & Zillmer, E. A. (Eds.). (2006). *Military psychology: Clinical and operational applications.* New York: Guilford Press.

Moore, B. A. (Ed.). (in press). *Handbook of counseling military couples.* New York: Routledge/Taylor & Francis.

Moore, B. A., & Jongsma, A. E. (2009). *The veterans and active-duty military psychotherapy treatment planner.* New York: Wiley.

Moore, B. A., & Kennedy, C. H. (2010). *Wheels down: Adjusting to life after deployment.* Washington, DC: American Psychological Association.

Morgillo-Freeman, S., Moore, B. A., & Freeman, A. (2009). *Living and surviving in harm's way: A psychological treatment handbook for pre-and post-deployment of military personnel.* New York: Routledge/Taylor & Francis.

Squier-Kraft, H. (2007). *Rule number two: Lessons I learned in a combat hospital.* Boston: Little, Brown.

Military Regulations

Department of the Army. (2007). *Military occupational classification and structure* (Pamphlet 611-21). Washington, DC: Author.

Department of the Army. (2006). *Combat and operational stress control* (FM 4-02.51 [FM 8-51]). Washington, DC: Author.

Department of the Army. (2009). *Combat and operational stress control manual for leaders and soldiers* (FM 6-22.5). Washington, DC: Author.

Department of Defense. (1997). *Department of Defense directive 6490.1: Mental health evaluations of members of the armed forces.* Washington, DC: Author.

Department of Defense. (1997). *Department of Defense instruction 6490.4: Requirements for mental health evaluations of members of the armed forces.* Washington, DC: Author.

Journal Articles

Adler, A., Bliese, P., McGurk, D., Hoge, C., & Castro, C. (2009). Battlemind debriefing and battlemind training as early interventions with soldiers returning from Iraq: Randomization by platoon. *Journal of Consulting and Clinical Psychology, 77*(5), 928–940.

Brenner, L., Terrio, H., Homaifar, B., Gutierrez, P., Staves, P., Harwood, J., et al. (2010). Neuropsychological test performance in soldiers with blast-related mild TBI. *Neuropsychology, 24*(2), 160–167.

Chaumba, J., & Bride, B. (2010). Trauma experiences and posttraumatic stress disorder among women in the United States military. *Social Work in Mental Health, 8*(3), 280–303.

Dausch, B., & Saliman, S. (2009). Use of family-focused therapy in rehabilitation for veterans with traumatic brain injury. *Rehabilitation Psychology, 54*(3), 279–287.

Evans, L., Cowlishaw, S., & Hopwood, M. (2009). Family functioning predicts outcomes for veterans in treatment for chronic posttraumatic stress disorder. *Journal of Family Psychology, 23*(4), 531–539.

Gahm, G., & Lucenko, B. (2008). Screening soldiers in outpatient care for mental health concerns. *Military Medicine, 173*(1), 17–24.

Greene-Shortridge, T., Britt, T., & Andrew, C. (2007). The stigma of mental health problems in the military. *Military Medicine, 172*(2), 157–161.

Huebner, A., Mancini, J., Bowen, G., & Orthner, D. (2009). Shadowed by war:

Building community capacity to support military families. *Family Relations*, *58*(2), 216–228.

Johnson, W., & Kennedy, C. (2010). Preparing psychologists for high-risk jobs: Key ethical considerations for military clinical supervisors. *Professional Psychology: Research and Practice*, *41*(4), 298–304.

Jordan, R. (2007). Reflecting on the military's best practices. *Human Resource Management*, *46*(1), 143–146.

Kennedy, C., & Moore, B. A. (2008). Evolution of clinical military psychology ethics. *Military Psychology*, *20*, 1–6.

LeardMann, C., Smith, T., Smith, B., Wells, T., & Ryan, M. (2009). Baseline self-reported functional health and vulnerability to posttraumatic stress disorder after combat deployment: Prospective U.S. military cohort study. *British Medical Journal*, *338*(7701), 1–9.

Linnerooth, P. J., Mrdjenovich, A. J., & Moore, B. A. (in press). Professional burnout in clinical military psychologists: Challenges and recommendations, before, during, and after deployment. *Professional Psychology: Research and Practice*, *42*(1), 87–93.

Maguen, S., Cohen, G., Cohen, B., Lawhon, G., Marmar, C., & Seal, K. (2010). The role of psychologists in the care of Iraq and Afghanistan veterans in primary care settings. *Professional Psychology: Research and Practice*, *41*(2), 135-142.

Manguno-Mire, G., Sautter, F., Lyons, J., Myers, L., Perry, D., Sherman, M., et al. (2007). Psychological distress and burden among female partners of combat veterans with PTSD. *Journal of Nervous and Mental Disease*, *195*(2), 144–151.

Moore, B. A., & Krakow, B. (2007). Imagery rehearsal therapy for acute posttraumatic nightmares among combat soldiers in Iraq. *American Journal of Psychiatry*, *164*, 683–684.

Moore, B. A., & Krakow, B. (2010). Imagery rehearsal therapy: An emerging treatment for nightmares in service members. *Psychological Trauma: Theory, Research, Practice, and Policy*, *2*(3), 232–238.

Moore, B. A., & McGrath, R. E. (2007). How prescriptive authority for psychologists would help service members in Iraq. *Professional Psychology: Research and Practice*, *38*, 191–195.

Moore, B. A., & Reger, G. M. (2006). Combating stress in Iraq. *Scientific American Mind*, *17*, 30–37.

Moore, B. A., & Reger, G. M. (2006). Clinician to frontline soldier: A look at the roles and challenges of Army clinical psychologists in Iraq. *Journal of Clinical Psychology*, *62*(3), 395–403.

Reger, G. M., & Moore, B. (2006). Combat operational stress control in Iraq: Lessons learned during Operation Iraqi Freedom. *Military Psychology*, *18*(4), 297–307.

Reger, M. A., Etherage, J. R., Reger, G. M., & Gahm, G. A. (2008). Civilian psychologists in an Army culture: The ethical challenge of cultural competence. *Military Psychology*, *20*(1), 21–35.

Seal, K., Metzler, T., Gima, K., Bertenthal, D., Maguen, S., & Marmar, C. (2009). Trends and risk factors for mental health diagnoses among Iraq and Afghanistan veterans using Department of Veterans Affairs health care, 2002–2008. *American Journal of Public Health, 99*(9), 1651–1658.

Shaw, M., & Hector, M. (2010). Listening to military members returning from Iraq and/or Afghanistan: A phenomenological investigation. *Professional Psychology: Research and Practice, 41*(2), 128–134.

Shiner, B., Watts, B. V., Pomerantz, A., Groft, A., Scott, D., Street, B., et al. (2009). Access to what? An evaluation of the key ingredients to effective advanced mental health access at a VA medical center and its affiliated community-based outreach clinics. *Military Medicine, 174*(10), 1024–1032.

Staal, M., & King, R. (2000). Managing a multiple relationship environment: The ethics of military psychology. *Professional Psychology: Research and Practice, 31*(6), 698–705.

Theeler, B., & Erickson, J. (2009). Mild head trauma and chronic headaches in returning U.S. soldiers. *Headache: The Journal of Head and Face Pain, 49*(4), 529–534.

Tuerk, P., Grubaugh, A., Hamner, M., & Foa, E. (2009). Diagnosis and treatment of PTSD-related compulsive checking behaviors in veterans of the Iraq war: The influence of military context on the expression of PTSD symptoms. *American Journal of Psychiatry, 166*(7), 762–767.

Wright, K., Cabrera, O., Bliese, P., Adler, A., Hoge, C., & Castro, C. (2009). Stigma and barriers to care in soldiers postcombat. *Psychological Services, 6*(2), 108–116.

Military Organizations and Programs

Air Force Aid Society

www.afas.org

Incorporated in 1942 as a nonprofit organization, the AFAS is the official charity of the United States Air Force. Its mission is to help relieve financial distress of Air Force members and their families and to assist them in financing their higher education goals.

American Red Cross

www.redcross.org

The American Red Cross sends emerging communications to deployed service members on behalf of their families. In addition, Red Cross Armed Forces Emergency Services personnel serve in 700 chapters in the United States, in military installations around the world, and alongside U.S. troops in Kuwait, Afghanistan, and Iraq.

Books for Soldiers

www.booksforsoldiers.com

This service enables anyone who visits the website to fill a request from deployed military personnel for books, DVDs, CDs, video games, and relief supplies. All packages must be requested by the soldier, according to Department of Defense guidelines.

List compiled by Kenneth S. Pope, PhD, ABPP. A current list of references can be found at *www.kspope.com*.

Children of Fallen Soldiers Relief Fund
www.cfsrf.org

This organization provides college grants and financial assistance to surviving children and spouses of U.S. military service members who have lost their lives in the Iraq and Afghanistan wars. Its financial assistance program assists families of disabled service members as well.

Defense Centers of Excellence for Psychological Health and Traumatic Brain Injury
www.dcoe.health.mil

The DCoE provides help to service members and their families with psychological health and traumatic brain injury issues. It partners with the Department of Defense, the Department of Veterans Affairs, and a national network of military and civilian agencies, community leaders, advocacy groups, clinical experts, and academic institutions to establish best practices and quality standards for psychological problems and traumatic brain injury. Its work includes clinical care, education and training, prevention, research, and patient, family, and community outreach. In addition, the DCoE is working to tear down the stigma that still deters some from seeking treatment for problems such as PTSD and traumatic brain injury with its Real Warriors campaign.

Department of Homeland Security
www.dhs.gov

The mission of the Department is to guard against terrorism; secure national borders; enforce immigration laws; and improve readiness for, response to, and recovery from disasters.

Family Advocacy Program
www.militaryhomefront.dvd.mil [go to "Troops & Families"]

The FAP provides services to troops and family members experiencing domestic abuse and child abuse through prevention efforts, early identification and intervention, support for victims, and treatment for abusers. The website provides a link to a directory of FAP representatives at Army, Marine Corps, Navy, and Air Force installations around the world.

Federal Benefits for Veterans, Dependents and Survivors
www1.va.gov/opa/publications/benefits_book.asp

This online guide from the Department of Veterans Affairs informs veterans and their dependents of the variety of federal benefits available.

Find State Resources for Veterans
wwwmaps.servicelocator.org/military/select_state.aspx

On this website one selects his or her state to find job search, educational, National Guard/Reserve, and homeless veteran resources.

Fisher House
www.fisherhouse.org

Fisher House provides a "home away from home" that enables family members to be close to a loved one at the most stressful time—during hospitalization for an illness, disease, or injury.

GI Bill Web Site
www.gibill.va.gov

This VA website provides comprehensive information about the GI Bill. One can search for approved programs at colleges, non-college-degree-granting institutions, licensing and certification granting providers, and national testing providers.

Give an Hour
www.giveanhour.org

Give an Hour is dedicated to meeting the mental health needs of the troops and families affected by the ongoing conflicts in Iraq and Afghanistan. It provides counseling to individuals, couples and families, and children and adolescents, and offers treatment for anxiety, depression, substance abuse, PTSD, traumatic brain injuries, sexual health and intimacy concerns, and loss and grieving. Mental health professionals who join Give an Hour are giving an hour of their time each week to provide free mental health services to military personnel and their families.

Hooah4Health
www.hooah4health.com

This is the U.S. Army health promotion and wellness website. It is specifically designed to address the force health protection and readiness requirements of the Army, particularly its Reserve component.

Legal Information and Resources for Military Personnel and Their Families
www.jag.navy.mil

The Judge Advocate General's Corps provides online legal information and resources in such areas as family matters, financial issues (including taxes), insurance, immigration, housing (including landlord–tenant issues), estates, the Soldiers and Sailors Civil Relief Act, and consumer and contract issues.

Coming Home Project
www.cominghomeproject.net

This is a nonprofit organization devoted to providing compassionate care, support, and stress management tools for Iraq and Afghanistan veterans and their families. Its programs address the mental, emotional, spiritual, and relationship challenges faced by veterans and families before, during, and after deployment. A group of veterans, psychotherapists, and interfaith leaders help veterans and family members rebuild the connectivity of mind, heart, body, and spirit that combat trauma can unravel, renew their relationships with loved ones, and create new support networks. Its free services include workshops and retreats, psychological counseling, training for care providers, and community forums.

Military Homefront
www.militaryhomefront.dvd.mil

This is the official Department of Defense website for reliable quality-of-life information designed to help troops and their families, leaders, and service providers.

Military Sentinel
www.ftccomplaintassistant.gov/military_home.htm

This joint project of the Federal Trade Commission and the Department of Defense provides information and resources about consumer protection issues that affect members of the United States Armed Forces and their families, including from auto leasing, identity theft, and work-at-home scams. It also provides an easy, formal way to enter consumer complaints directly into a database that is immediately accessible by over 500 law enforcement organizations throughout the United States, Canada, and Australia. These law enforcement agencies use these complaint data to target cases for prosecution and other enforcement measures. The information from Military Sentinel can also be used by members of the JAG staff and others in the Department of Defense to help protect armed services members and their families from consumer protection-related problems.

Military Spouse Career Center
www.military.com/spouse

This website helps military spouses find jobs.

National Center for PTSD
www.ptsd.va.gov

The mission of this program, which is within the Department of Veterans Affairs, is to advance the clinical care and social welfare of America's veterans through research, education, and training in the science, diagnosis, and treatment of PTSD and stress-related disorders.

National Coalition for Homeless Veterans
www.nchv.org

The NCHV is the resource and technical assistance center for a national network of community-based service providers and local, state, and federal agencies that provide emergency and supportive housing, food, health services, job training and placement assistance, legal aid, and case management support for homeless veterans.

National Military Family Association
www.nmfa.org

Among this organization's primary purposes is to educate military families concerning their rights and the benefits and services available to them and to inform them regarding the issues that affect their lives.

National Personnel Records Center—Military Personnel Records
www.archives.gov/st-louis/military-personnel

This site is provided for those seeking information regarding military personnel, health, and medical records stored at NPRC (MPR). A veteran or next of kin of a deceased veteran may use *vetrecs.archives.gov* to order a copy of the veteran's military records.

Operation Dear Abby
www.OperationDearAbby.net

Dear Abby, the U.S. Department of Defense, and the U.S. Department of the Navy's LifeLines Services Network provide this private and secure online resource that allows individuals to send a sailor, Marine, soldier, airman, or Coast Guardsman a holiday greeting or message of support.

Operation Family Fund
www.operationfamilyfund.org

This program provides financial grants for immediate or long-term needs to the families of soldiers who have been killed or severely disabled as part of the worldwide war on terrorism.

Operation Military Support
www.operationmilitarysupport.com

This program receives names of military personnel who are not receiving mail or packages from home and assigns them a volunteer who wants to write and send packages to them.

Operation Uplink
www.vfw.org/Assistance/National-Military-Services

This program keeps military personnel and hospitalized veterans in touch with their families and loved ones by providing them with a free phone card.

Operation USO Care Package
www.uso.org/oucp

This USO program enables individuals to financially support care packages that will be delivered to service members en route to overseas destinations. The care packages contain an assortment of items specifically requested by the military, such as prepaid international calling cards, disposable cameras, toiletries, and sunscreen.

Seamless Transition
www.oefoif.va.gov

This Department of Veterans Affairs (VA) website provides resources for active-duty, National Guard, and Reserve service members who are returning from Iraq and Afghanistan. It includes a locator for the local VA hospital.

SOFAR: Strategic Outreach to Families of All Reservists
www.sofarusa.org

This is a pro bono mental health project that provides free psychological support, psychotherapy, psychoeducation, and prevention services to extended family of Reserve and National Guard members deployed during the worldwide war on terrorism from time of alert through the period of reunion and reintegration.

Soldiers Project
www.thesoldiersproject.org

The Soldiers Project is a component of the Ernest S. Lawrence Trauma Center of the Los Angeles Institute and Society for Psychoanalytic Studies (LAISPS). The Center's projects are run by volunteer licensed clinicians who provide free psychoanalytically informed psychological services to "at-risk" populations, as well as educational presentations to the community.

Tragedy Assistance Program for Survivors
www.taps.org

TAPS is a national nonprofit organization made up of, and providing services to, all those who have lost a loved one who was serving in the Armed Forces. The heart of TAPS is its national military survivor peer support network. They also offer grief counseling referral, caseworker assistance, and crisis information, all available to help families and military personnel cope and recover. These services are provided 24 hours a day free of charge.

TriWest Healthcare Alliance Behavioral Health Resources
www.triwest.com/provider/behavioralhealth.aspx

This site offers practice guidelines, assessment tools, and a number of other resources to help clinicians assist patients experiencing depression, stress, PTSD, substance use disorders, and more.

VeteranEmployment.com
veteranemployment.com

In partnership with Monster.com, veterans, active-duty personnel, and Guard and Reserve personnel can search among thousands of jobs for veterans from employers who value military experience. There is a special section for security clearance jobs.

Vets4Vets
www.vets4vets.us

The primary goal of Vets4Vets is to help Iraq and Afghanistan-era veterans understand the value of peer support and to regularly use peer support to express their emotions, manage their challenges, and ease their reintegration into society. Anytime a veteran needs to talk with someone who really understands, a local Vets4Vets peer support group is available at no cost.

Virtual Naval Hospital
www.vnh.org

This site is a digital collection of naval medicine and military medicine texts.

APPENDIX C

Select Common
Military Abbreviations

AD—active duty
AGR—active Guard/Reserve
BDE—brigade
BN—battalion
CBRNE—chemical, biological, radiological/nuclear, and explosive
CIV—civilian
CONUS—continental United States
DoD—Department of Defense
ENL—enlisted
FM—Field Manual
FRG—family readiness group
JAG—Judge Advocate General
MEDCOM—Medical Command
MEPS—Military Entrance Processing Station
MOA—memorandum of agreement
MOS—military occupational specialty
MTF—Medical/Military Treatment Facility
MWR—morale, welfare, and recreation
NGO—nongovernmental organization
OCONUS—outside the continental United States
OFF—officer
OTSG—Office of the Surgeon General
PCS—permanent change of station
POC—point of contact
POV—privately owned vehicle
RC—reserve component
SOFA—Status of Forces Agreement
TDY—temporary duty
TM—technical manual
TOE—Table of Organization and Equipment (unit)
TRADOC—Training and Doctrine Command

See *www.dtic.mil/doctrine/dod_dictionary* for a comprehensive list of military abbreviations and terms.

Author Index

359

Subject Index

Page numbers followed by *t* or *f* indicate tables or figures.